'An excellent new book.'   *New Yorker*

'A remarkable, compassionate "biography" of Alzheimer's . . . poignant and haunting'   DUNCAN HAMILTON, *Nottingham Evening Post*

'Deeply affecting . . . a fascinating meditation on the scientific, political and cultural history of Alzheimer's disease.' *Washington Post*

'A graceful, masterful portrait of the illness . . . Readers can't help but be taken by Shenk's humanity and compassion, which brim throughout.'   *Los Angeles Times*

'Written with a researcher's attention to detail and a storyteller's ear.'
                                                                New York Times

'Destined to be a classic . . . Shenk's guided tour is free of medical jargon, and filled instead with clear and memorable phrasing.'
                                                                Seattle Times

'A brilliant and quirky new book on Alzheimer's that offers food for thought on the unthinkable and a new, deeper understanding of the coming epidemic.'   *Salon.com*

'Compelling and immensely humane . . . Shenk's integration of historical and scientific information and personal stories makes for an absorbing read.'   *Newsday*

'A fascinating mix of medical history, the voices of patients and their families, and accounts of the search for a cure . . . Shenk makes the science understandable and recounts personal stories that are both moving and illuminating.'   *Business Week*

'A dazzling literary and scientific history of Alzheimer's disease.'
                                                                Detroit Free Press

'Carefully researched and engagingly written.'   *Wall Street Journal*

THE FORGETTING

Understanding Alzheimer's:
A Biography of a Disease

❧

DAVID SHENK

Flamingo
An Imprint of HarperCollins*Publishers*

For Lucy

Flamingo
An Imprint of HarperCollins*Publishers*
77–85 Fulham Palace Road,
Hammersmith, London W6 8JB

www.**fire**and**water**.com

Published by Flamingo 2003
9 8 7 6 5 4 3 2 1

First published in Great Britain by
HarperCollinsPublishers 2002

First published in the US by Doubleday 2001

ISBN 0 00 653208 X

Author photograph by Jon Shenk

Printed and bound in Great Britain by
Clays Ltd, St Ives plc

CONTENTS

❧

Preface by Adam Phillips   *ix*

Prologue   *1*

PART I
EARLY STAGE

1. I Have Lost Myself   11
2. Bothered   28
3. The God Who Forgot and the Man
   Who Could Not   44
4. The Race   62
5. Irrespective of Age   72
6. A Most Loving Brother   86

PART II
MIDDLE STAGE

7. Fumbling for the Name of My Wife   101
8. Back to Birth   112

9. National Institute of Alzheimer's 132

10. Ten Thousand Feet, at Ten O'Clock at Night 148

11. A World of Struldbruggs 162

12. Humanize the Mouse 178

13. We Hope to Radio Back to Earth Images
of Beauty Never Seen 192

PART III

END STAGE

14. Breakthrough? 209

15. One Thousand Subtractions 216

16. Things to Avoid 228

17. The Mice Are Smarter 242

Epilogue 253

Acknowledgments 257

Resources for Patients and Families 261

Sources 265

Index 281

LEAR: Does any here know me? This is not Lear.

Does Lear walk thus, speak thus? Where are his eyes?

Either his notion weakens, his discernings

Are lethargied—Ha! Waking? 'Tis not so.

Who is it that can tell me who I am?

FOOL: Lear's shadow.

—William Shakespeare, *King Lear*

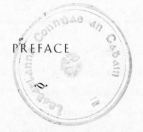

It is easy to forget just how much we need to remember in order to do the simplest things. We don't think of ourselves as having to remember our own names, or where we live, or how to eat or read. And yet, memory—all the skills and impressions we so carefully acquired in the past—informs much of what we do. We know how to play a game when we know the rules; and knowing the rules means not having to bother to remember what they are. It is always a sign of success when we can do things without thinking; when, for example, we can read without having to go back over the alphabet. And we call this second nature, presumably, because we think of natural things, such as recognising your mother's face, or knowing where to sleep as virtually automatic. It is only when things begin to go wrong that we begin to notice just what it is we have been taking for granted. Our incompetence is a revelation.

* * *

It is forgetting—absurdly, perhaps, as this remarkable book shows—that reminds us so vividly about the provenance of memory (we talk of forgetting ourselves, but not of remembering ourselves). Alzheimer's as a disease—and as a disease we should remember that it is as natural as the lives it so insidiously disrupts—reveals just how unforgiving forgetting can be. And just how dependent we are on our memory: and so, how dependent we are on others when we lose it. Impaired memory sabotages self-reliance. Other people have to do our remembering for us. Adults who begin to lose their memory as they age, like infants before they have acquired memories, cannot conceal their need for other people. With the advent of Alzheimer's we have to face the fact of there being, for many people, an adult infancy. That we will no longer be able to conceive of our lives as a journey from utter dependence to relative independence; but rather as a series of intense and mostly unchosen involvements with other people. It is the quieter implication of this startling book that the new long-term dependence of the old who have Alzheimer's—and because there are, and will be, greater numbers of older people than ever before: and therefore more people with the disease—will radically change our notions of looking after people, and our assumptions about independence. If looking after each other is one of the best things we do, looking after people with Alzheimer's makes it plain that it can also be the hardest thing we do. The fact that we find it so hard may be more of a problem than the disease itself. What we do willingly for the young we do grudgingly for the old. It has become one of the basic assumptions of our culture that we should grow out of the need to be looked after—as though the vulnerability of our bodies is itself a disease. *The Forgetting* thus reminds us of so much more than the epidemic it so tellingly documents.

* * *

As a "biography of a disease" *The Forgetting* is inevitably a story of ravaged lives; and the brief accounts by sufferers and their carers have a heartbreaking immediacy. But Shenk never shirks the fact that, when it comes to Alzheimer's, to be forewarned is not to be forearmed. Indeed *The Forgetting* is itself so heartening because it tells us the facts, as stark as they are, without shying away from the cost in human terms. In this book you will find the most shocking and pertinent statistics—the life-expectancy in modern Western societies, the sheer number of older people and what proportion of the population they now are, the percentage of people suffering from, or likely to suffer from Alzheimer's, and the cost of treating and caring for those who suffer from the disease. But you will also find a web of stories that illuminate the harsher knowledge we now seem to have of this daunting disease. And also an unwillingness on the author's part to entrust the disease too entirely to the scientists. Shenk believes that our need for comfort and inspiration is every bit as urgent as our need for truth. He doesn't want the facts of life without the romance of hope. He doesn't want knowledge for its own sake, but for ours.

So there is in this book the history of the discovery, of the gradual recognition, of this disease and of the contending scientific explanations for it. Stories, that is to say, of the inspired ingeniousness of scientists; and, of course, of careerism and financial opportunism (science as a democratic and disinterested pursuit is one of the book's more dismaying casualties). And there are also astonishingly lucid accounts, in the best tradition of so-called popular science, of how the disease itself works; despite the havoc it wreaks, one can't help but be struck by the sheer force and ingenuity of the disease process as it works its way through the brain. It is part of Shenk's subtlety as a writer to be as eloquently awestruck by the intricate competencies of the brain, as he is by the (so far) unstoppable drive and resilience of the disease. Nature degenerates as inventively as it generates. Disease is, as it were, a worthy antagonist.

Like most popular science books, *The Forgetting* wants us to be impressed by the way nature works; unlike most popular science books it is unusually mindful of what might happen to us—of what we might begin to feel—if we stopped being quite so impressed. It is perhaps our greatest gift to be able to see the wonder of nature where we might only be seeing its horror. Is it possible, to write a book about Alzheimer's that leaves us with any kind of hope? What Shenk suggests is that Alzheimer's—as *the* modern disease that, apart from cancer, haunts our lives—can help us revise our very sense of ourselves. Either a cure will be found— and *The Forgetting* has its inevitable (and reassuring) cast of optimistic scientists—or many of us will have to grow up with the knowledge that aging will involve the gradual dismantling of our memories, and a regression to virtual infancy. Instead of growing out of dependence we will have to grow into it. And some of those who don't have the disease will have to become dependable in new ways. So what exactly is there to look forward to?

There is, Shenk proposes, an opportunity in our acknowledging a new-found vulnerability. The devastation of Alzheimer's has mobilised resources—scientific, communal and individual resources—that we would never have known about. And as a disease of remembering it compels us to reconsider our relationship to time; Alzheimer's, as one of the heroic sufferers Shenk quotes, is about living in (and so, for) the moment. We are what we can make out of what we have to live with. In the age of information technology we have discovered the pathologies of memory. Alzheimer's, Shenk says, "is not only a disease, but also a prism through which we can view life in ways not normally available to us". It is part of a more realistically humane natural history to think of diseases as new ways of life: to describe illness, however catastrophic, as part of ordinary life. Out of fear of mortality we have idealised health and youth and competence. *The Forgetting* reminds us, among many other things, that there is more to life than all that.

Adam Phillips, 2001

PROLOGUE

❦

"When I was younger," Mark Twain quipped near the end of his life, "I could remember anything, whether it had happened or not; but my faculties are decaying now and soon I shall be so I cannot remember any but the things that never happened."

At age seventy-two, Twain's memory and wit were intact. But behind his remark lay a grim recollection of another celebrated writer's true decline. In December 1877, Twain had come to Boston at the invitation of William Dean Howells, editor of the *Atlantic Monthly,* to satirize a group of Brahmin intellectuals. Among Twain's targets that night was the father of American Transcendentalism, Ralph Waldo Emerson.

It was after midnight when Twain finally took to the floor at the Hotel Brunswick to spin his yarn. He told the venerable crowd about a lonely miner who had been victimized by three tramps claiming to be famous American writers. The literary outlaws stormed into the miner's cabin, ate his beans and bacon, guzzled his whiskey, and stole his only pair of boots. They played cards and fought bitterly. One of the tramps called himself Emerson.

The point of the skit was to poke some harmless fun at Emerson by corrupting some of his noble expressions. As they played cards at the climax of the story, the Emerson hobo spat out contorted fragments of his poem "Brahma." A mystical paean to immortality, the original included these stanzas:

> If the red slayer think he slays,
> Or if the slain think he is slain,
> They know not well the subtle ways
> I keep, and pass, and turn again.
>
> They reckon ill who leave me out;
> When me they fly, I am the wings;
> I am the doubter and the doubt,
> And I the hymn the Brahmin sings.

Twain twisted the verse into drunken poker banter:

> I am the doubter and the doubt—
> They reckon ill who leave me out,
> They know not well the subtle ways I keep,
> I pass and deal again.

An elegant master of spoof, Twain was revered around the world as the funniest living man. But on this important night, his material bombed. From the start, Twain drew only silence and quizzical looks, most prominently from Emerson himself. At the finish, Twain later recalled, there "fell a silence weighing many tons to the square inch." He was humiliated. Shortly afterward, he sent a letter of apology to Emerson.

Only then did Twain learn of the hidden backdrop to his performance: Emerson had been present only in body, not in mind. Emerson's dead silence and flat affect, Twain discovered, was a function of neither offense nor boredom. As his daughter Ellen wrote to Twain in reply, it was simply that he had not understood a word of what Twain was saying.

At age seventy-four, this was no longer the Ralph Waldo Emerson who had written "Self-Reliance" and *Nature;* who had said, "Insist on yourself; never imitate"; who had mentored Henry David Thoreau; the Emerson of whom James Russell Lowell had said, "When one meets him the Fall of Adam seems a false report."

This was now a very different man, a waning crescent, caught in the middle stages of a slow, progressive memory disorder that had ravaged his concentration and short-term memory and so dulled his perceptions that he was no longer able to understand what he read or follow a conversation.

"To my father," Ellen wrote to Twain of the performance, "it is as if it had not been; he never quite heard, never quite understood it, and he forgets easily and entirely."

One of the great minds in Western civilization was wasting away inside a still vigorous body, and there was nothing that anyone could hope to do about it.

～

Taos, New Mexico: March 1999

They came from Melbourne, Mannheim, St. Louis, London, and Kalamazoo; from Lexington, Stockholm, Dallas, Glasgow, Toronto, and Kuopio. From Tokyo, Zurich, and Palo Alto.

Some took two flights, others three or four, followed by a winding three-hour van ride from the floodplains of Albuquerque, up through the high desert terrain of Los Alamos, past the Sandia mountains, past the Jemez volcanic range, past the Camel Rock, Cities of Gold, and OK casinos, up near the foothills of the Sangre de Cristo mountains.

More than two hundred molecular biologists gathered in the small but sprawling city of Taos, amidst the adobe homes and green-chile quesadillas, to share data and hypotheses. This high-altitude, remote desert seemed like a strange place to fight a threatening disease. But specialists at the biannual conference "Molecular Mechanisms in Alzheimer's Disease" needed a refuge from their routine obligations.

For four and a half days they met in Bataan Hall, an old ballroom converted into a civic center. The room had once been used as a shipping-off point for soldiers in World War II, and later named in memory of those same soldiers' wretched ordeal in the infamous Bataan Death March. Some five hundred prisoners died each day on that trek, about the same number now dying each day in the U.S. from Alzheimer's disease.

At 8:00 P.M. on the first evening, Stanley Prusiner, a biologist at the University of California at San Francisco and a 1997 recipient of the Nobel Prize in medicine, rose to give the keynote address. "I can't compete with Monica," he began with a shrug. "But I think we all know that we wouldn't learn anything new."

Barbara Walters' much-anticipated TV interview with Monica Lewinsky was starting to air on ABC at that very moment, which further fueled the sense of isolation. The local support staff had just raced home to their televisions to catch the well-lighted promotion for the million-dollar book about the sordid affair with the needy President.

No TVs here. The scientists in this large, windowless chamber were distracted by something else: Alzheimer's disease was about to become an epidemic. Known as senility for thousands of years, Alzheimer's had only in the past few decades become a major health problem. Five million Americans and perhaps 15 million people worldwide now had the incurable disease, and those numbers would soon look attractive. Beginning in 2011, the first of the baby boomers would turn sixty-five and start to unravel in significant numbers. By 2050, about 15 million people in the U.S. alone would have Alzheimer's, at an annual cost of as much as $700 billion.

Other industrialized nations faced the same trends. In Japan, one in three would be elderly by 2050. In Canada, the number of elderly would increase by 50 percent while the working-age population increased by just 2 percent. In Britain and elsewhere in industrialized Europe, eighty-five-and-over would continue to be the fastest growing segment of the population. "We have to solve this problem, or it's going to overwhelm us," said Zaven Khachaturian, former director of the Alzheimer's Research Office at the National Institutes of Health. Alzheimer's had already become a costly and miserable fixture in society. Unless something was done to stop the disease, it would soon become one of the defining characteristics of civilization, one of the cornerstones of the human experience.

They were here to solve this problem.

PART I

&

EARLY

STAGE

The other day I was all confused in the street for a split second. I had to ask somebody where I was, and I realized the magnitude of this disease. I realized that this is a whole structure in which a window falls out, and then suddenly before you know it, the whole façade breaks apart.

This is the worst thing that can happen to a thinking person. You can feel yourself, your whole inside and outside, break down.

—M.
New York, New York

Chapter 1

I HAVE LOST MYSELF

∾

A healthy, mature human brain is roughly the size and shape of two adult fists, closed and pressed together at the knuckles. Weighing three pounds, it consists mainly of about a hundred billion nerve cells—neurons—linked to one another in about one hundred *trillion* separate pathways. It is by far the most complicated system known to exist in nature or civilization, a control center for the coordination of breathing, swallowing, pressure, pain, fear, arousal, sensory perception, muscular movement, abstract thought, identity, mood, and a varied suite of memories in a symphony that is partly predetermined and partly adaptable on the fly. The brain is so ridiculously complex, in fact, that in considering it in any depth one can only reasonably wonder why it works so well so much of the time.

Mostly, we don't think about it at all. We simply take this nearly silent, ludicrously powerful electrochemical engine for granted. We feed it, try not to smash it too hard against walls or windshields, and let it work its magic for us.

Only when it begins to fail in some way, only then are we surprised, devastated, and in awe.

On November 25, 1901, a fifty-one-year-old woman with no personal or family history of mental illness was admitted to a psychiatric hospital in Frankfurt, Germany, by her husband, who could no longer ignore or hide quirks and lapses that had overtaken her in recent months. First there were unexplainable bursts of anger, and then a strange series of memory problems. She became increasingly unable to locate things in her own home and began to make surprising mistakes in the kitchen. By the time she arrived at Städtische Irrenanstalt, the Frankfurt Hospital for the Mentally Ill and Epileptics, her condition was as severe as it was curious. The attending doctor, senior physician Alois Alzheimer, began the new file with these notes in the old German Sütterlin script.

> She sits on the bed with a helpless expression.
> "What is your name?"
> *Auguste.*
> "Last name?"
> *Auguste.*
> "What is your husband's name?"
> *Auguste, I think.*
> "How long have you been here?"
> (She seems to be trying to remember.)
> *Three weeks.*

It was her second day in the hospital. Dr. Alzheimer, a thirty-seven-year-old neuropathologist and clinician from the small Bavarian village of Markbreit-am-Main, observed in his new patient a remarkable cluster of symptoms: severe disorientation, reduced comprehension, aphasia (language impairment), paranoia, hallucinations, and a short-term memory so incapacitated that when he spoke her full-name, *Frau Auguste D———*, and asked her to write it down, the patient got only as far as "Frau" before needing the doctor to repeat the rest.

He spoke her name again. She wrote "Augu" and again stopped.

When Alzheimer prompted her a third time, she was able to write her entire first name and the initial "D" before finally giving up, telling the doctor, "I have lost myself."

Her condition did not improve. It became apparent that there was nothing that anyone at this or any other hospital could do for Frau D. except to insure her safety and try to keep her as clean and comfortable as possible. Over the next four and a half years, she became increasingly disoriented, delusional, and incoherent. She was often hostile.

"Her gestures showed a complete helplessness," Alzheimer later noted in a published report. "She was disoriented as to time and place. From time to time she would state that she did not understand anything, that she felt confused and totally lost. Sometimes she considered the coming of the doctor as an official visit and apologized for not having finished her work, but other times she would start to yell out of the fear that the doctor wanted to operate on her [or] damage her woman's honor. From time to time she was completely delirious, dragging her blankets and sheets to and fro, calling for her husband and daughter, and seeming to have auditory hallucinations. Often she would scream for hours and hours in a horrible voice."

By November 1904, three and a half years into her illness, Auguste D. was bedridden, incontinent, and largely immobile. Occasionally, she busied herself with her bed clothes. Notes from October 1905 indicate that she had become permanently curled up in a fetal position, with her knees drawn up to her chest, muttering but unable to speak, and requiring assistance to be fed.

What was this strange disease that would take an otherwise healthy middle-aged woman and slowly—very slowly, as measured against most disease models—peel away, layer by layer, her ability to remember, to communicate her thoughts and finally to understand the world around her? What most struck Alzheimer, an experienced diagnostician, was that this condition could not fit neatly into any of the standard psychiatric boxes. The symptoms of Auguste D. did not present themselves as a case of acute delirium or the consequence of a stroke; both would have come on more suddenly. Nor was this the general paresis—mood changes, hyperactive reflexes, hallucinations—that can set in during the late stages of syphilis. She was clearly not a victim of dementia praecox (what we now call schizophrenia), or Parkinson's palsy, or Friedreich's ataxia, or Huntington's disease, or Korsakoff's syndrome, or any of the other well-recognized neurological disorders of the day, disorders that Alzheimer routinely treated in his ward. One of the fundamental elements of diagnostic medicine has always been the exercise of exclusion, to systematically rule out whatever can be ruled out and then see what possibilities are left standing. But Alzheimer had nothing left.

What the fifty-one-year-old Auguste D.'s condition did strongly evoke was a well-known ailment among the elderly: a sharp unraveling of memory and mind that had, for more than five thousand years, been accepted by doctors and philosophers as a routine consequence of aging.

History is stacked with colorful, poignant accounts of the elderly behaving in strange ways before they die, losing connection with their memories and the world around them, making rash decisions, acting with the impetuousness and irresponsibility of children. Plato insisted that those suffering from "the influence of extreme old age" should be excused from the commission of the crimes of sacrilege, treachery, and treason. Cicero lamented the folly of "frivolous" old men. Homer, Aristotle, Maimonides, Chaucer, Thackeray, Boswell, Pope, and Swift all wrote of a distressing feebleness of mind that infected those of advancing years.

"Old age," wrote Roger Bacon, "is the home of forgetfulness."

Known as *morosis* in Greek, *oblivio* and *dementia* in Latin, *dotage* in Middle English, *démence* in French, and *fatuity* in eighteenth-century English, the condition was definitively termed *senile dementia* in 1838 by the French psychiatrist Jean Étienne Esquirol. In a depiction any doctor or caregiver would recognize today, Esquirol wrote: "Senile dementia is established slowly. It commences with enfeeblement of memory, particularly the memory of recent impressions."

But that was *senile* dementia. What was this? Alois Alzheimer wanted to know. Why did a fifty-one-year-old appear to be going senile? How could Auguste D. be suffering from the influence of extreme old age?

We are the sum of our memories. Everything we know, everything we perceive, every movement we make is shaped by them. "The truth is," Friedrich Nietzsche wrote, "that, in the process by which the human being, in thinking, reflecting, comparing, separating, and combining . . . inside that surrounding misty cloud a bright gleaming beam of light arises, only then, through the power of using the past for living and making history out of what has happened, does a person first become a person."

The Austrian psychiatrist Viktor Frankl made much the same point in *Man's Search for Meaning,* his memoir of experiences as a concentration camp inmate. Frankl recalled trying to lift the spirits of his fellow camp inmates on an especially awful day in Dachau: "I did not only talk of the future and the veil which was drawn over it. I also mentioned the past; all its joys, and how its light shone even in the present darkness. [I quoted] a poet . . . who had written, *Was Du erlebst, kann keine Macht der Welt Dir rauben.* (What you have experienced, no power on earth can take from you.) Not only our experiences, but all we have done, whatever great thoughts we may have had and all we have suffered, all this is not lost, though it is past; we have brought it into being. Having been is a kind of being, and perhaps the surest kind."

Emerson was also fascinated by memory—how it worked, why it failed, the ways it shaped human consciousness. Memory, he offered about a decade or so before his own troubles first appeared, is "the cement, the bitumen, the matrix in which the other faculties are embedded . . . without it all life and thought were an unrelated succession." While he constructed an elaborate external memory system in topical notebooks, filling thousands of pages of facts and observations that were intricately cross-referenced and indexed, Emerson was also known for his own keen internal memory. He could recite by heart all of Milton's "Lycidas" and much of Wordsworth, and made it a regular practice to recite poetry to his children on their walks. His journal entries depict an enchantment with the memory feats of others.

He kept a list:

- Frederic the Great knew every bottle in his cellar.
- Magliabecchi wrote off his book from memory.
- Seneca could say 2,000 words in one hearing.
- L. Scipio knew the name of every man in Rome.
- Judge Parsons knew all his dockets next year.
- Themistocles knew the names of all the Athenians.

"We estimate a man by how much he remembers," Emerson wrote.

Ronald Reagan was never particularly admired for his memory. But in the late 1980s and early '90s, he slowly began to lose his grasp on ordinary function. In 1992, three years after leaving the White House, Reagan's forgetting became impossible to ignore. He was eighty-one.

Both his mother and older brother had experienced senility, and he had demonstrated a mild forgetfulness in the late years of his presidency. Like many people who eventually suffer from the disease, Reagan may have had an inkling for some time of what was to come. In his stable of disarming jokes were several about memory troubles afflicting the elderly. He shared one at a 1985 dinner honoring Senator Russell Long.

An elderly couple was getting ready for bed one night, Reagan told the crowd. The wife turned to her husband and said, "I'm just so hungry for ice cream and there isn't any in the house."

"I'll get you some," her husband offered.

"You're a dear," she said. "Vanilla with chocolate sauce. Write it down—you'll forget."

"I won't forget," he said.

"With whipped cream on top."

"Vanilla with chocolate sauce and whipped cream on top," he repeated.

"And a cherry," she said.

"And a cherry on top."

"Please write it down," she said. "I know you'll forget."

"I won't forget," he insisted. "Vanilla with chocolate sauce, whipped cream, and a cherry on top."

The husband went off and returned after a while with a paper bag, which he handed to his wife in bed. She opened up the bag, and pulled out a ham sandwich.

"I told you to write it down," she said. "You forgot the mustard."

It seems clear enough that Reagan was increasingly bothered by personal memory lapses. In a regular White House checkup late in his second term, the President began by joking to his doctor, "I have three things that I want to tell you today. The first is that I seem to be having a little problem with my memory. I cannot remember the other two."

Did Reagan have Alzheimer's disease in office? Yes and no. Without a doubt, he was on his way to getting the disease, which develops over many years. But it is equally clear that there was not yet nearly enough decline in function to support even a tentative diagnosis. Reagan's mind was well within the realm of normal functioning. Even if his doctors had been looking intently for Alzheimer's, it is still likely that they would not have been able to detect the disease-in-progress. A slight deterioration of memory is so common among the elderly that even today it is considered to be a natural (if unwelcome) consequence of aging. About a third to a half of all human beings experience some mild decline in memory as they get older, taking longer to learn directions, for example, or having some difficulty recalling names or numbers.

Alzheimer's disease overtakes a person very gradually, and for a while can be indistinguishable from such mild memory loss. But eventually the forgetting reaches the stage where it is quite distinct from an absentminded loss of one's glasses or keys. Fleeting moments of almost total confusion seize a person who is otherwise entirely healthy and lucid. Suddenly, on a routine drive home from work, an intersection he has seen a thousand times is now totally unfamiliar. Or he is asking about when his son is coming back from his vacation, and his wife says: "What do you mean? We both spoke to him last night." Or he is paying the check after a perfectly pleasant night out and it's the strangest thing, but he just cannot calculate the 20 percent tip.

The first few slips get chalked up to anxiety or a lousy night's sleep or a bad cold. But how to consider these incidents of disorientation and confusion when they begin to occur with some frequency? What begin as isolated incidents start to mount and soon become impossible to ignore. In fact, they are not incidents; collectively, they are signs of a degenerative condition. Your brain is under attack. Months and years go by. Now you are losing your balance. Now you can no longer make sense of an analog clock. Now you cannot find the words to complain about your food. Now your handsome young husband has disappeared and a strange elderly man has taken his place. Why is someone taking your clothes off and pouring warm water over you? How long have you been lying in this strange bed?

By 1992, the signs of Reagan's illness were impossible to ignore. At the conclusion of a medical exam in September, as the *New York Times* would later report, Reagan looked up at his doctor of many years with an utterly blank face and said, "What am I supposed to do next?" This time, the doctor knew that something was very wrong.

Sixteen months later, in February 1994, Reagan flew back to Washington, D.C., from his retirement home in Bel Air, California, for what would turn out to be his final visit. The occasion was a dinner celebrating his own eighty-third birthday, attended by Margaret Thatcher and twenty-five hundred other friends and supporters.

Before the gala began, the former President had trouble recognizing a former Secret Service agent whom he had known well in the White House. This didn't come as a total shock to his wife, Nancy, and other close friends, but it did cause them to worry that Reagan might have problems with his speech that night.

The show went on as planned. After an introduction by Thatcher, Reagan strolled to the podium. He began to speak, then stumbled, and paused. His doctor, John Hutton, feared that Reagan was about to humiliate himself. "I was holding my breath, wondering how he would get started," Hutton later recalled, "when suddenly something switched on, his voice resounded, he paused at the right places, and he was his old self."

Back at his hotel after the dinner, Reagan again slipped into his unsettling new self, turning to Nancy and saying, "Well, I've got to wait a minute. I'm not quite sure where I am." Though the diagnosis and public announcement were both months away, Reagan was already well along the sad path already trod by his mother, his brother, and by Auguste D.

The doctors who diagnosed Reagan in 1994 knew with some specificity what was happening to his brain. Portions of his cerebral cortex, the thin layer of gray matter coating the outside of his brain, were becoming steadily clouded with two separate forms of cellular debris: clumpy brown spherical *plaques* floating between the neurons, and long black stringy *tangles* choking neurons from inside their cell membranes. As those plaques and tangles spread, some neurons were losing the ability to transmit messages to one another. Levels of glucose, the brain's sole energy source, were falling precipitously, weakening cell function; neurotransmitters, the chemicals that facilitate messages between the neurons, were becoming obstructed. The tangles in some areas of the brain were getting to be so thick it was like trying to kick a football through a chain-link fence.

Ultimately, many of the neurons would die, and the brain would begin to shrink. Because the brain is highly specialized, the strangulation of each clump of neurons would restrict a very specific function—the ability to convert recent events into reliable memories, for example, or the ability to recall specific words, or to consider basic math problems. Or, eventually, to speak at all, or recognize a loved one. Or to walk or swallow or breathe.

We know about plaques and tangles because of Auguste D. and Alois Alzheimer. After four and a half years in the hospital, Frau D. died on April 8, 1906. Her file listed the cause as "septicaemia due to decubitis"—acute blood poisoning resulting from infectious bed sores. In her last days, she had pneumonia, inflammation of the kidneys, excessive fluid in the brain, and a high fever. On the day of her death, doctors understood no more than they had on the first day she was admitted. They could say only this about Auguste D.: that a psychic disturbance had developed in the absence of epileptic fits, that the disturbance had progressed, and that death had finally intervened.

Alois Alzheimer wanted to learn more. He wanted to look at her brain.

Standing apart from most doctors at the time, Alzheimer was equally interested in both clinical and laboratory work. He was known for his tireless schedule, his devoted teaching, and his own brand of forgetfulness. An inveterate smoker, he would put a half-smoked cigar down on the table before leaning into a student's microscope for a consultation. A few minutes later, while shuffling to the next microscope, he'd light a fresh cigar, having forgotten about the smoke already in progress. At the end of each day, twenty microscopes later, students recalled, twenty cigar stumps would be left smoldering throughout the room.

But Alzheimer did not forget about the woman who had lost herself in Frankfurt. Though he had since moved to the Royal Psychiatric Clinic, in Munich, to work for the renowned psychiatrist Emil Kraepelin, he sent for Frau D.'s central nervous system as soon as she died. Her brain, brainstem, and spinal cord were gently removed from the elaborate bone casing, that flexible yet durable wrapper that allows us all to crouch, twist, and bump into things without much concern. The exposed contents were then likely wrapped in formalin-soaked towels, packed carefully in a wooden crate, and shipped by locomotive 190 miles southeast to Munich.

Imagine, now, that lifeless brain on a passenger train. A coconut-sized clump of grooved gelatinous flesh; an intricate network of prewired and self-adapting mechanisms perfected over more than a billion years of natural selection; powered by dual chemical and electrical systems, a machine as vulnerable as it is complex, designed to sacrifice durability for maximal function, to burn brightly—a human brain is 2 percent of the body's weight but requires 20 percent of its energy consumption—at the cost of impermanence. Enormously powerful and potato-chip fragile at the same time, the brain is able to collect and retain a universe of knowledge and understanding, even wisdom, but cannot hold on to so much as a phone number once the glucose stops flowing. The train, an elementary device by comparison, can, with proper maintenance, be sustained forever. The brain, which conceived of the train and all of its mechanical cousins, cannot. It is ephemeral by design.

But there was nothing in the brain's blueprint about this sort of thing, as far as Alzheimer could infer. This was a flaw in the design, a molecular glitch, a *disease process,* he suspected, and it was important to see what that process looked like up close.

It was also now actually possible to do this for the first time, thanks to a whirl of European innovation. Ernst Leitz and Carl Zeiss had just invented the first distortion-free microscopes, setting a standard in optics that survives today. Franz Nissl had revolutionized tissue-staining, making various cell constituents stand out, opening up what was characterized as "a new era" in the study of brain cells and tissues. (The "Nissl method" is still in use. Nissl, a close collaborator and friend of Alois Alzheimer, became a medical school legend with his instructions on how to time the staining process. "Take the brain out," he advised. "Put it on the desk. Spit on the floor. When the spit is dry, put the brain in alcohol.")

Dr. Alzheimer's assistants prepared for microscopic examination more than 250 slides from slivers of the outer lining (the meninges) of Frau D.'s brain; from the large cerebral vessels; from the frontal, parietal, and occipital areas of the cerebral cortex (locus of conscious thought); from the cerebellum (regulator of balance, coordination, gait) and the brainstem (breathing and other basic life functions); and from the spinal cord, all chemically preserved in a cocktail of 90 percent alcohol/10 percent formalin, and stained according to a half-dozen recipes of Alzheimer's contemporaries.

Having fixed, frozen, sliced, stained, and pressed the tissue between two thin pieces of glass, Alzheimer put down his cigar and removed his pince-nez, leaned into his state-of-the-art Zeiss microscope, and peered downward. Then, at a magnification of several hundred times, he finally saw her disease.

It looked like measles, or chicken pox, of the brain. The cortex was speckled with crusty brown clumps—plaques—too many to count. They varied in size, shape, and texture and seemed to be a hodgepodge of granules and short, crooked threads, as if they were sticky magnets for microscopic trash.

The plaques were nestled in amongst the neurons, in a space normally occupied by supporting tissue known as glial cells. They were so prominent that Alzheimer could see them without any stain at all, but they showed up best in a blend of magenta red, indigo carmine, and picric acid. Alzheimer had squinted at thousands of brain slides, but he found these clumps "peculiar" and had no idea what they could be.

A different stain, invented just four years earlier, revealed the other strange invasion of Auguste D.'s brain. In the second and third layers of the cortex, nearly a third of the neurons had been obliterated internally, overrun with what Alzheimer called "a tangled bundle of fibrils"—weedy, menacing strands of rope bundled densely together.

The tangles were just as foreign to Alzheimer as the plaques, but at least the ingredients looked familiar. They seemed to be composed of fibrils, an ordinary component of every neuron. It was as if these mild-mannered, or "Jekyll," fibrils had swallowed some sort of steroidal toxin and been transformed into "Hyde" fibrils, growing well out of proportion and destroying everything within their reach. Many affected neurons were missing a nucleus completely, and most of the rest of their cell contents. A good portion of the neurons in the upper cell layers of the cortex had disappeared. They just weren't there. Alzheimer's assistant Gaetano Perusini wrote of the neurofibrillary tangles in Frau D.'s brain:

> It is impossible to give a description of all the possible pictures: there are present all the variable and twisted formations that one can imagine; at times large fibrils seem to lie only on the periphery of the cell. But on focusing untangled fibrillar agglomerations are found. Changing the focus again one has the impression that the single dark-coloured fibrils unwind into an infinite number of

thinner fibrils . . . arranged as balls of twine or half-moons or baskets.

Connecting a camera lucida to the top of the microscope, Alzheimer and Perusini both drew pictures of the tangles.

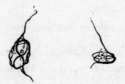

The menacing drawings perfectly convey the ghastly significance of their discovery. Here was the evidence that Auguste D. had not lost herself. Rather, her "self" was taken from her. Cell by cell by cell, she had been strangled by unwelcome, malignant intruders.

What were they, exactly, and where did they come from?

When my kids began to say they were worrying about my memory, I said to them, "Well, I've never had a photographic memory, and I have a lot more on my mind now. There's a lot more to remember with life being so complex. How can I remember everything? What do you want—total recall?" I always had an answer. I really was in denial, and it just didn't occur to me that I had a problem. But I also knew that they weren't totally exaggerating.

—D.
New York, New York

Chapter 2

BOTHERED

∾

Queens, New York: August 1998

It was lunch time in Freund House, in the village of Flushing. A small group of elderly Jews sat quietly at a round table. Not much was said as they ruffled open their brown paper bags and popped the lids off drinks. Someone brought in a big bottle of ginger ale and some plastic cups, and offered to pour.

Irving looked over at Greta and noticed that she was sitting still, her hands folded together on the bright red table cloth.

"Did you bring your lunch today, Greta?"

"I don't think so. I usually don't bring my lunch here."

"Yes, you do. You bring cereal."

Irving waited for Greta to recollect her routine, but she could not. An elegant, shrunken woman with short cropped hair, dark eyebrows, and a supple, leathery face, Greta did not look even remotely like someone in decline. Her eyes still sparkled and her voice had spunk. She spoke without hesitation and in full, clear sentences. There was no clue from her cadences that her brain was under attack.

Paying close attention, though, one could tell that something was not right. For example, in a conversation about Japan, Greta very clearly explained that she had been there a number of times. She discussed the temples of Kyoto, which she enjoyed, and the food, which she did not.

Then, about an hour later, the subject of Japan came up again. This time, she said matter-of-factly, "Japan—never did get there. Couldn't get in."

These hiccups in logic were typical, I now recognized, of someone beginning to advance past the very earliest stages of the disease. She wasn't very far along yet, and most of her brain was still working quite well; but her symptoms were no longer strictly limited to the classic short-term memory loss that usually signals the disease's onset. Occasionally, now, a queer incongruity would creep in.

Standing off to one side of the table was Judy Joseph, the co-leader, with Irving Brickman, of this support group. About a year earlier she had been introduced to Irving in the New York offices of the Alzheimer's Association, where each had come to see what, if anything, could be done about this ominous new social phenomenon. Suddenly, it seemed, Alzheimer's disease was everywhere. Nursing home dementia units were filling beyond capacity. Middle-aged children were moving back home to take care of their parents. Community police were regularly being phoned to help track down wandering relatives. The disease was cropping up continually in newspaper articles and everyday conversation. Perhaps most tellingly, a vibrant Alzheimer's consumer market was springing up—products like automatic medication dispensers (no memory required!), wireless tracking devices for wanderers, and even a stovetop fire extinguisher designed explicitly for people who might forget to turn off the range.

All of a sudden, everyone seemed to know someone touched by Alzheimer's. Partly, this was due to a shift in public conception of senile dementia. Only in the mid-1970s had doctors started to realize that senility is not an inevitable process of brain aging and decay but a recognizable—and perhaps one day treatable—disorder. Gradually, this perception also started to seep into the general consciousness: *Senility is a disease.*

Since then, there had been a staggering rise in actual cases of Alzheimer's, corresponding to a vast increase in the elderly population. People were now living much longer lives. Longer lives meant more cases of Alzheimer's. Since 1975, the estimated number of Alzheimer's cases in the U.S. had grown tenfold, from 500,000 to nearly 5 million. Worldwide, the total was probably about three times that figure. In the absence of a medical breakthrough, the gloomy trend would not only continue, but would also get much, much worse.

The Roman poet Virgil wrote in the first century B.C., "Time wastes all things, the mind, too." He was partly right. Scientists do not believe that Alzheimer's is an *inevitable* consequence of aging. Many people will never get the disease regardless of how long they live. But aging is by far the greatest risk factor. It is almost unheard of in people aged 20–39, and very uncommon (about one in 2,500) for people aged 40–59. For people in their sixties, the odds begin to get more worrisome. An estimated

- 1 percent of 65-year-olds
- 2 percent of 68-year-olds
- 3 percent of 70-year-olds
- 6 percent of 73-year-olds
- 9 percent of 75-year-olds
- 13 percent of 77-year-olds

and so on have Alzheimer's or a closely related dementia. The risk accelerates with age, to the point where dementia affects nearly half of those eighty-five and over.

So, as the twentieth century came to a close, a shadow legacy was rapidly becoming apparent—the dark, unintended consequence of the century's great advances in hygiene, nutrition, and medicine. Life spans in industrialized nations had nearly doubled over the previous one hundred years, and the percentage of elderly among the general population had more than tripled. In the process, the number of cases of senile dementia mushroomed. A hundred years before, it had not even been a statistical blip. Paradoxically, in the full blush of medical progress of the twentieth century, it had blossomed into a major public health problem.

Most strikingly to social workers like Judy and Irving, the number of people who had Alzheimer's *and who knew they had Alzheimer's* had exploded. A huge portion of the newly diagnosed cases were in the very early stages of the disease. "This is something new in the field," Irving explained. "Most people never before realized that there *is* an early stage of Alzheimer's. I had worked with the more advanced stages, but when I came into this it was overwhelming for me. It's very hard to get used to a normal person who happens to have dementia. It's a whole different ballgame."

Judy and Irving recognized, along with many others in the national Alzheimer's community, that something had to be done to help this emerging new constituency: early-stage dementia sufferers still functioning well enough to fully understand what lay ahead. With the assistance of the Alzheimer's Association, they formed a support group at Freund House. "Our goal," explained Irving, "is to try to help these people live a quality life, to help them gain some coping mechanisms for their deficits, and to help them feel better as human beings." While scientists did battle with this disease, victims and their families had the opposite task: to make a certain peace with it, to struggle to understand the loss, come to terms with it, create meaning out of it.

Alzheimer's is what doctors call a disease of "insidious onset," by which they mean that it has no definitive starting point. The plaques and tangles proliferate so slowly—over decades, perhaps—and silently that their damage can be nearly impossible to detect until they have made considerable progress. Part of the function of any early-stage support group must be to try to make sense of this strange new terrain that lies between *healthy* and *demented*. Where, in specific behavioral terms, is the person overshadowed by the disease?

Individually and collectively, the Freund House group was trying to find out, and to make sense of the answer. "My wife gets frustrated with me," Arnie related to his fellow group members, "and she is right to be frustrated. She asks me to put a can in the recycling . . . and I don't do it. She says, 'I know this is because of your illness, that this is not you.' "

Sadie nodded her head in recognition. "My mother had this, too," she said. "Now I know what it was like for my father to take care of her. We used to get so mad at him when he would be short with her."

Coping with a particular disability was one thing; trying to cope with an ever-shifting invisible illness, though, was a challenge unique to Alzheimer's disease. In this early period, the insidiousness itself was often the most troubling thing about the disease—arguably even a disease unto itself. As a group, these new patients could gain a more confident understanding of their disease, and tackle issues that would seem impossibly difficult to one isolated, failing person.

Driving, for instance. The first big question they confronted right after forming the group was: Should they continue, in this blurry period of semi-normalcy, to pilot massive steel boxes at thirty and forty and fifty miles per hour down roads lined with bicycles and toddlers? Studies showed conclusively that Alzheimer's is, overall, a major driving hazard. Bystanders had been killed by Alzheimer's patients making a lapse in judgment or being overcome momentarily by confusion. But the law had not yet caught up with this reality. Even with a diagnosis, no doctor or judge had ever confiscated a license. Families were forced to decide on their own when driving was no longer appropriate.

Together, after much deliberation, the group decided that it had already become too dangerous. Collectively, they gave up this highly charged symbol of autonomy and competence. On this shaky new terrain, a person's independence could no longer be taken for granted.

In the summer of 1984, at the age of eighty-five, E. B. White, the tender essayist and author of *Charlotte's Web*, became waylaid by some form of dementia. It came on very swiftly. In August, he began to complain of some mild disorientation. "We didn't pay much attention," recalls his stepson, Roger Angell, "because he was a world-class hypochondriac." But just a few weeks later, White was severely confused much of the time. By the following May, he was bedridden with full-on dementia, running in and out of vivid hallucinations and telling visitors, "So many dreams—it's hard to pick out the right one." He died just a few months after that, in October 1985.

An obituary in the *New York Times* reported White as having Alzheimer's disease, but that appeared to miss the mark. In fact, he was never even informally diagnosed with the disease, and his symptoms strongly suggested another illness. The rapid onset of the confusion and the abrupt shift from one stage to the next were classic signs of multi-infarct dementia, the second-most common cause (15 percent) of senile dementia after Alzheimer's (60 percent). Multi-infarct dementia is caused by a series of tiny strokes. Its victims can have much in common with those of Alzheimer's, but the experience is not as much of an enigma. Its cause is known, somewhat treatable, and, to a certain extent, preventable (diet, exercise, and medication can have an enormous impact on risk of strokes). Its jerky, stepwise approach is easier to follow and understand as symptoms worsen.

Alzheimer's disease is not abrupt. It sets in so gradually that its beginning is imperceptible. Creeping diseases blur the boundaries in such a way that they can undermine our basic assumptions of illness. Alzheimer's drifts from one stage to the next in a slow-motion haze. The disease is so gradual in its progression that it has come to be formally defined by that insidiousness. This is one of the disease's primary clinical features, one key way that Alzheimer's can be distinguished from other types of dementia: those caused by strokes, brain tumor, underactive thyroid, and vitamin deficiency or imbalance in electrolytes, glucose, or calcium (all treatable and potentially reversible conditions).

It is also nearly impossible to officially diagnose. A definitive determination requires evidence of both plaques and tangles—which cannot be obtained without drilling into the patient's skull, snipping a tiny piece of brain tissue, and examining it under a microscope. Brain biopsies are today considered far too invasive for a patient who does not face imminent danger. Thus—Kafka would have enjoyed this—as a general rule, Alzheimer's sufferers must die before they can be definitively diagnosed. Until autopsy, the formal diagnosis can only be "probable Alzheimer's."

These days, a decent neuropsychologist can maneuver within this paradox—can make a diagnosis of probable Alzheimer's with a confidence of about 90 percent—through a battery of tests. The process almost always begins with this simple quiz:

What is today's date?
What day of the week is it?
What is the season?
What country are we in?
What city?
What neighborhood?
What building are we in?
What floor are we on?
I'm going to name three objects and I want you to repeat them back to me: street, banana, hammer.
I'd like you to count backwards from one hundred by seven. [Stop after five answers.]

Can you repeat back to me the three objects I mentioned
    a moment ago?

[Points at any object in the room.] What do we call this?

[Points at another object.] What do we call this?

Repeat after me: "No ifs, ands, or buts."

Take this piece of paper in your right hand, fold it in half,
    and put it on the floor.

[Without speaking, doctor shows the patient a piece of pa-
    per with "CLOSE YOUR EYES" printed on it.]

Please write a sentence for me. It can say anything at all,
    but make it a complete sentence.

Here is a diagram of two intersecting pentagons. Please
    copy this drawing onto a plain piece of paper.

This neurological obstacle course is called the Mini Mental
State Examination (MMSE). Introduced in 1975, it has been a
part of the standard diagnostic repertoire ever since. The MMSE is
crude but generally very effective in detecting problems with time
and place orientation, object registration, abstract thinking, recall,
verbal and written cognition, and constructional praxis. A person
with normal functioning will score very close to the perfect thirty
points (I scored twenty-nine, getting the date wrong). A person
with early-to-moderate dementia will generally fall below twenty-
four.

The very earliest symptoms in Alzheimer's are short-term
memory loss—the profound forgetting of incidents or conversations from just a few hours or the day before; fleeting spatial
disorientation; trouble with words and arithmetic; and some impairment of judgment. Later on, in the middle stages of the disease, more severe memory problems are just a part of a full suite of

cognitive losses. Following that, the late stages feature further cognitive loss and a series of progressive physical disabilities, ending in death.

One brilliantly simple exam, the Clock Test, can help foretell all of this and can enable a doctor to pinpoint incipient dementia in nine out of ten cases. In the Clock Test, the doctor instructs the patient to draw a clock on a piece of paper and then draw hands to a certain time. Neurologists have discovered that patients in the early stages of dementia tend to make many more errors of omission and misplacing of numbers on the clock than cognitively healthy people. They're not entirely sure why this is, but the accuracy of the test speaks for itself.

A battery of other performance tests can help highlight and clarify neurological deficiencies. The Buschke Selective Reminding Test measures the subject's short-term verbal memory. The Wisconsin Card Sorting Test gauges the ability to deduce sorting patterns. In the Trail Making Test, psychomotor skills are measured by timing a subject's attempt to draw a line connecting consecutively numbered circles. Porteus Mazes measure planning and abstract-puzzle-solving ability.

If the patient performs poorly in a consistent fashion, the next step will likely involve elaborate instruments. Conveniently for physicians, Alzheimer's disease always begins in the same place: a curved, two-inch-long, peapod-like structure in the brain's temporal lobes called the hippocampus (the temporal lobes are located on either side of the head, inward from the ear). Doctors can get a good look at the hippocampus with a magnetic resonance imaging (MRI) scanner, which bombards the body with radio waves and measures the reflections off tissue. A simple volume measurement of the hippocampus will often show, even in the very early stages of Alzheimer's, a pronounced decrease in volume, particularly in contrast with other brain structures. By itself, the MRI cannot diagnose Alzheimer's. But it can add one more helpful piece to the diagnostic puzzle.

Other advanced measurements might also help: A positron emission tomography (PET) scan may detect a decrease in oxygen flow or glucose metabolism in the same area. A single photon emission computed tomography (SPECT) scan may catch decreases in blood flow. A moderate to severe amount of slowing in the alpha rhythm in an electroencephalogram (EEG) is often characteristic of dementia. But such measurements are generally not required for a tentative diagnosis. In the face of convincing results from memory and performance tests, and in the absence of any contravening evidence—disturbance in consciousness, extremely rapid onset of symptoms, preponderance of tremors or other muscular symptoms, difficulties with eye movements or reports of temporary blindness, seizures, depression, psychosis, head trauma, a history of alcoholism or drug abuse, any indication of diabetes, syphilis, or AIDS—a diagnosis of *probable Alzheimer's* is rendered.

Alzheimer's disease. The diagnosis is a side-impact collision of overwhelming force. It seems unreal and unjust. After coming up for air, the sufferer might ask, silently or out loud, "What have I done to deserve this?" The answer is, simply, *nothing.* "I remember walking out of the clinic and into a fresh San Diego night feeling like a very helpless and broken man," recalled Bill, a fifty-four-year-old magazine editor, to writer Lisa Snyder. "I wondered if there was anything for me to live for."

It can take a while to sink in. Experienced doctors know not to try to convey any other important information to a patient or family member on the same day that they disclose the diagnosis. They put some helpful information into a letter, and schedule a follow-up.

There is no cure for Alzheimer's at the present time, and not much in the way of treatment. Historically, the one saving grace of the disease over the years has been that many, if not most, of the people who acquire the disease do not comprehend what is about to happen to them and their families. Now, for better or worse, that has changed. More and more are learning at the earliest possible opportunity what they have, and what it means.

What will they do with the advance knowledge? It is not an easy question. Will they use the time left to get their affairs in order and to prepare themselves emotionally for the long fade? Or will the knowledge only add to the frustration and force them into a psychological spiral to accompany the physiological one?

The Freund House early-stage support group was one experimental approach to tackling such unknowns. When Judy and Irving created it in 1997, they weren't sure it would work. Could people struggling with memory loss, spatial disorientation, and confusion actually strike up a meaningful relationship with a group of strangers? They had to assemble just the right team. "We had to turn many people away," said Judy, "because we didn't feel they were right for a support group. They weren't introspective enough. They weren't *bothered* enough."

The group was also temporary by design. As participants lost the ability to contribute, they would be eased out of the group, and perhaps admitted to a middle-stage group like the one that Judy ran down the hall. In that group, volunteer caregivers always accompanied patients to the restroom and back, because otherwise they would get lost. Most, not all, still responded to their own name. After a cafeteria-style lunch, everyone came together in a circle to sing fun songs together, like the theme from *Barney:*

> I love you
> You love me
> We're a happy family

Members of the early-stage group occasionally caught a glimpse of the middle-stage group as they passed by to get a cup of coffee. The quiet, desperate hope of everyone in this group was not to end up in the other group. Barring a scientific miracle, though, there would be no avoiding it. The average interval from diagnosis to death in Alzheimer's disease is eight years.

In the meantime, there were a hundred small consolations. The early-stage group members had quickly come to rely on one another for help through this very strange ordeal. Sometimes barely able to remember from week to week, they had nevertheless become friends. They shared memories of movie stars and kosher butchers. They talked about travel and passed around pictures of grandchildren. They even talked politics.

"Greta, any comments on Giuliani?" Judy asked one afternoon.

Greta swatted an invisible bug away from her face. "Oh don't get me started about him," she said. "You know I can't stand him."

"Clinton, then? What does everyone think about Monica?"

Opinions ran the gamut. Ted, his hands shaking with a Parkinsonian tremor (it is not unusual for people to suffer from both Parkinson's and Alzheimer's), suggested that Clinton should resign because he lied directly to the American people. Greta, a lifelong subscriber to *The Nation,* thought that Clinton probably kissed Monica but that the whole issue was overblown. Sadie thought it was all a Republican scheme.

Doris had an opinion, too, but with her severe expressive aphasia—an inability to retrieve words—she had great difficulty making it known.

"Gore . . . President . . . I think . . . good leader . . . lies . . ."

She appeared to be aware of her thoughts and very clear on what she wanted to say. But the words were no longer accessible. This was especially painful to watch because, as everyone in the group knew by now, Doris had a forty-year-old son with cerebral palsy who was deaf. The two were very close, and, as it happened, she was the only one in the family to have ever learned sign language. Now Doris's aphasia was also wiping away that second and more vital language. She could no longer speak to her son, leaving him marooned.

It was now a few minutes after one o'clock, time to say goodbye for the week. Rides were arranged. Someone went to fetch William's wife, a volunteer in the middle-stage group.

Robert seemed to be having a hard time of it. Just a moment before, he had been lucidly telling me about his family and his past. He'd had no problem relating how he was spirited out of Nazi Germany as a young boy, turned over to relatives in England and later in New York. I learned all about his children, their occupations and families, the cities they lived in. But now he was struggling to understand a piece of paper his wife had written out for him about getting home. To the undamaged brain, the instructions were fairly straightforward—*Robert will be picked up by the car service at 1:15, and should be driven to his home at* _____

Street. . . . —but he was having a lot of trouble making sense of it. Then there was the other problem. In the last half hour, he had told me how he eventually came to live in the Bronx, where he was introduced to his wife, a distant cousin. He had described how crowded that Bronx apartment was, and where else he had lived in the city as he'd grown older. But now, for the life of him, Robert could not remember where he had put his jacket.

It was on the back of his chair.

～

Very often I wander around looking for
something which I know is very pertinent, but then
after a while I forget about what it is I was looking
for. . . . Once the idea is lost, everything is lost and
I have nothing to do but wander around trying to
figure out what it was that was so important earlier.
You have to learn to be satisfied with what comes
to you.

—C.S.H.
Harrisonburg, Virginia

～

Chapter 3

THE GOD WHO FORGOT AND
THE MAN WHO COULD NOT

◦

There could be no happiness, cheerfulness, hope, pride,
immediacy, without forgetfulness. The person in whom this
apparatus of suppression is damaged, so that it stops working, can
be compared . . . to a dyspeptic; he cannot "cope" with anything.

—FRIEDRICH NIETZSCHE

As found in the *Pyramid Texts,* from 2800 B.C., *Ra* was the Sun God, the creator of the universe and of all other gods. From his own saliva came air and moisture. From his tears came humankind and the river Nile. He was all-powerful and, of course, immortal— but still not immune to the ravages of time: Ra, the supreme God, became old and senile. He began to lose his wits, and became easy prey for usurpers.

Throughout recorded history, human beings have been cele-brating the powers of memory and lamenting its frailties. "Worse than any loss in body," wrote the Roman poet Juvenal in the first century A.D., "is the failing mind which forgets the names of slaves, and cannot recognize the face of the old friend who dined with him last night, nor those of the children whom he has begotten and brought up."

It took several thousand years, though, for anyone to figure out how memory actually worked. Plato was among the first to suggest a mechanism. His notion was of a literal impression made upon the mind. "Let us suppose," he wrote, "that every man has in his mind a block of wax of various qualities, the gift of Memory, the mother of the Muses; and on this he receives the seal or stamp of those sensations and perceptions which he wishes to remember. That which he succeeds in stamping is remembered and known by him as long as the impression lasts; but that, of which the impression is rubbed out or imperfectly made, is forgotten, and not known."

Later came the ventricular theory of cognition, from Galen (129–ca. 199 A.D.), Nemesius (fourth century), and St. Augustine (354–430). According to this notion, the three major functions of the brain—sensation, movement, and memory—were governed from three large, round fluid-filled sacs. Vital Spirit, a mysterious substance that also contained the human soul, was harbor to the swirl of memories.

From this model came *cerebral localization,* the theory that the various functions of the brain were each controlled by specialized "modules." This model of specialization turned out to be generally correct (if radically different in the details from what Galen had imagined). In the early twentieth century, it emerged that the brain wasn't really an organ so much as a collection of organs, dozens of structures interacting with one another in dazzling complexity. Deep in the center of the brain the amygdala regulates fear while the pituitary coordinates adrenaline and other hormones. Visual stimulus is processed in the occipital lobe, toward the rear of the skull. Perception of texture is mediated by Area One of the parietal lobe near the top of the head, while, just to the rear, the adjacent Area Two differentiates between the size and shape of objects and the position of joints. The prefrontal cortex, snuggled just behind the forehead, spurs self-determination. Broca's area, near the eyes, enables speech. Wernicke's area, above the ears, facilitates the understanding of speech.

The more researchers discovered about localization, though, the more they wondered about the specialized zone for memory. Where was it? If vision was in the back of the brain, texture on top, and so on, what region or regions controlled the formation of lasting impressions and the retrieval of those impressions?

Part of the answer came in 1953, when a Harvard-trained neurosurgeon named William Beecher Scoville performed experimental surgery on a twenty-seven-year-old patient known as H.M. He had been suffering from violent epileptic seizures since childhood, and in a last-ditch effort to give him a chance at a normal life, Scoville removed a small collection of structures, including the hippocampus, from the interior portion of his brain's two temporal lobes. The surgery was a great success in that it significantly reduced the severity of H.M.'s epilepsy. But it was also a catastrophe in that it eliminated his ability to lay down new memories. The case revolutionized the study of memory, revealing that the hippocampus is essential in consolidating immediate thoughts and impressions into longer-lasting memories (which are in turn stored elsewhere).

Time stopped for H.M. in 1953. For the rest of his long life, he was never again able to learn a new name or face, or to remember a single new fact or thought. Many doctors, researchers, and caregivers got to know him quite well in the years that followed, but they were still forced to introduce themselves to him every time they entered his room. As far as H.M. was concerned, he was always a twenty-five-year-old man who was consulting a doctor about his epilepsy (he had also lost all memory of the two years immediately prior to the surgery). H.M. became perhaps the most important neurological subject in history and was subject to a vast number of studies, but he remembered none of the experiments once they were out of his immediate concentration. He was always in the Now.

In the clinical lexicon, this was a perfect case of *anterograde amnesia,* the inability to store any new memories. Persons with incipient Alzheimer's disease exhibit a slightly less severe form of the same problem. The memory of leaving the car keys in the bathroom isn't so much *lost* as it was never actually *formed.*

In a healthy brain, sensory input is converted into memory in three basic stages. Before the input even reaches consciousness, it is held for a fraction of a second in an immediate storage system called a *sensory buffer.*

Moments later, as the perception is given conscious attention, it passes into another very temporary system called *short-term (working) memory.* Information can survive there for seconds or minutes before dissolving away.

Some of the information stirring in working memory is captured by the mechanism that very slowly converts into a *long-term memory* lasting years and even a lifetime.

Long-term memories can be either *episodic* or *semantic.* Episodic memories are very personal memories of firsthand events remembered in order of occurrence. *Before the baseball game the other day, I put on my new pair of sneakers, which I had gotten ear-*

lier that morning. Then we drove to the stadium. Then we parked. Then we gave the man our tickets. Then we bought some hot dogs. Then we went to our seats . . .

Now, days later, if I notice a mustard stain on my shoe, I can plumb my episodic memory to determine when and how it happened. If my feet start bothering me, my episodic memory will help me figure out whether it happened before or after I bought my new shoes.

Semantic memories are what we know, as opposed to what we remember doing. They are our facts about the world, stored in relation to each other and not when we learned them. The memory of Neville Chamberlain's "peace in our time" is semantic.

They are separate systems—interrelated, but separate. An early-stage Alzheimer's patient who cannot retain memories of where she put her keys has not forgotten what keys are for, or what kind of car she drives. That will come much, much later, when she starts to lose old semantic memories.

The experience with H.M. taught researchers that the hippocampus is key to long-term memory formation. Without that tiny organ, he was totally incapable of forming new, lasting memories. Alzheimer's patients suffer the exact same systemic loss, but over several years rather than one surgical afternoon. For H.M., there were no new memories after 1953, period. In later years, he was unable to recognize his own face in the mirror. Real time had marched on, 1955 . . . 1962 . . . 1974, but as far as he was concerned, he was still twenty-five years old. If you are a young man, alert and intelligent, and you look into an ordinary mirror only to discover the face of a sixty-year-old perfectly mimicking your expressions, perhaps only then do you know the real meaning of the word *horror*. Fortunately, the extreme distress H.M. suffered during such world-shattering incidents was always immediately and completely forgotten as soon as his attention could be distracted by something happening in the new moment. Not remembering can sometimes be a great blessing.

The discovery of hippocampus-as-memory-consolidator was critical. What memory specialists have been trying to figure out ever since then is, once formed, where do these long-term memories actually reside? Are memories stored up in the front of the brain in the prefrontal cortex? On top, in the parietal lobe? In the brainstem at the base of the brain? Where?

One tantalizing theory emerged in the late 1950s: memories were everywhere, stored in discrete molecules scattered throughout the brain. A stampede to confirm this notion was set off by a 1962 *Journal of Neuropsychiatry* article, "Memory Transfer Through Cannibalism in Planaria," in which the University of Michigan's James McConnell eagerly reported that worms could capture specific memories of other worms simply by eating those worms. McConnell had trained a group of flatworms to respond to light in a noninstinctive way. He then killed these worms, chopped them up, and fed them to untrained flatworms. After eating their brethren, McConnell claimed, the untrained worms proceeded to behave as though they had been trained—they had somehow acquired the memory of the trained worms. It was the unexpected apotheosis of the old saying, "You are what you eat."

Out of this report numerous research grants were born, some of which yielded tantalizing results. Three years after McConnell's initial study, four California scientists reported in the journal *Science* that when cells extracted from the brains of trained rats were injected into the guts of untrained rats, the untrained rats picked up the learned behavior of the trained rats. These experiments apparently showed that specific, concrete individual memories were embedded as information in discrete molecules in the same way that genetic information is embedded in DNA, and that these memories were transferable from brain to brain. A later experiment by Baylor University's Georges Ungar was the most vivid yet: Brain cells from rats that had been trained to fear the dark were transferred to untrained mice (ordinarily, neither mice nor rats fear the dark), who suddenly took on this new fear. Ungar even isolated a peptide comprising fifteen amino acids that he said contained the newly created memory. He called the transmissible fear-of-the-dark memory molecule *scotophobin*.

The theory that emerged out of these experiments was of memory as a distinct informational molecule that could be created organically in one brain, isolated, and then transferred to another brain—even to the brain of another species. Its implications were immense. Had this cold fusion of an idea been validated rather than widely discredited not long after Ungar's paper was published in *Nature* in 1972, it is clear that ours would be a very different world today: Memory swaps. Consciousness transfers. Neurochemical behavioral enhancements that would make Prozac seem like baby aspirin. The rapid decoding of a hidden science of memory molecules might well have spawned a new type of biochemical computer that could register, react to, and even *create* memory molecules of its own. Laptops (or cars or stuffed animals) could be afraid of the dark or partial to jazz or concerned about child abuse. Memories and feelings could be bottled and sold as easily as perfume.

But that world did not, and cannot, emerge. The memory transfer experiments, while entertaining and even seductive—DNA pioneer Francis Crick was among the many prestigious scientists on board for a while—were ultimately dismissed as seriously misguided). The idea of transferable memories strained credulity to begin with; to suggest that one animal's specific fear could travel through another animal's digestive tract, enter its bloodstream, find its way to the brain, and turn itself on again in the new host mind was an even further stretch.

And then there was the problem of physical mass. Skeptics calculated that if specific memories were contained in molecules the way Ungar suggested, the total number of memories accumulated over a lifetime would weigh somewhere in the vicinity of 220 pounds. The brain would literally be weighed down by thought and ideas.

After a decade or so, the notion and burgeoning industry of memory molecules crumbled into dust. It is now one particularly humiliating memory that many neuroscientists would just as soon not retain. What has grown up out of that rubble over the last thirty years is a very different understanding of memory—not as a substance but as a *system*. Memories are scattered about; that part the memory molecularists had right. Memory *is* everywhere. But it is everywhere in such a way that it is impossible to point to any one spot and identify it with an explicit memory. We now know that memory, like consciousness itself, isn't a thing that can be isolated or extracted, but a living process, a vast and dynamic interaction of neuronal synapses involved in what Harvard's Daniel Schacter elegantly terms "a temporary constellation of activity." Each specific memory is a unique network of neurons from different regions of the brain coordinating with one another. Schacter explains:

> A typical incident in our everyday lives consists of numerous sights, sounds, actions, and words. Different areas of the brain analyze these various aspects of an event. As a result, neurons in the different regions become more strongly connected to one another. The new pattern of connections constitutes the brain's record of the event.

The power of the constellation idea is reinforced by the understanding of just how connected the 100 billion neurons in the brain actually are. A. G. Cairns-Smith, of the University of Glasgow, observes that no single brain cell is separated from any other brain cell by more than six or seven intermediaries.

The molecular basis for these synaptic constellations that can be reignited again and again (though never in precisely the same configuration), is a biochemical process called long-term potentiation (LTP) that intensifies the affinity between specific neurons after a significant connection is made. Think of an ant farm, with worker ants constantly building new tunnels among one another; once a tunnel is built, transport becomes many times easier; an easy, natural connection has been created between those two points. With memory formation and retrieval, pathways are at first built and later simply used. Each notable experience causes a unique set of neurons to fire in conjunction with one another. As a result, those connections become chemically more sensitive to one another so that they can more easily trigger each other again. With that unique constellation of synapses, one has created a permanent physical trace of the original sensation. Neurologists call these memory traces "engrams."

The ant farm analogy also applies in another important way: Neurobiologists have found that memory formation is *slow*. Long-term memories can take many months or even years to fully form.

Long-term memories are durable, but not unassailable. They can last a lifetime, but from the first moments are subject to influences from other memories and experience. Inevitably, as they age and are evoked again and again, all memories change in character.

This is part of the brain's famous plasticity, its ability to adapt to life's events. Plasticity makes us as much creatures of our own experience as we are products of evolution. Not everything in the brain is adaptable, of course; much of it comes "hard-wired," genetically preprogrammed to specialize and perform specific tasks such as processing light and sound, regulating heart rate and breathing, and so on. But the regions reserved for fine motor skills, intelligence, and memory are more like soft clay, able to take on a definite shape and yet remain constantly responsive to new stimuli.

Memory constellations, then, are not fixed, immutable collections of memories, but ever-variable collections of memory fragments that come together in the context of a specific conscious moment. Any common free-association experiment is a vivid illustration of this point. For me, at this moment, the word "cat" prompts ⟶ a thought of Brownfoot, my boyhood feline friend ⟶ the garage roof she used to leap from ⟶ the 1971 T-top Corvette my father used to drive ⟶ the tragicomic month in which Mom wrecked this car twice ⟶ a feeling of malaise associated with my parents' divorce years later. This instant montage of memories is neither chronological nor predictable, even by me. If someone were to prompt me with "cat" tomorrow, depending on my mood or recent experience, I might think of the cat that my daughter called to yesterday outside our house. Or it could be that Brownfoot will come to mind, but that from there I will shift to an image of my playing her dentist, and then I might think of my own current dentist and how I'm way overdue for a cleaning. That guilty feeling might then trigger another distant idea, related only by a parallel feeling of guilt. And so on.

Taken together, this interconnected universe of constellations in each of us forms the core of who we are. Our life's ocean full of memory waves wash against one another to create a complex and ever-adapting character.

The director Martin Scorsese is an interesting memory-character study, mostly because he seems to forget very little compared to others. He remembers not just every shot and crew credit from each of the thousands of movies he's seen, observes the *New Yorker*'s Mark Singer, but also every detail of every book, song, and personal experience he's had in fifty-plus years—"all of it," Singer writes, "seemingly instantly retrievable."

Singer depicts the Scorsese memory constellation in action. After a colleague criticizes a piece of film dialogue as "too piercing," Scorsese is instantly thrown into an interconnected memory odyssey:

> He was reminded of the old Harry Belafonte calypso tune "The Banana Boat Song"—or, rather, a parody of same by Stan Freberg, which included a reference to "piercing," and that reminded him of another Freberg routine, a parody of the television series *Dragnet,* which in turn reminded him of *Pete Kelly's Blues,* a feature film directed by Jack Webb, the star of *Dragnet.* The production designer of *Pete Kelly's Blues,* in which Webb played a bandleader during the twenties, was a Disney veteran who brought to it a remarkably vivid palette, a reality-heightening Technicolor glow reminiscent of the live-action Disney children's films of the forties. . . . And, Scorsese further recalled, *Pete Kelly's Blues* had a screenplay by Richard L. Breen, whose name, curiously, Webb had heralded before the title. When the picture was released, in 1955, the year Scorsese turned thirteen, he fol-

lowed it from theatre to theatre, as was his habit. . . . [He then recalled all the specific theaters he used to frequent.] One particular Saturday afternoon double-feature at the Orpheum came to
mind: *Bomba the Jungle Boy* and *Great White Hunter.* . . .

The pathways linking engrams can be built on temporal, intellectual, or aesthetic associations, and when the mind really wan-
ders, during daydreams or at night before sleep sets in, it's amazing
what sort of involuntary memory leaps one makes, from impressions that often have no logical or logistical relationship but which
share a texture or smell or emotional fragment. What's more—and
this may be the single most important point to understand about
memory—*every time a memory is recalled, new trails are made.*

The act of remembering itself generates new memories. Which
means that Emerson was exactly right when he noted in his journal: "Most remembering is only the memory of memories, & not
a new & primary remembrance . . . HDT [Henry David Thoreau]
noticed this to me some time ago." Overlap, in other words, is not
only built into the biology of memory. It is the very basis of memory—and identity. New memory traces are laid down on top of a
foundation of old memories, and old memories can only be recalled in a context of recent experiences. Imagine a single painting
being created over the course of a lifetime on one giant canvas.
Every brush stroke coming into contact with many others can be
seen only in the context of those prior strokes—and also instantly
alters those older strokes. Because of this, no recorded experience
can ever be fully distinct from anything else. Whether one likes it
or not, the past is always informed by the present, and vice versa.

Scores of experiments confirm the malleability of old memories, and horror stories of False Memory Syndrome are by now widespread. The psychologist Elizabeth Loftus has spent the better part of her career documenting the ease with which false memories can be planted—accidentally or on purpose. Often, these false memories lead to wrongful convictions. In 1979, twenty-two-year-old marine corporal Kevin Green was convicted of second-degree murder for the brutal beating of his wife and the death of their full-term fetus. His wife had testified after coming out of a coma that Green, her own husband, was the attacker. Sixteen years later, the real attacker, a total stranger, confessed to police about that and six other murders. It turned out that Green's guilt had been suggested to his wife early on in her rehabilitation. By the time it came to trial, she had created a memory so clear that she was able to confidently testify against her husband.

"Eyewitness misidentification . . . is known as the single greatest cause of the conviction of the innocent," says attorney Barry Scheck. He describes a typical scenario: "You can have as many as five witnesses who begin in kind of a soft way, saying, 'That *might* be the guy,' and then, like wet concrete hardening, the [memories] get fixed to the point that by the time they get to the courtroom, they're saying '*That's* the man.' "

Part of the deep attraction to the idea of distinct memory molecules was that it connoted the ability to *replay* old memories like videotapes on a VCR—just as they were originally recorded. But the biology of memory constellations dictates that there is no such thing as pure memory. *Recall* is never *replay.*

But why? Why would millions of years of evolution produce a machine so otherwise sophisticated but with an apparent built-in fuzziness, a tendency to regularly forget, repress, and distort information and experience?

The answer, it turns out, is that fuzziness is not a severe limitation but a highly advanced feature. As a matter of engineering, the brain does not have any physical limitations in the amount of information it can hold. It is designed specifically to forget most of the details it comes across, so that it may allow us to form general impressions, and from there useful judgments. Forgetting is not a failure at all, but an active metabolic process, a flushing out of data in the pursuit of knowledge and meaning.

We know this not just from brain chemistry and inference, but also because psychologists have stumbled upon a few individuals over the years who actually could not forget *enough*—and were debilitated by it.

In his *New Yorker* profile, Mark Singer wonders if Martin Scorsese is such a person—burdened by too good a memory.

> Was it, I wondered, painful to remember so much? Scorsese's powers of recall weren't limited to summoning plot turns or notable scenes or acting performances; his gray matter bulged with camera angles, lighting strategies, scores, sound effects, ambient noises, editing rhythms, production credits, data about lenses and film stocks and exposure speeds and aspect ratios. . . . What about all the sludge? An inability to forget the forgettable—wasn't that a burden, or was it just part of the price one paid to make great art?

For some perspective on the inability to forget, consider the case study that psychologists call *S*. In the 1920s, S. was a twenty-something newspaper reporter in Moscow who one day got into trouble with his editor for not taking notes at a staff meeting. In the midst of the reprimand, S. shocked his boss by matter-of-factly repeating everything that had been said in the meeting—word for word.

This was apparently no stretch at all for S., who, it emerged upon closer examination, remembered virtually every detail of sight and sound that he had come into contact with in his entire life. What's more, he took this perfect memory entirely for granted. To him, it seemed perfectly normal that he forgot nothing.

The editor, amazed, sent S. to the distinguished Russian psychologist A. R. Luria for testing. Luria did test him that day, and for many other days over a period of many decades. In all the testing, he could not find any real limit to his capacity to recall details. For example, not only could he perfectly recall tables like this one full of random data after looking at them for just a few minutes:

6	6	8	0
5	4	3	2
1	6	8	4
7	9	3	5
4	2	3	7
3	8	9	1
1	0	0	2
3	4	5	1
2	7	6	8
1	9	2	6
2	9	6	7
5	5	2	0
x	0	1	x

And not only could he efficiently recite these tables backwards, upside down, diagonally, etc., but after years of memorizing thousands of such tables he could easily reproduce any particular one of them, without warning, whether it was an hour after he had first seen it, or twenty years. The man, it seemed, quite literally remembered everything.

And yet he understood almost nothing. S. was plagued by an inability to make meaning out of what he saw. Unless one pointed the obvious pattern out to him, for example, the following table appeared just as bereft of order and meaning as any other:

1	2	3	4
2	3	4	5
3	4	5	6
4	5	6	7

"If I had been given the letters of the alphabet arranged in a similar order," he remarked after being questioned about the 1–2–3–4 table, "I wouldn't have noticed their arrangement." He was also unable to make sense out of poetry or prose, to understand much about the law, or even to remember people's faces. "They're so changeable," he complained to Luria. "A person's expression depends on his mood and on the circumstances under which you happen to meet him. People's faces are constantly changing; it's the different shades of expression that confuse me and make it so hard to remember faces."

Luria also noted that S. came across as generally disorganized, dull-witted, and without much of a sense of purpose or direction in life. This astounding man, then, was not so much gifted with the ability to remember everything as he was cursed with the inability to forget detail and form more general impressions. He recorded only information, and was bereft of the essential ability to draw meaning out of events. "Many of us are anxious to find ways to improve our memories," wrote Luria in a lengthy report on his unusual subject. "In S.'s case, however, precisely the reverse was true. The big question for him, and the most troublesome, was how he could learn to forget."

What makes details hazy also enables us to prioritize information, recognize and retain patterns. The brain eliminates trees in order to make sense of, and remember, the forests. Forgetting is a hidden virtue. Forgetting is what makes us so smart.

＊

One of the worst things that I have to do is put on my pants in the morning. This morning I kept thinking there is something wrong because my pants just didn't feel right. I had put them on wrong. I sometimes will have to put them on and take them off half a dozen times or more. . . . Setting the washing machine is getting to be a problem, too. Sometimes I'll spend an hour trying to figure out how to set it.

—B.
San Diego, California

＊

Chapter 4

THE RACE

❧

Taos

"Ten years to a cure," a Japanese scientist whispered to me in our hotel lobby as we waited for the shuttle bus to the Taos Civic Plaza.

The whisper was as telling as the words. He couldn't contain his optimism, and yet he also couldn't afford to put it on display.

Other Alzheimer's researchers had lately been adopting a similar posture. As scientists, they were reserved by nature. But the recent acceleration of discovery had made them a little giddy. Hundreds of important discoveries had come in recent years, and funding for research was way up. The study of Alzheimer's was now in the top scientific tier, alongside heart disease, cancer, and stroke research. This seemed fitting, since the disease was emerging as one of the largest causes of death in the U.S., not far behind those other three.

There was now even an Alzheimer's drug on the market, Aricept, introduced in 1997, which boosted the brain's supply of the neurotransmitter acetylcholine. Some of the functional loss in early Alzheimer's involves a deficiency of acetylcholine; replenishing it with this drug seemed to help about half of early and middle-stage patients to slow or even arrest the progression of symptoms for a year or more.

On the one hand, this was a giant advance: a real treatment that often made a tangible difference. But it was also a frustrating baby-step: Aricept did *not* slow the advance of the actual disease by a single day. It only worked on the symptoms. Scientists couldn't stop Alzheimer's yet—only put a thick curtain in front of it for a while.

More ambitious advances were brewing. An electronic update service named *Alzheimer's Weekly* had been launched in 1998. Neurologists in the 1960s would have considered this phrase a sarcastic reference to the drudging nature of discovery: Understanding of the disease was practically frozen for more than half a century. But after a thaw in the 1970s and a renewed effort in the '80s, genetic and molecular discoveries started to cascade so quickly by the mid-1990s that the excavation of Alzheimer's seemed to be moving at the same clip as sporting events and financial markets.

Now a weekly update was not only useful but essential. In fact, updates on other Web sites came almost daily:

News from the Research Front

3 September 1998. H. J. Song et al. report that they are able to manipulate growth cones . . .

5 September 1998. Puny polymer pellets show promise as a vehicle for delivering nerve-growth factor to the basal forebrain . . .

6 September 1998. A novel brain-imaging agent promises to open up a window on the functioning of the brain's dopamine system . . .

10 September 1998. Findings published in *Nature Neuroscience* indicate that the accumulation of calcium in the mitochondria triggers neuronal death . . .

10 September 1998. C. Y. Wang et al. report they have identified four genes that are targets of NF-kB activity . . .

11 September 1998. E. Nedivi et al. describe CPG15, a molecule that enhances dendritic arbor growth in projection neurons . . .

—from the *Alzheimer Research Forum* (at www.alzforum.org)

The research was so intensely specialized that few individual scientists appeared to even be working on the problem of Alzheimer's disease *per se.* It was more like each was unearthing a single two-inch tile in a giant mosaic. By themselves, these individual experiments were so narrowly focused that they were far removed from a comprehensive understanding of the disease. But the minutiae had a purpose. If the great challenge of Alois Alzheimer had been to distinguish a general pathology of dementia from the normal cells of the brain, the task of contemporary scientists—employing exotic techniques with names like fluorescent protein tagging, immuno-lesioning, and western blot analysis—was to try to see what the process looked like in flux. Alzheimer glimpsed a mono-colored, silver-stained microscopic snapshot. Contemporary scientists, crunching and exchanging data with parallel processors and fiber optics, were trying to patch together more of a motion picture. Once they understood the actual disease *process,* particularly the early molecular events, they hoped they would be able to proceed toward genuine therapies.

The research had expanded in every direction, and had also gone global. Thousands of scientists from every continent now worked on the problem, as time became critical. In a little over a decade, the much-anticipated "senior boom" would begin, eventually quadrupling the number of Alzheimer's cases and making it the fastest-growing disease in developed countries. In addition to the sheer misery, the social costs of such a slow, progressive disease would be staggering. In the U.S., the costs of doctor's visits, lab tests, medicine, nursing, day care, and home care was already estimated to be $114.4 billion annually. That was more than the combined budgets for the U.S. Departments of Commerce, Education, Energy, Justice, Labor, and Interior.

"We have to solve this problem, or it's going to overwhelm us," Zaven Khachaturian said. "The numbers are going to double every twenty years. Not only that: The duration of illness is going to get much longer. That's the really devastating part. The folks who have the disease now are mostly people who came through the Depression. Some had college education, but most did not. The ones who are going to develop Alzheimer's in the next century will be baby boomers who are primarily much better educated and better fed. The duration of their disability is going to be much longer than the current crop. That's going to be a major factor.

"See, in considering the social impact of the disease, it's not so much the pain and suffering that matters. From the point of view of the individual, that is of course the important factor. But from the point of view of society, what's important is how long I am disabled and how much of a burden I am to society. With cancer and heart disease, the period where I cannot function independently is fairly short—three to five years. With Alzheimer's, it's going to be extremely long—like twenty years, where you are physically there, you don't have any pain, you appear normal, and yet you have Alzheimer's. You *cannot* function independently."

If Khachaturian was correct, and the average duration of the disease was set to more than double, then the problem would be even worse than epidemiologists were predicting. Either way, it was clear that if Alzheimer's disease was not conquered reasonably soon, it would become one of the most prominent features of our future. Nationally, the number of nursing home beds would at least quadruple. (The stay of Alzheimer's sufferers in a nursing home is, on average, twice as long as that of other patients.) We would need vastly more home health care workers, elder-care nurses and physicians, assisted living facilities, day-care programs and support groups. (There was already a grave shortage of qualified professional caregivers—and, due to the low pay, a shocking annual turnover rate of 94 percent.) Family leave would also have to be redefined. Progressive nations would likely adopt a system of employee flexibility for senior care (extended leave, flexible work hours, and so on) similar to the one recently implemented for new parents in the U.S.—with the added caveat that *reverse parenthood* lasts significantly longer and is more draining than conventional parenthood.

All this would cost money, and would require a painful shift in resources away from other public needs. Public officials would be forced into difficult decisions. Would the U.S. government, for example, continue to allow an Alzheimer's patient to give away all assets to his children in order to qualify for government-sponsored care? Would governments require citizens to have some sort of dementia or frailty insurance?

And what about public safety issues? With as many as fifteen million people suffering from insidious (and largely invisible) cognitive decline, how would we insure street and highway safety without automatically invalidating all driver's licenses of senior citizens?

There was a dual race on, then. Researchers were racing against one another, and against time. The prize for the winner of this race—if there was to be a winner—would be worldwide fame, nearly unparalleled professional esteem, enormous wealth, and the pride of knowing that you were personally responsible for preventing an ocean of future human suffering.

One glimpse into the magnitude of an Alzheimer's cure: In the nearly fifty years since Jonas Salk and Albert Sabin introduced their vaccines against polio, somewhere between 1 and 2 million lives have been saved. Curing Alzheimer's disease sometime in the first decade of the twenty-first century would save as many as 100 million lives worldwide in the same length of time.

The far-flung researchers kept in touch by E-mail, phone, and fax, and accomplished much in their labs spread out all over the world. Still, every so often, they needed to come together physically, to be in the same room to check their progress, to goad each other, critique and criticize each other, to energize.

In 1999, the gathering place was Taos. They came from everywhere, a global convergence of neuromolecular intelligentsia sitting on fold-out chairs in Bataan Hall to share knowledge and probe their ignorance. There was still so much they didn't know: Why are women more susceptible to Alzheimer's than men? Why are Cree and Cherokee Indians less susceptible than the rest of us? What is it about the environment in Hawaii, as contrasted with Japan, that apparently doubles one's chances of getting Alzheimer's? Why do a third of Alzheimer's victims develop Parkinson's disease but not the other two-thirds? Why do some cigarette smokers seem to be *less* likely to develop Alzheimer's than nonsmokers?

After ninety-plus years, the field was littered with half-answers to these questions—and far more basic ones: Does Alzheimer's have one cause or many? Is it really one disease or a collection of very similar diseases? Which come first—plaques or tangles? Why do they always originate in the same part of the brain? How long do they proliferate before they begin to affect brain performance? Why do some people accrue a brain full of plaques and tangles but never display any symptoms of the disease? Is anyone naturally immune to Alzheimer's?

So, humbly, they gathered. With respect for the vexing nature of this disease, the molecular biologists and geneticists spent thirty hours listening to theories of plaque and tangle formation, and intervention strategies. After each short talk, they quickly lined up behind a microphone in the aisle to poke the presenter with questions, looking for holes in the research and analysis. The tone was alternately respectful and suspicious, and occasionally hostile.

Hostile because of the billions of dollars at stake, and also because of a fracturing debate within the community about which aspect of research mattered most. A nearly one-hundred-year-old question still had not been answered: Which are closer to the root of the problem—the plaques or the tangles?

Alois Alzheimer thought it was the tangles. "We have to conclude," he wrote in 1911, "that the plaques are not the cause of senile dementia but only an accompanying feature."

Most, however, now said the plaques. In a field where there were so many open questions and possible approaches, the vast majority of researchers in this room and elsewhere were focused tightly on the issue of plaque formation, while relatively few were concerned with tangles and only a handful of others busied themselves with important issues like inflammation, viruses, and possible environmental factors.

The disparity bothered many. "When I was a little girl, I wanted to go into science because I thought it was a very open community," Ruth Itzhaki, a biologist from the University of Manchester, told me one morning in Taos. "I learned better. It is, in fact, a very cynical community layered with politics and filled with people who just want to follow the herd." Itzhaki was herself embittered by her struggle to fund research linking the herpes simplex virus 1 (HSV1) with Alzheimer's.

Could Alzheimer's be herpes of the brain? It was not the most prominent theory of the day, but no one could rule it out. Nearly all humans are infected by HSV1 by the time they reach middle age. The virus mostly seems to lie dormant but can become active and create cold sores and other hazards in times of stress. Whether or not HSV1 does any damage depends largely on individual levels of immune response and on genetic makeup.

In her presentation, Itzhaki said she had found evidence of HSV1 presence in the temporal and frontal cortex of the brain, as well as in the hippocampus—three areas closely associated with Alzheimer's. She posited that the virus might be interacting with a particular gene to set the disease process in motion. If proven true, a massive new global infant immunization project would be in order.

But the crowd in Taos did not seem very interested. Her talk drew little in the way of response. The focus quickly shifted back to plaques.

One evening I got a telephone call from a friend. He was telling me what a tough day he'd had on the job; he'd made several mistakes. "If you have Alzheimer's, I must have a double dose of it," he said.

I could feel myself entering a state of rage. "Do you forget simple words, or substitute inappropriate words, making your sentences incomprehensible? Do you cook a meal and not only forget you cooked it, but forget to eat it? Do you put your frying pan in the freezer, or your wallet in the sugar bowl, only to find them later and wonder what in the world is happening to you? Do you become lost on your own street? Do you mow your lawn three or four times a day? When you balance your checkbook, do you completely forget what the numbers are and what needs to be done with them? Do you become confused or fearful ten times a day, for no reason? And most of all, do you become irate when someone makes a dumb statement like you just made?"

"No."

"Then you don't have Alzheimer's," I said, and hung up.

—L.R.
Lafayette, Louisiana

Chapter 5

IRRESPECTIVE OF AGE

⌒

Late one night in the early 1950s, Meta Neumann, a neuropathologist at St. Elizabeth's Hospital in Washington, D.C., got word that an elderly colleague of hers, the clinical psychiatrist Dr. P., had died. It came without warning. That very morning, Dr. P. had ably led a vigorous meeting of hospital staff.

Situated on a three-hundred-acre campus across the Anacostia River in the southeast quadrant of the District, St. Elizabeth's was at the time the premier mental hospital in the United States. It had been founded a century earlier, in 1855, the first national mental health facility, as part of a massive effort throughout the Western world to rehabilitate the mentally ill. By the mid-twentieth century, St. Elizabeth's housed between seven and eight thousand patients. The poet Ezra Pound was confined there from 1946 to 1958 for his pro-Fascist broadcasts from Italy during World War II. In 1981, it became the home of John Hinckley, Jr., Ronald Reagan's would-be assassin.

St. Elizabeth's also had the oldest pathology lab of any mental health institution, including an unmatched archive of twenty-three hundred brains taken from deceased residents. These preserved brains floated in formaldehyde inside large clear glass jars. For more than a decade, Neumann had been the curator of the brain bank, regularly adding specimens to it and using it for research.

Now Dr. P.'s brain would become an unexpected addition to the collection. The morning after his sudden death, Neumann performed an autopsy on him. She was a specialist in neurodegenerative disorders, and so it didn't take her long to notice something unsettling about the brain of Dr. P. It was badly sclerotic. The arteries in his brain were severely clogged with fatty deposits, much like heart vessels before a major heart attack.

In itself, the cerebral arteriosclerosis was not unusual; indeed, Dr. P. had a classic case. What made it curious was that prior to his death he had not exhibited any of the symptoms of senile dementia. At the time, the medical establishment believed senile dementia—dementia in old age—was caused by cerebral arteriosclerosis, the slow buildup of fat in the brain's arteries over time. Medical schools in the early and mid-twentieth century taught as gospel that there were two clearly distinct types of dementia, easily separated by the age of onset:

Alzheimer's disease—
A very rare disease afflicting people in their forties and fifties, characterized by plaques and tangles. Cause unknown.

Senile dementia—
A relatively common condition affecting the elderly (sixties and older), caused by cerebral arteriosclerosis.

Senile dementia was not regarded as a disease, just an unfortunate side effect of getting old. Few had questioned this distinction, but in Meta Neumann's autopsy lab on that particular morning in 1952, it didn't hold up. According to what she saw in his brain, Dr. P. should have died in a senile fog. But Neumann and her husband, Robert Cohn—also a neuropathologist at St. Elizabeth's (they had met during an autopsy)—had spoken with Dr. P. just before his death, and found him to be perfectly lucid.

If Dr. P. had fatty deposits in his brain, and he wasn't senile, logic dictated that fatty deposits must not cause senility. So, Neumann wondered, what does?

It was a question she could seriously explore on her own. With her own in-house brain bank, she had all the resources she needed at her disposal to examine a large number of cases of diagnosed senile dementia and see if the brains did, in fact, show sclerotic changes. She and Cohn began the hard digging.

Two hundred and ten brains later, her hunch was confirmed. Just as Neumann had suspected, few of the dementia brains showed sclerosis. Instead, they showed plaques and tangles. These were *Alzheimer's* brains.

Alzheimer's was not a rare disease after all. It was the leading cause of dementia, by far, in people of all ages. "The clinical picture was the same," says Cohn, "irrespective of age."

The question of what Alzheimer's disease was, exactly, had been a great sad muddle for many decades, ever since Alois Alzheimer first shared details of his remarkable five-year interaction with Auguste D. as both patient and lab specimen. If the case of Frau D. was destined to be an important part of the history of neuroscience, it was impossible to tell by the initial hearing. Alzheimer discussed his findings at a regional conference for German psychiatrists in November 1906, where he was met with indifference. At the lecture's conclusion, conference chairman Alfred Hoche, a leading psychiatrist from Freiburg, called for questions or comments. No one spoke a word. After a long silence, Hoche called again for questions. Again, nothing. Dementia, death, plaques, tangles—no one in the room seemed to much care. Hoche himself couldn't even muster a comment as a courtesy. "So then, respected colleague Alzheimer, I thank you for your remarks," Hoche said finally. "Clearly there is no desire for discussion."

But the following year, Alzheimer's written report of the autopsy, "A Peculiar Disease of the Cerebral Cortex," was published to a more enthusiastic audience: his boss, Emil Kraepelin.

Kraepelin was the most ambitious and authoritative psychiatrist of the day. In his *Handbook of Psychiatry*, he published the first psychiatric nosology, or classification of diseases. By the early 1890s, it had become an international bestseller, a seminal text. Kraepelin published new editions every few years, and his colleagues regarded his updates and modifications with close attention. By the time of Auguste D.'s death in 1906, Kraepelin was nearly unrivaled in his influence, and not shy about using it.

But Kraepelin was also a man in need. The radical contention of his *Handbook* was that a vast number of mental illnesses were actually organic diseases, with distinct pathologies. The trouble was, he had no proof—no recorded link between mental distress and the alteration of brain tissue. With no evidence to back up his claim, many of Kraepelin's peers loudly doubted his central notion, arguing that brain diseases would never be so easily classifiable from the study of structural changes in the brain. At a 1906 conference in Munich, three prominent psychiatrists confronted him. "There can be no talk of nosological specificity," insisted the distinguished Berlin academic Karl Bonhoeffer.

Robert Gaupp, the new director of the University Hospital for Psychiatry and Psychotherapy in Tübingen, agreed, stating unequivocally, "No psychological symptoms can be explained from anatomical findings."

Alfred Hoche twisted the knife a bit further, poking fun at Kraepelin for what he saw as foolishness. "The search for illness types is a hopeless hunt for a phantom!" teased Hoche.

Only Kraepelin's protégé Alois Alzheimer came to his defense. He did so not only out of loyalty, but also because he had the perfect ammunition. "I can *verify* [this] anatomical doctrine," Alzheimer told the critics flatly. "Twelve days ago, on April 8, a Frankfurt patient, Auguste D., died. I have had the clinical history and the brain sent to Munich, and I have undertaken to document in this case that there is indeed an anatomical doctrine."

Kraepelin's most formidable rival, Viennese neurologist Sigmund Freud, was not at the Munich conference. Freud was fashioning the new school of psychoanalysis out of the proposition that an enormous number of mental problems were neuroses of the mind, not organic diseases of the brain. Where Kraepelin saw the brain as a cell-based organ at the mercy of biological processes, internal mishaps caused by what he called "autotoxins," Freud saw it as a reservoir of thoughts and emotions that played off against one another and competed for dominance. Further, Freud insisted that mental health was not a simple matter of healthy vs. diseased, but more of a continuum. He saw no clear line of demarcation between emotionally healthy and emotionally sick persons.

These competing views would eventually come to be embraced as dually legitimate and coexistent, but in the first decade of the twentieth century, Kraepelin's organic psychiatry and Freud's psychoanalysis were a pair of sumo wrestlers on a small bamboo raft: two ideologies aggressively competing for the hearts and minds of Central Europe. Co-existence was not considered acceptable to either side.

Kraepelin wrote scathingly of Freud as early as 1899, sarcastically calling his ideas "highly remarkable conceptions" and dismissing what he and his colleagues saw as an obsession with sex. "If . . . our much-plagued soul can lose its equilibrium for all time as a result of long-forgotten unpleasant sexual experiences," Kraepelin remarked, "that would be the beginning of the end of the human race." To the organic psychiatrists standing with Kraepelin, Freud's ideas were little more than *Schweinerei*—"smut." In 1906, Walther Spielmeyer, one of Kraepelin's colleagues, called Freud's work "mental masturbation."

Freud responded with equal acidity. When Otto Gross, one of Kraepelin's clinical assistants, wrote a book that attempted to synthesize both sides of the debate, Freud commented, "What interests me most about Gross's book is that it comes from the clinic of the Super-Pope, or at least was published with his permission."

The critically important brain physiology vs. psychology debate was really just beginning, and would last through the twentieth century and beyond. Along the way, Alzheimer made a significant contribution. As both the physician at Auguste D.'s side and the pathologist examining her brain, Alzheimer established a direct link between her dementia and the plaques and tangles clouding her cortex. This wasn't irrefutable *proof* of an organic brain disease, but it was the first solid evidence. "Alzheimer . . .

offered a causal relation between neuropathological and psychopathological alterations," says psychiatrist and historian Matthias M. Weber. ". . . For this reason, Alois Alzheimer was perhaps the most important coworker of Emil Kraepelin."

After Kraepelin read Alzheimer's article, he immediately seized on the detailed descriptions and moved quickly to formalize the discovery. Grateful to Alzheimer for bolstering his organic doctrine, he probably also wanted to reward him. So he named the disease after him. In the 1910 edition of his *Handbook,* Kraepelin mentioned Alzheimer and his work numerous times before blurting out a surprising and indistinct reference to *Morbus Alzheimer:*

"The clinical interpretation of this Alzheimer's disease is still confused."

Alzheimer's disease was born.

Every disease needs a name. As a matter of social reality, no disease exists until it has one.

Acquired Immunodeficiency Syndrome • Acrocephalosyndactylia • Adams-Stokes Disease • Bell's Palsy • Beriberi • Bloom Syndrome • Blue Rubber Bleb Nevus Syndrome • Bronchitis • Bronchopulmonary Dysplasia • Canavan Disease • Candidiasis • Cherubism • Chicken Pox • Cholangitis • Depression • Dermatofibroma • Dyslexia • Epilepsy • Erb's Palsy • Esotropia • Evans Syndrome • Fibromyalgia • Fuchs' Endothelial Dystrophy • Furunculosis • Giardiasis • Gilbert Disease • Glycogen Storage Disease • Gonorrhea • Goodpasture Syndrome • Hashimoto's Disease • Hematospermia • Hemophilia A • Herpes Simplex • Influenza • Irritable Bowel Syndrome •

Isaac's Syndrome • Job's Syndrome • Keratosis Follicularis • Klinefelter's Syndrome • Klippel-Feil Syndrome • Kuru • Labyrinth Diseases • Laurence-Moon Syndrome • Lemierre's Syndrome • Lentigo • Leukemia • Lyme Disease • Malaria • Malignant Hyperthermia • Measles • Moyamoya Disease • Multiple Myeloma • Multiple Sclerosis • Noonan Syndrome • Nystagmus • Obesity • Oculomotor Nerve Diseases • Osteoarthritis • Pellagra • Pertussis • Pleurisy • Pneumonia • Poland Syndrome • Proctitis • Q Fever • De Quervain's Tendinitis • Reye's Syndrome • Rhabdoid Tumor • Rhinitis • Rocky Mountain Spotted Fever • Romano-Ward Syndrome • Rubella • Sarcoma • Scabies • Scarlet Fever • Scheie Syndrome • Sezary Syndrome • Smallpox • Sprengel's Deformity • Supraglottitis • Syringomyelia • Takayasu's Arteritis • Tay-Sachs Disease • Tinea • Toxic Shock Syndrome • Trichinosis • Typhoid • Undulant Fever • Vasculitis • Volvulus • West Syndrome • Von Willebrand Disease • Wilms' Tumor • Xerostomia • Yaws • Yellow Fever • Zoonoses • Zygomycosis

The disease name is public recognition of a shared affliction. The name says, *THIS is what you are suffering from. You are not alone. Others are suffering from the same thing.*

The name also says, *We're going to fight this thing.* "Choosing to call a set of phenomena a disease," writes medical philosopher H. Tristram Engelhardt, Jr., "involves a commitment to medical intervention, the assignment of the sick-role, and the enlistment in action of health professionals." Naming a disease is tantamount to launching an assault against that disease.

Finally, the name is also a necessary tag for an otherwise intangible phenomenon. A disease is not a *thing* but a *process;* it is neither the cause of the problem nor its visible effects—neither the virus infecting the tissue nor the damaged tissue itself—but the interaction between the two. Because of the elusive nature of disease, the name is often the only available emblem. Once accepted, specific names quickly come to dominate social reality. The flavor of the name can make a real difference in how the disease is perceived and acted on.

Any casual observer can easily see that the history of disease-naming is a haphazard one, four thousand years of jigs and jags that have left us with appellations ranging from the vaguely mythological ("influenza" originally referred to the vast influence of the gods) to the icily clinical (acquired immunodeficiency syndrome). A disease might be named after the major symptom (smallpox), a side effect (yellow fever), a known or suspected cause (schistosomiasis, tuberculosis), or might instead be a vague reference to a social consequence (the plague).

The sporadic tradition of naming a disease after the identifying physician seems to have started in the mid-nineteenth century, when French neurologist Jean-Martin Charcot coined the name *"la maladie de Parkinson"* after London physician James Parkinson's 1817 "Essay on the Shaking Palsy." Thomas Addison earned the honor of "Addison's disease" in 1855 by characterizing a complex disorder involving the destruction of the adrenal glands. Huntington's disease is named after George Huntington, who in 1872 detailed the hereditary chorea that begins with muscle spasms and ends in dementia.

Kraepelin followed in this nascent tradition by naming what seemed to be a new discovery after the discoverer. It was also a political maneuver with two obvious payoffs for the namer. By bringing attention to this new disease, he ensured the maximum possible exposure for the emerging evidence of organic brain disease. And in fashioning a formal new disease after a staff member, Kraepelin also gained additional glory for his own institute.

But what was the disease, exactly? Kraepelin wrote:

> The clinical interpretation of this Alzheimer's disease is still confused. While the anatomical findings suggest that we are dealing with a particularly serious form of senile dementia, the fact that this disease sometimes starts already around the age of fifty does not allow this supposition. In such cases we should at least presume a "senium praecox" [premature aging] if not perhaps a more or less age-independent unique disease process.

The words dropped onto the medical community like a giant crop circle—it was a powerful, resonant event, but what exactly did it mean? Even as the term "Alzheimer's disease" quickly gained currency throughout the world, largely on the strength of Kraepelin's formidable reputation (he would eventually come to be known as the "Linnaeus of psychiatry" for his importance in mental disease classification), it confused many.

On the one hand, it seemed that he intended Alzheimer's disease to refer only to a rare form of so-called presenile dementia that affected a tiny number of people in their forties and fifties. On the other hand, he included his description in the "senile dementia" section of his book, not the presenile section. Also, his suggestion that this was "perhaps a more or less age-independent unique disease process" seemed to imply that the disease could affect anyone, irrespective of age.

Kraepelin's suggestion was strangely jumbled for a man whose life's work had been orderly classification. In one short sentence, he somehow managed both to brazenly introduce a new disease and to undermine it.

On the surface, it seemed like sloppiness. But it could not have been. Kraepelin wasn't blind to the ricochet effect of his words. Far from it: he was as much a political animal as a medical man, running the highest-profile psychiatric clinic in Germany (and arguably in all of Europe). Nor was he known for carelessness. Medical scholars looking back over the span of a century to particulars of his work are continually impressed with his precision and intelligence.

He did it on purpose, as a way of recognizing Alois Alzheimer's genuine discovery but sidestepping the question of how it challenged thousands of years of thinking about old age. For whatever reason, Kraepelin did not want to be the one to suddenly insist that senility was a disease to be fought. "Accepting Alzheimer's disease as a separate disease prevented the coming about of another, more complicated question, i.e., the question whether senile dementia is a disease entity to be distinguished from aging," suggests Dutch physician and historian Rob Dillman.

So Kraepelin left it as "perhaps."

He left it fuzzy, proposing Alzheimer's as a middle-age dementia—and "perhaps" a senile dementia.

Still, it was the first strong hint that senility was not a reasonable part of aging. For all of human history, senile dementia had been tacitly accepted as merely a lamentable stage of life. "But if I am to live on," the Greek historian Xenophon wrote in *Memorabilia* (fourth century B.C.), "haply [by chance] I may be forced to pay the old man's forfeit—to become sand-blind and deaf and dull of wit, slower to learn, quicker to forget, outstripped now by those who were behind me."

In Ecclesiasticus 3.12–13 (second century B.C.) we find these words: "O son, help your father in his old age, and do not grieve him as long as he lives/even if he is lacking in understanding, show forbearance."

Most prominently of all, Shakespeare defined senility as one of life's natural stages. In *As You Like It,* Jaques declares:

> . . . one man in his time plays many parts. . . .
> Last scene of all,
> That ends this strange eventful history,
> Is second childishness and mere oblivion. . . .

Even as recently as Ralph Waldo Emerson's steady sinking into what a biographer called his "soft oblivion," through the 1870s and up to his death in 1882, his condition was lamented but accepted with an unwavering fatalism. This isn't particularly surprising, given that in his own notebook Emerson had noted his admiration for a remark by his friend Bronson Alcott on the subject of senility: "That as the child loses, as he comes into the world, his angelic memory, so the man, as he grows old, loses his memory of this world."

The voluminous records of Emerson's life suggest that he saw a doctor about his failing memory only once; apparently, nothing noteworthy came from it. And Edward Emerson, a physician, made no medical observations of his father's condition. Though the disorder attacked Emerson's single greatest asset, his mind, there was no public or private suggestion of *treating* his memory loss, *fighting* it, or in any way considering it a disease. Indeed, when a friend inquired about Emerson's health late in his life, he replied, "Quite well; I have lost my mental faculties but am perfectly well." It is striking to see, through the prism of modern medicine, the stark separation of Emerson's senility from his physical health.

Now, less than three decades after Emerson's ordeal, Kraepelin was suggesting that *perhaps* senile dementia was not just a matter of aging or accelerated aging. *Perhaps* it was a disease; *perhaps* doctors now had a moral obligation to do something about it.

Years passed and the world forgot about Kraepelin's "perhaps." Alzheimer's disease congealed in medical circles as a rare, middle-aged disorder. It came to Meta Neumann and Robert Cohn in 1953 to challenge that thinking with new and convincing evidence. "There is no difference in the clinical or pathological picture in the various age groups," they wrote in their article, published that year in the *Archives of Neurology and Psychiatry.*

The data were meticulous and compelling, but not nearly enough to force a change in convention. Proof or no proof, people weren't ready to call senility a disease. "They didn't believe it," Cohn recalled of colleagues' reactions to the paper they published. "They felt that Meta was talking nonsense."

In the eyes of the psychiatric community, "Alzheimer's" remained a designation for a very rare presenile disease. Senility remained a natural part of aging.

The confusion endured.

⊷

A.P.: *On the kitchen door, I have little yellow
Post-it Notes. So when I leave the house I know I
have to do certain things. I can't go out until I
see that note on the door.*

M.W.: *I do the same sort of thing, except that I have a
big calendar in my kitchen.*

T.R.: *I have a book I write in every day.*

J.J.: *Well, I make a list in the kitchen and then one
in the bedroom. They are the same.
Sometimes in the bathroom I put a different list.*

H.K.: *I never thought of that. That sounds so good, to
have two lists—one on one end of the house and
another on the other end—because by the time
I get back to the other end I think, "Why have I
come?"*

—Houston, Texas

⊷

Chapter 6

A MOST LOVING BROTHER

∽

In 75 A.D., Plutarch chronicled the exuberant life and gloomy decline of the great Roman warrior-diplomat Lucius Licinius Lucullus, who fought in Italy and Asia under the emperor Sulla and subsequently governed Africa. After retiring to a life of extravagance, he slid into full-blown dementia. Lucullus's intellect, said Plutarch, "failed him by degrees . . . so disabled and unsettled his mind, that while he was yet alive, his brother took charge of his affairs."

Of the ordeal, Plutarch seemed most impressed by the burden cast on Lucullus's brother Marcus. It was Marcus who had to manage Lucullus's slow decline, as well as his estate. And when Lucullus died (at age fifty-three), it was Marcus who stood up to popular pressure to bury the body in the Field of Mars alongside Sulla. Marcus instead honored Lucullus's specific request that he be buried on his own family grounds. A short time later, Marcus himself was buried in the same spot, no doubt worn down by his tireless duties in service to his ailing brother. Admiring Marcus's sacrifice, Plutarch closed his long essay with a benediction not for the famous victim but his caregiver. "In all respects," he wrote, "a most loving brother."

The unique curse of Alzheimer's is that it ravages several victims for every brain it infects. Since it shuts down the brain very slowly, beginning with higher functions, close friends and loved ones are forced not only to witness an excruciating fade but also increasingly to step in and compensate for lost abilities. We all rely on the assistance of other people in order to live full, rich lives. A person with dementia relies increasingly—and, in the fullness of time, *completely*—on the care of others. Lucullus had his brother. Reagan has his wife and Secret Service agents. Greta, Arnie, and Doris have their doctors, nurses, spouses, siblings, children, and friends.

The caregiver must preside over the degeneration of someone he or she loves very much; must do this for years and years with the news always getting worse, not better; must every few months learn to compensate for new shortcomings with makeshift remedies; must negotiate impossible requests and fantastic observations; must put up sometimes with deranged but at the same time very personal insults; and must somehow learn to smile through it all. The work shift in this literally thankless job lasts for twenty-four hours a day, seven days a week. On-the-job training includes basic neurology, an introduction to nursing, and mind reading. Caregivers must be able to diagnose a wide variety of ordinary ailments—toothache, nausea, urinary tract infection, and so on—under extraordinary circumstances. Imagine a patient suddenly upset about something but completely unable to communicate the problem, or even to understand it himself. Is he hungry? Exhausted? Sore? Does he have a bad headache or did he break his toe? Is his back in spasms or is his appendix inflamed? Can he point to the problem? No, he cannot.

The stress facing caregivers is so extraordinary that it commonly leads to very serious problems on its own. "Caregiver's dementia" is widely used to describe the overpowering symptoms of fatigue and forgetfulness that often come with the role of Alzheimer's caregiver—staying up all hours, going days or weeks without a break, and so on. The term is half tongue in cheek, not intended to refer to a biological dementia. Still, this stress-induced psychological condition can be very, very serious. One estimate has roughly half of all Alzheimer's caregivers struggling with clinical depression.

In the late 1990s, some 10–15 million Americans were called to duty. More often than not they were women, often in their forties or early fifties, often recently retired from the more conventional parenting role after nearly two decades. The kids had just gone off to work or started college; life was supposed to begin all over again—and then a call came in: Mom or Dad had been acting a little strange lately.

There are no wages for this grueling job, of course, and depending on the patient's health insurance and the size of her estate, the illness can actually cost the caregiver tens of thousands of dollars every year. Neither Medicare nor private health insurance covers the type of long-term care most patients need. The average out-of-pocket costs for Alzheimer's patients are $12,500 per year. Nursing home care averages more than $40,000 annually.

If estranged family members don't happen to be sensitive to the burdens of Alzheimer's disease, there might also be substantial legal bills. The very slow fade of a parent often tends to knock pegs out from under already shaky families. In Shakespeare's rendition of *King Lear*, written in 1605–1606, Lear's two elder daughters take cruel advantage of their father's weakening state of mind while the third daughter, Cordelia, suffers for her loyalty and lack of guile. The play is about a family's dissolution through misunderstanding and distrust. Senility is the playwright's device.

It was a striking plot choice. There had been at least fifty versions of the Lear (or "Leir") story prior to Shakespeare's, but his was the first to put the king in a deep senile fog. Throughout Shakespeare's play, Lear hallucinates, doesn't recognize old friends, and cannot remember who he is. "My wits begin to turn," he remarks in one scene; in another, "I am cut to the brains." With a few exceptions (most notably his plot-driven mental recovery in the last act), his complaints are perfectly in synch with the Alzheimer's experience:

> I fear I am not in my perfect mind.
> Methinks I should know you, and know this man;
> Yet I am doubtful; for I am mainly ignorant
> What place this is; and all the skill I have
> Remembers not these garments; nor I know not
> Where I did lodge last night. . . .
>
> —KING LEAR, ACT IV, SCENE 3

Shakespeare's decision to incorporate dementia may have been inspired by the real-life case of Bryan Annesley, a wealthy palace attendant to Shakespeare's patron, Queen Elizabeth. In 1603—two years before Shakespeare wrote *King Lear*—Annesley's senility became a public spectacle in the English court. Annesley was in the late stages of progressive dementia: "Fallen into such imperfection and distemperature of mind and memory," reported an observer, "[and] altogether unfit to govern himself." His youngest daughter (of three), named Cordell, the only one not yet married, remained at home to care for him. By contrast, the eldest daughter, Grace, kept her attentions focused on the sizable estate, suing to have her father declared a lunatic so she could take immediate custody of his possessions.

Under the law at that time, a lunatic was deprived of all civil and human rights and was subject to the whims of the family property owner. Cordell's successful defense of her father's rights—she convinced the royal minister Lord Cecil to place the estate into the custody of a loyal family friend—very likely insured that he would have the most comfortable and dignified descent possible. Annesley died the next year, still under Cordell's care.

Four centuries later, Cordell Annesleys could be found in every city of the world. "My sister-in-law visited for a few days while my mother-in-law was in the hospital," reported Sally D., from Logansport, Indiana. "When I went over to mow the lawn, I found she had rearranged the china cabinet. A lot of stuff was not there. I suppose we should take an inventory of everything in the house, so when the time comes, we can see what has walked away during the interim. We should not have to do this."

Longer lives and the proliferation of Alzheimer's were colliding with yet another modern circumstance—the scattering of families. As if there were not enough layers of sadness already, the disease too often also became a wedge, driving already fractured families further apart. "Things are going from bad to worse here," said Jean B. from Lexington, Massachusetts. "I just got a letter from my sister's law firm about the estate and having to inventory everything in this house. First, they said everything here is Dad's, conveniently ignoring the fact that Ashley and I brought things here and have acquired things subsequently. It also said I was 'staying with' Dad—which has a far different connotation than 'taking care of' Dad—like I am here mooching off him because of some deficiency in my own life."

Though they lived a thousand miles apart, Sally and Jean were able to find and support each other, and hundreds of other caregivers scattered throughout the world, via the Alzheimer List, on the Internet at http://www.adrc.wustl.edu/alzheimer. A virtual support group created by the Alzheimer's Disease Research Center at Washington University in St. Louis in 1994, the list helped more than a thousand caregivers, social workers, clinicians, and researchers form a community through E-mail dispatches. Discussions ranged from whether/how to tell already demented loved ones about their disease, to appropriate dosage levels of medications, to which air fresheners best remove the smell of human feces from a room. For pixels on a screen, the talk was surprisingly warm and intimate.

13 Aug 2000
From: Carla Flaherty
Subject: Visiting Dad at Primrose

Thank you Kathy, Geri, Michelle, Eveline, and Connie for your responses to my sad visits with Dad. You are all, as always, a great help and gave me good thoughts—which made Friday's visit much easier on me.

Yes—two of you mentioned this—what I REALLY want is for Dad to come back for a minute and say, "Hey, you did good, kiddo. I know you didn't want this, and I didn't either, but you did the best you could and I'm satisfied with it." Getting clear that I wanted the impossible made it easier. So I will tell myself these things instead. And pick pears for Dad, knowing I HAVE done the best I could.

Luck & hope,
Carla

Perhaps the Internet was the perfect medium for Alzheimer's caregivers: millions of them sprinkled across the earth, stuck in their homes taking care of their loved ones, rarely able to break away. Then, with little warning, a free moment popped up in the early afternoon or the middle of the night. Down the stairs in a cluttered basement office, a screen and keyboard provided the connection to countless others with similar concerns.

At 2:30 A.M., Diane wrote in from San Diego with a question about her mother's sleeplessness. At 9:00 A.M., a response came from Jerry in Spokane. He patiently recalled his own experience with "sundowning," passing on the array of tactics and tools used, and assuring her that the night restlessness would eventually pass.

Nina from Adrian, Michigan, needed some advice on how to handle her mother's stubborn refusal to allow a nurse into the home. Geri from Minneapolis piped in: She had been through exactly the same thing with her husband, and explained the legal Catch-22: If Nina's mother was already so impaired that she couldn't take care of herself, she was probably also too impaired to give Nina legal authority to make key decisions on her behalf. If so, Nina would have to ask a judge to declare her mother incompetent (the modern equivalent of the Elizabethan "lunatic").

Focused exchanges like this continued twenty-four hours a day, in a never-ending swap of empathy, camaraderie, and advice. After several years and some 14 million words, the group had covered a lot of ground: room monitors, mini-strokes, drug trials, spending sprees, wandering, day care, power of attorney, stages of grieving, assisted living, door knob covers, incontinence, corporate insensitivity, family reunions, caregiver's depression, sadness, terror, relief, betrayal, even attempted murder. Hanging over all the painful details like a wide porch roof was a rich poignancy, a sense that these family members had been tested and dredged for all their depth of feeling. Here were people in the throes of a slow, horrible loss, aggravating and draining, and yet many seemed to be experiencing the fullness of life in a way that made me as a distant observer feel perversely envious. No one in this group seemed dead to the world, stuck in old habits, numb and sleepwalking through daily chores. These people were buzzing with life.

Following their conversations, I realized that while medical science gives us many tools for staying alive, it cannot help us with the art of living—or dying. Life, in its precious transience, is something we can only define on our own terms. With Alzheimer's disease, the caregiver's challenge is to escape the medical confines of *disease* and to assemble a new humanity in the loss.

One realization that popped up over and over again on the List, for example, was the importance of not forcing "reality" onto someone living with Alzheimer's. "During the early years," recalled Rolfe S. from Fairfield, Vermont, "I tried to have Phyllis live life the . . . 'normal' . . . way—my way or our pre-Alzheimer's way of life. It did not work. When I corrected her or tried to 'normalize' her she became agitated, which in turn agitated me and made life hell. She was unhappy. I was unhappy.

"I finally realized that whatever I said or did to correct her made no difference. I realized that life would be easier if I let her do what she wanted (within safety limits). I no longer scolded her but thanked her for bringing the frying pan into the bathroom. After that, life changed very much for the good. She is happy but still declining. I am happy and have adjusted to my new 'life.' It will change some day but if it doesn't, so be it. Enjoy life as best you can."

Over the years, List participants had discussed it all, it seemed. But there were still occasional surprises. In late February 1999, an extraordinary dispatch came in from Morris Friedell, a quiet, bushy-bearded, tweed-coated sociologist from Southern California.

"I first subscribed to this list because of my mother's probable Alzheimer's," Morris wrote. "A neurologist and a neuropsychologist told me my own forgetfulness was probably benign aging plus Caregiver's Dementia. Unfortunately, another neurologist, with the help of an MRI, a PET, and a qEEG, diagnosed me as having Alzheimer's myself."

A patient—on the List? This was something new. The community was well-versed in talking *about* Alzheimer's sufferers, not *to* them.

And that was only half the surprise.

Morris had not come to kvetch. He was no helpless Lear, flailing about, but part of the new class of Alzheimer's sufferers, diagnosed so early as to still be able to speak for themselves, to eloquently describe their experience, and to champion their rights. More than that, even, Morris wanted to talk about *rehabilitation*.

Not long before, this fifty-nine-year-old college professor had been planning his early retirement, hoping to read and write books free from the commitments of teaching. Then memory troubles intervened. During his final year with students, he began to have trouble remembering what his students said in class. Later, he couldn't remember a conversation he'd just had with his mother. At the neuropsychologist's office, he couldn't tell the doctor about a movie he'd seen just the night before. They ran the usual tests. He got a perfect score on the MMSE. On the brain scans, he didn't fare so well.

The diagnosis hit Morris like an ice bath. At a decidedly unelderly age, his "mid-life" was suddenly very late-life. He was now on a slow but certain trajectory toward forgetting and death. In the turmoil, his on-and-off relationship with a girlfriend fizzled out. He was home alone with his books and his dreary thoughts.

At the University of California at Santa Barbara, Morris taught a course called "Human Dignity" and had written his own book on the subject. He crafted a career out of interpreting authors like Viktor Frankl, Martin Buber, and Elie Wiesel. In a superstitious way, Morris hoped that teaching about human suffering might give him a personal bye. "I now see," Morris wrote after his diagnosis, "I thought that teaching this stuff meant, magically, that I'd die by being run over by a truck and never have to face a dramatic challenge to my own human dignity. Oh, well."

His teaching did not shield him from personal tragedy, but it did, evidently, prepare him for it. "For a couple of weeks after the MRI I was struggling with clinical depression. Fortunately, the advice helpful to cancer victims and prisoners-of-war worked for me: Control what you can control, communicate—express your feel-

"There is pain in forgetfulness," he wrote, "but sometimes there is something delicious in oblivion. Recently I spent some time with the three-year-old grandson of a friend of mine. He has Down's syndrome. I could enjoy sharing with him his friendly little non-verbal world in a way that I never could have before. Not only was my aphasia not a problem—it was like the absence of street noise so I could better savor the music."

Something delicious in oblivion. Could Morris help bridge the widening chasm between the optimistic world of science and the despairing world of sufferers? He knew full well that, as a disease, Alzheimer's is degenerative and incurable. He chose instead to face it as a human condition. In his own forgetting, Morris wanted to find meaning, and hope.

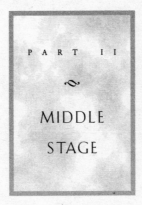

PART II

&

MIDDLE

STAGE

Chapter 7

FUMBLING FOR
THE NAME OF MY WIFE

On November 12, 1879, two years after he never quite heard, never quite understood, and then entirely forgot Mark Twain's tale of the three famous tramps, Ralph Waldo Emerson, age seventy-six, gave a lecture at the home of Harvard Divinity School professor C. C. Everett. Though Emerson's dementia had steadily progressed over the decade, and he had not written an original lecture in four years, he still occasionally read aloud from old works.

On this particular night, the aging Transcendentalist made a sharply ironic choice of material. Of all things, he read from his twenty-two-year-old essay, "Memory." "Without it," Emerson intoned, "all life and thought were an unrelated succession. As gravity holds matter from flying off into space, so memory gives stability to knowledge; it is the cohesion which keeps things from falling into a lump or flowing in wave. . . .

"Memory performs the impossible for man by the strength of

his divine arms; holds together past and present, beholding both, existing in both, abides in the flowing, and gives continuity and dignity to human life. It holds us to our family, to our friends. Hereby a home is possible; hereby only a new fact has value."

How poignant, and how awful, that as Emerson read aloud these evocative words, his own memory was broken. Much like H.M., he could form no new memories at all. His life from moment to moment *was* an unrelated succession. There was no more continuity except that provided for him by friends and family. At this particular reading, his daughter and caregiver Ellen stood by as a sort of Seeing Eye memory guide. He continually looked up at her to be sure he did not repeat words or sentences.

This was not just an exercise in caution. Without her help, Emerson had recently lost his place many times in lectures, skipped or repeated sentences, and even reread entire pages over again without noticing. In at least one public reading, he had stopped suddenly in the middle of his material and stood silently at the lectern, oblivious. "His words are either not all written or not well remembered," ran a typically disappointed review of these years from the *New Brunswick Daily Times*. ". . . He shows a want of fluency in language, and frequently descends to a tone even fainter than the conversational, and a manner unpleasantly hesitant."

We will never know for sure, of course, whether Emerson was beset with what we now call "Alzheimer's disease." No one bothered to look at the folds of his brain after he died, and if they had they would not have been able to discern anything as detailed as plaques and tangles. Alois Alzheimer was, at the time of Emerson's decline, still a raucous Bavarian youth. Franz Nissl had not yet invented his important tissue stains. Emil Kraepelin had not proposed his radical ideas about autotoxins and organic brain diseases.

We do know from the voluminous record of the details of his life that Emerson had a slow, progressive dementia that in every way appears consistent with the course of typical Alzheimer's disease (albeit on the slower side of the average progression). His illness crept in over time and engendered a slow, almost imperceptible decline. For several years after the trouble first appeared, he was able to hold on to his essential self and treat the memory impairments as disabilities to be worked around, not necessarily any more severe than a broken leg requiring crutches or a wheelchair.

But by the mid-1870s, according to the description of biographer Phillips Russell, Emerson (in his early seventies) had passed into what we now refer to loosely as the middle stages of the disease: "He lived in an internal quietude not to be shattered even by the loudest noises. Outlines and edges were no longer perceptible, and he dwelt in a dreamlike mist which hid from his vision everything that was not intimate and immediately recognizable. . . .

"His love for reading continued, but words ceased to have any intrinsic meaning, and books were sought only for their general tone or flavor. Personality disappeared from all names, and when he sometimes took down from his shelves his own books they possessed a novelty for him exactly like that he would have found in the works of an unknown author. One day when his daughter entered his study, she found him reading very intently in one of his own books. His face revealed his pleasure, and looking up at her, he exclaimed, 'Why, these things are really very good.'"

Because his progression was so slow, Emerson was aware of his deficits for many years. For all of the imperceptible, incremental declines over the months and years in Alzheimer's, one meaningful way to view the disease is as a two-stage disorder: the *awareness* stage and the *postawareness* stage. Regardless of when (or whether) the actual diagnosis takes place, the sufferer is usually aware for several years that something is not quite right. He knows that he is forgetting. Then, at a certain point, usually years into the disease, he no longer knows.

For a long while, Emerson certainly knew. Even before others perceived any symptoms at all, in fact, he shocked his friends and family in 1866 (age sixty-three) with a very personal announcement of his imminent decline in the poem "Terminus."

TERMINUS

It is time to be old,
To take in sail:—
The god of bounds,
Who sets to seas a shore,
Come to me in his fatal rounds,
And said: "No more!
No farther shoot
Thy broad ambitious branches, and thy root.
Fancy departs: no more invent,
Contract thy firmament
To compass of a tent.
There's not enough for this and that,
Make thy option which of two;
Economize the failing river,
Not the less revere the Giver,
Leave the many and hold the few.
Timely wise accept the terms,
Soften the fall with wary foot;
A little while

Still plan and smile,
And—fault of novel germs—
Mature the unfallen fruit. . . ."

As the bird trims her to the gale,
I trim myself to the storm of time,
I man the rudder, reef the sail,
Obey the voice at eve obeyed at prime:
"Lowly faithful, banish fear,
Right onward drive unharmed;
The port, well worth the cruise, is near,
And every wave is charmed."

"There he sat," his son Edward later recalled of the chilling moment his father first read the finished poem aloud, "with no apparent abatement of bodily vigor, and young in spirit, recognizing with serene acquiescence his failing forces; I think he smiled as he read. He recognized, as none of us did, that his working days were nearly done."

Sure enough, soon after this formal declaration of decline, expressive aphasia and short-term memory problems surfaced. Groping for the names of famous writers and close friends, for everyday words like "umbrella," and "chair," for new ideas to fill his notebooks and lectures, Emerson gradually settled into a slower, more sheltered life for himself. He cut back on lectures, limited his travel, and worked on a final few projects. "Father has sat quiet in a chair all the forenoon," Ellen wrote to her mother in November 1872, "declaring that idlesse is the business of age, and he loves above all things 'to do noshing' [sic], and that he never before had discovered this privilege of seventy years. . . . also bragging that Edward was a lion over at the

Cathedral yesterday, knew dates and facts like an antiquary, and saying he was glad to have him go to dinners with him, 'so that when I am fumbling for the name of my wife he can remember it for me.'"

Because of who he was and who his friends and colleagues were, Emerson's forgetting was often both personally poignant and historically significant. In a visit by Walt Whitman to Emerson's home in the early 1870s, Emerson turned to Ellen at one point and discreetly asked her, "What is the name of this poet?" Many years later, at the funeral for Henry Wadsworth Longfellow, he is reported to have said of his friend of fifty years, "The gentleman who lies here was a beautiful soul, but I have forgotten his name."

It is a powerful irony that Emerson, of all people, should have lost his memory, not just because he contributed so much to the public discourse on the subjects of intellect, identity, imagination, and the human spirit, but also because he spent his entire life constructing one of the most elaborate external memory systems—in the form of books and journals—of any writer in history. His "Wide World" journals, which he inaugurated in his junior year at Harvard College as "a receptacle of . . . all the luckless raggamuffin Ideas which may be collected & imprisoned hereafter in these pages," ended up filling hundreds of pages and being organized into many distinct subjects and meticulously cross-referenced.

The young Emerson explicitly referred to his brand-new journal as a "tablet to save the wear & tear of weak Memory." It is almost as if Emerson was in conscious preparation throughout his life for the time when he would lose his memory, constructing an elaborate mechanism to fall back on. In his later years, he withdrew to his precious notebooks and more formal writings in order to sustain him as a public figure for the fifteen years that followed the onset of his illness. "I cannot remember anybody's name; not even my recollections of the Latin School," he announced at the centennial celebration of his alma mater. "I have therefore guarded against absolute silence by bringing you a few reminiscences which I have written."

It takes memory, though, to make memory. Once his illness began, his life's work of creating a reservoir of external memory was effectively over. His fertile notebook entries and evocative letters became fewer and terser, accompanied by steady acknowledgments of how his "broken age" had "tied my tongue and hid my memory." His late letters are saturated with basic spelling errors ("som" for some, "claimess" for claims, "tahat" for that), missing words, and repeated words. In sum, he was, by his own third-person declaration, "a man who has lost his wits."

And yet he rarely let on that he was bothered by it. The decision to continue speaking in public perfectly illustrates his exceptional poise. "Things that go wrong at these lectures don't disturb me," Emerson said, "because I know that everyone knows I am worn out and passed by; and that it is only my friends come for friendship's sake to have one last season with me." On another occasion, preparing for a speech, he remarked to Ellen, "A funny occasion it will be—a lecturer who has no idea what he's lecturing about." In light of what Emerson had lost, and *knew* that he had lost, the good humor was remarkable. As Edward had noticed on first hearing "Terminus," the world-famous Emersonian serenity had only intensified, it seemed, with the onset of his dementia.

"Memory" was not an isolated work, but had been conceived and written in his earlier years as a part of what Emerson told his close friend and literary executor James Elliot Cabot was the "chief task" of his life: a series of essays and lectures he called "Natural History of the Intellect." Originally imagined in the 1830s, undertaken in earnest in 1847–48, and reworked in the 1850s, Emerson finally seized the chance to finish the lifelong project as a lecture series for Harvard in the spring of 1870.

Because of their importance, Emerson made sure to invest the necessary time to get them just right. He devised a plan for sixteen lectures, and took most of the winter and spring to organize them. The overall goal was to integrate Transcendentalism with traditional philosophy and science, to bring a spirit of scientific inquiry to the consideration of the nature of mind, of imagination and creativity. "I wish to know the laws of this wonderful power," he wrote, "that I may domesticate it. I observe with curiosity its risings and its settings, illumination and eclipse; its obstructions and its provocations, that I may learn to live with it wisely, court its aid, catch sight of its splendor, feel its approach, hear and save its oracles and obey them."

Alas, he had waited too long. Even with eighteen months of work—he reworked and redelivered the lectures the following spring—he couldn't get it right. After a lifetime of masterly organization, Emerson complained to Thomas Carlyle that he was now finding his work "oppressive." He had lots of good source material, he said, and some good ideas, "but in haste they are misplaced and spoiled." His son Edward observed bluntly that it was "too late for the satisfactory performance of the duty." Emerson wanted desperately to define the parameters of intellect, but his own intellect was no longer up to the task.

After the Harvard ordeal, Emerson was treated to a luxurious seven-week trip westward by John Forbes, the wealthy father of his new son-in-law. A party of twelve piled into a private Pullman train car in Chicago, and were seen off by George Pullman himself. As reported later in a detailed journal by fellow excursioner James Bradley Thayer, Emerson was thrilled to do nothing on this trip but read, relax, talk, eat, and smoke cigars. He developed a happy morning ritual of eating pie before any other foods, and attempted to seduce others into joining him. When, one morning, he was unable to convince anyone within earshot, Emerson playfully slid a knife underneath a slice of pie and, gently tilting it up toward a companion, asked with exaggerated face and voice, "But Mr. ———, what is pie for?"

The first stop was Salt Lake City, where Emerson was introduced to (but was unimpressed by) Mormon leader Brigham Young. Then on to San Francisco, where he admired the sea lions and the California wine. At the San Francisco Unitarian Church, he read aloud his address "Immortality." From there the group traveled to Yosemite. In the Mariposa Grove, Emerson was overwhelmed by the majesty of the giant sequoias, which he called "those gentleman trees."

He was particularly moved by their ability to age with grace, to survive the indignities of fire and other abuse. In thirteen hundred years of life, he remarked, the trees "must have met that danger and every other in turn. Yet they possess great power of resistance."

Continuing their tour of Yosemite, the group came to the majestic Vernal Fall, where someone recited from Longfellow's "Wreck of the Hesperus":

She struck where the white and fleecy waves
Looked soft as carded wool . . .

Emerson was very glad to hear the verse of his friend, but he found it impossible to retain the words in his mind for more than a few moments. "Mr. Emerson gave a pleased nod, and desired it said over again," noted Thayer, evidently oblivious to Emerson's incipient decline. "And then he wished a reference to it when we should get to the hotel. Had he then let Longfellow's poetry pass by him so much?"

In Yosemite, the party on horseback was joined by the young environmentalist John Muir, a great admirer of Emerson. Muir, who would go on to convince Congress to establish Yosemite National Park in 1890, observed that Emerson was as "serene as a sequoia." Emerson was delighted to discover a western protégé. As his group left Yosemite on horseback, Muir recalled: "Emerson lingered in the rear . . . and when he reached the top of the ridge, after all the rest of the party were over and out of sight, he turned his horse, took off his hat and waved me a last good-bye."

﹏

I'm blessed to have a wonderful daughter. . . . I
sent her to school and to college, and now she knows
how to take care of all my business. I depend on her.
I'm in her hands. I'm in my baby phase now, so to
speak. So sometimes I call her my "mumma." Yes,
she's my mumma now.

—B.
San Diego, California

﹏

Chapter 8

BACK TO BIRTH

❦

Old men are children twice over.

—Aristophanes, 419 b.c.

Queens, New York: Fall 1999

The decline was sure and steady at Freund House, in Queens.

After two years in the group, Doris was now facing more severe aphasia. Her sentences were now so pockmarked with "yeah" in place of other words that it was difficult to tell what she was trying to say much of the time. Even the most productive conversations with Doris involved almost no exchange of information. Over lunch one afternoon, someone mentioned tuna fish. Doris's eyes lit up.

"My mother had a . . . a . . ."

"A recipe?" someone offered.

"Yes . . . she . . . yeah . . . she . . ."

"She had a recipe for tuna fish salad?"

"Yes . . . wonderful."

The thread of conversation ended there. Doris clearly had much more to say on the subject, but translating these thoughts into spoken words was no longer possible. Her world did not collapse entirely on her inability to discuss tuna fish, but to have all potential conversations restricted to a handful of words effectively extinguished her ability to communicate any real thoughts out loud. (One suspected that the intended subject of this un-conversation was not tuna fish, but Doris's mother.)

Rachel, another veteran member of the group, was also deteriorating, and—perhaps blessedly—oblivious to the decline. At the end of one week's session, Irving felt the need to be blunt with her. "Rachel, please talk to your son about getting a review, a medical update. I think it's extremely important."

"On what?"

"On the progression of your dementia."

"Why—do you see something?"

Irving paused briefly to check his frustration. "Yes—I mentioned it to you before that we see a little more progression."

"About remembering? Really?"

"Well, what's happening is that there's even a little bit more of the not-remembering that you're forgetting."

"Not remembering forgetting?"

"Not remembering that *you're* forgetting. In the beginning, you used to come in and say, 'Oh, I forgot.' Now you don't even remember in some of the cases that you forgot."

"Oh."

William was much more confused than before. He got lost on bathroom breaks. Greta had also deteriorated and seemed headed to soon join the middle-stage group for which she had once volunteered.

The group was collapsing. The original vision had been to cycle individual members out of the group as they progressed into the middle stages of the disease—once they were no longer "bothered enough," in Judy's words, to contribute. In practice, this had proven very tough to do, a lot tougher than Irving or Judy had anticipated. Whenever they tried to discuss the exit of one or another member, Irving explained, "The other members jumped on us. They were horrified. 'He's not hurting the group!' they would say."

Even as minds slipped away, the group still held a lot of meaning for these people. They didn't want to let go of their friends, or to acknowledge decline. Shortly before the group disbanded, there was a frank discussion about the future. Or rather, there was an *attempt* by the group leaders at a frank discussion. Stefanie, another group facilitator, tried to prepare the group for what was in store. "This group is a temporary group," she said. "Things may get worse. And you may not remember if they get worse." She raised the possibility of the group retaining the same members, but beginning to meet for a good portion of each day instead of once weekly. This would mark a transition from *self-help* to *day care*.

The group would hear none of it. Even in their impairment, they were sharp enough to know what she was driving at. She was warning them that the early stages were coming to an end.

They weren't ready. The group had been working on coping mechanisms for two years, but simply could not confront the wretched truth head-on. "A lot of people are worse off than me," William protested. "For me, it hasn't changed since I walked in the door. My wife would back me up in that."

"That's right," Greta said, in effect demonstrating her own deteriorating memory and judgment. "He has improved tremendously. He can express himself much better than before." Turning to the issue of her own decline, Greta disputed claims that she had recently been seen walking around Freund House in a state of confusion. "That's just crazy," she insisted. Doris also claimed she wasn't getting any worse.

Denial is an important part of the Alzheimer's experience, very commonly employed as symptoms first appear, or at the time of diagnosis, or at any juncture where a truth is so horrifying that the most emotionally healthy choice is to pretend that it does not exist. The poisonous reality is pushed back into the recesses of the mind and only slowly, in small drips, is it allowed to seep back into consciousness.

It's also customary for denial to fade away and then return again sometime later. This psychological mechanism of last resort can be invoked as often as need be, and in Freund House most of the group members now apparently needed to fall back on it again. For the time being, it didn't matter that they had bravely faced down their disease together for two years. It didn't matter that they had accepted their decreased functioning and voluntarily given up liberties like driving. It didn't matter that they had brought much frustration and despair to the surface. A new awful truth was emerging that was too hard to confront. What they each had glimpsed, if only briefly before suppressing, were the *middle stages*. It wouldn't be so long now before *they* were singing the Barney song and being escorted to the bathroom.

In effect, without anyone quite realizing it, the group had already become a middle-stage group. They no longer knew what had brought them there in the first place, could no longer examine the implications of their own deficits. Of the six of them, Arnie was the only one left still bothered enough to talk about the problems with some candor.

"I think we need to own up to the fact that change occurs," Arnie finally said to his friends in one of their last meetings together. "And in the main, these changes are not positive."

He paused for a moment. "I think I'll leave it at that for now."

Bel Air, California: Fall 1999

Ronald Reagan was also slipping well past the early stages. "Not good" was how Reagan's daughter Maureen characterized his condition in the fifth year following the diagnosis.

The mythic significance of the once "Great Communicator" now steadily unraveling was felt even by Reagan's detractors: Once the most powerful man on earth, he famously confronted the Soviet empire. Now he was caught in a humbling downward spiral, so powerless that he no longer even knew who he was. On the *Today* show, Ann Curry asked Maureen, "Does he remember being President?" She evaded the painful question.

Earlier in the illness, supporters had made much of the fact that Reagan was continuing to go to his office in downtown Los Angeles every day. He played the occasional game of golf and took casual walks in public parks, making himself accessible to passers-by.

Those visits and games were now over, and the Reagans had sold their beloved "Rancho del Cielo" mountaintop retreat. They were hunkering down for some more difficult times. As expected, Reagan's descent had progressed steadily. Friends and family watched his memory lapses become the rule rather than the exception. There was, for example, the day that former Secretary of State George Shultz visited his old boss. In the midst of a casual discussion about politics, Reagan briefly left the room with a nurse. When he returned a few moments later, he took the nurse aside and pointed to Shultz. "Who is that man sitting with Nancy on the couch?" he asked quietly. "I know him. He is a very famous man."

Incidents like these drove him into further isolation. Partly out of simple courtesy to Reagan and partly due to their own personal discomfort, many of his friends stopped visiting when he started having trouble recognizing them.

Then came language stumbles. Over the course of a few years, aphasia crept steadily in and eventually took from him the ability to articulate his thoughts. He could, for a time, still read others' words out loud from a children's storybook. But then that too slipped away.

In visits just after the diagnosis, Maureen and her father would tackle large, three-hundred-piece puzzles. "He and I do jigsaw puzzles together," she said. "He loves doing that. When I was a little girl he used to tell me, 'Do the border first.' Now I sit there and say, 'Dad, do the border first.'"

When the intricate puzzles got too difficult, she brought him simpler puzzles of a hundred pieces or so; then simpler puzzles still, with farm animal scenes. Finally, even those became too challenging. In other homes all over Southern California and elsewhere, tiny children were, day by day, learning to distinguish colors and shapes, gaining in depth perception, improving their hand-eye coordination, slowly gaining confidence as their brains developed to full capacity. Here at 668 St. Cloud Drive, the former President of the United States was heading through that same developmental process in reverse.

The middle stages bring the end of ambiguity. The subtle cues that something was not quite right—so easy to miss a few years ago—

are now bright, self-reflecting signposts of decline, impossible to avoid. Conversation is now pockmarked with lost names and empty recollections. Time and dates have become fungible. Concentration wanes. The mind is now clearly ebbing.

Inside the folds of the brain, the progression is marked by a precise trail of pathology. Now the plaques and tangles have spread well beyond their starting point in the hippocampus. It is not clear how long they germinated there to begin with—*five years? twenty-five years?*—but in a rather short time they have now spread throughout the limbic system and leeched into the temporal, parietal, and frontal lobes of the cerebral cortex. Throughout much of the thinking brain, gooey plaques now crowd neurons from outside the cell membranes, and knotty tangles mangle microtubule transports from inside the cells. All told, tens of millions of synapses dissolve away.

Because the structures and substructures of the brain are so highly specialized, the precise location of the neuronal loss determines what specific abilities will become impaired, and when—like a series of circuit breakers in a large house flipping off one by one:

In the very beginning, when the hippocampus begins to degrade, memory formation fails.

Then, when the nearby amygdala becomes compromised, control over primitive emotions like fear, anger, and craving is disrupted; hostile eruptions and bursts of anxiety may occur all out of proportion to events, or even out of nowhere.

From there, tangles spread outward through much of the rest of the brain, following exactly the same pathways that sensory data travel in a healthy brain. One tangled neuron leads to another tangled neuron leads to another, like a pileup of cars after an accident.

A preponderance of neurons in the brain, 80 percent, are devoted to so-called higher-order processing—finely tuned perception, analysis, comparison, recollection, anticipation, and abstraction—with the small remainder left for perceiving stimuli and behavioral response. Of the higher-order association areas, the temporal lobes, just inside from the ear on either side of the brain, are the closest to the hippocampus and therefore the next to bear the brunt of Alzheimer's. Temporal lobes are responsible for primary organization of sensory input, for processing language, and for ecstatic feelings of spiritual transcendence. A healthy temporal lobe stimulated by an electrical probe can spontaneously produce powerful religious images, along with specific memories of songs and vivid hallucinations of friends' faces. Not surprisingly, auditory and visual hallucinations are not uncommon in the middle and later stages of Alzheimer's.

Next in line are the parietal and frontal lobes. The parietal lobes, on top of the brain, extending to the rear, handle touch, vibration, pain, and spatial awareness. They enable the control of limbs and eyes, and the recognition of objects by physical contact. Damage to the sensory portions of the parietal lobe can cause *astereognosis,* the inability to understand the source or meaning of touch. The patient becomes an island, floating apart from the external world.

When tangles finally reach the frontal lobes, which help to manage the retrieval of already formed memories, identity itself begins to vanish. A lifetime of memories exists in constellations all throughout the brain, but without a reliable system of retrieval, they'll sit dormant forever. (The temporal lobe also plays a crucial role in accessing semantic—intellectual—memories.)

The frontal lobes are also where most of what we consider intelligent thought takes place. Here is where massive amounts of sensory data are brought together, integrated and analyzed, where the brain makes sense of unfolding events, contrasts them with previous experience, adapts future plans based on that contrast. Once the frontal lobes come under heavy fire, the will itself begins to unravel, and, as one Alzheimer's text puts it, "the chain of mental contents is no longer guided by a logically valid executive program." The sufferer and her family cannot continue to treat her forgetfulness as a liability that can be overcome with Post-it Notes. It now becomes the dominant force in the patient's life, a major disability.

The list of cognitive abilities that dwindle in the middle stages of the disease is difficult for a cognitively healthy person to fully comprehend, because the functions lost are so basic. Memories are erased not just of specific events (grocery shopping last night), but general concepts learned long ago (what groceries *are*). Other central competencies that wither include:

The ability to understand simple questions, instructions, gestures

The ability to follow a conversation, or even to keep track of one's own words or thoughts

The ability to place oneself in the right time of day, or the right time of year

The ability, even the desire, to plan for the future

The ability to choose one's own clothes and draw one's own bath

The ability to recognize one's friends and relatives, or even one's spouse

The capacity for awareness (In these years, the sufferer loses all awareness of his or her condition. Introspection vanishes. This is known as *anosognosia*.)

Perhaps the only practical way to understand such a catastrophic loss is to imagine oneself as a very young child who has not yet developed these abilities in the first place. "All actions of the bodie and minde are weakened and growne feeble," a physician of King Henry IV of France said of old age in 1599. "The senses are dull, the memorie lost, and the judgment failing so that they become as they were in the infancie." That same century, Erasmus suggested even more fully:

> Old men are more eagerly delighted with children, and they, again, with old men. . . . For what difference between them, but that the one has more wrinkles and years upon his head than the other? Otherwise, the brightness of their hair, toothless mouth, weakness of body, love of mild, broken speech, chatting, toying, forgetfulness, inadvertency, and briefly, all other their actions agree in everything. And by how much the nearer they approach to this old age, by so much they grow backward into the likeness of children, until like them they pass from life to death, without any weariness of the one, or sense of the other.

Five hundred years later, caregivers use the same comparisons. "Not long after my [recently diagnosed] mother came to live with us, our daughter also came with her fourteen-month-old son," Daisy from Raceland, Kentucky, told fellow caregivers via the Alzheimer List. "I find that what works with him also works with Mom, and they give the same angelic smile when pleased. On the downside, there is also the same tantrum at times and stamp of the foot. What I do to safety-proof the house for the baby also works as Nana-proofing, for the most part. The same behavior-addressing works as well. Often when he is cranky, it is due to some other influence—just like her. I have learned to read between the lines at both ends of the age spectrum. Sadly enough, he is learning to potty train at the time when my mom is losing that ability."

In 1980, New York University neurologist Barry Reisberg realized that the Alzheimer's-childhood analogy is not just anecdotal—that it could be measured scientifically. Reisberg was a pioneer in defining stages and substages of Alzheimer's, trying to gain a much more precise understanding of the disease's trajectory. The more he drilled down on the exact order of abilities lost, the more he was impressed by the comparison to child development. He began to notice that there were precise inverse relationships between stages of Alzheimer's disease and phases of child development in the areas of cognition, coordination, language, feeding, and behavior.

He documented these observations in comparison charts. Placed side by side, the sequences of abilities gained and lost nearly perfectly mirror one another.

CHILD DEVELOPMENT

Age	Acquired Ability
1–3 months	Can hold up head
2–4 months	Can smile
6–10 months	Can sit up without assistance
1 year	Can walk without assistance
1 year	Can speak one word
15 months	Can speak 5–6 words
2–3 years	Can control bowels
3–4.5 years	Can control urine
4 years	Can use toilet without assistance
4–5 years	Can adjust bath water temperature
4–5 years	Can put on clothes without assistance

5–7 years	Can select proper clothing for occasion or season
8–12 years	Can handle simple finances
12+ years	Can hold a job, prepare meals, etc.

ALZHEIMER'S DISEASE

Stage	Lost Ability
1	No difficulty at all
2	Some memory trouble begins to affect job/home
3	Much difficulty maintaining job performance
4	Can no longer hold a job, prepare meals, handle personal finances, etc.
5	Can no longer select proper clothing for occasion or season
6a	Can no longer put on clothes properly
6b	Can no longer adjust bath water temperature
6c	Can no longer use toilet without assistance
6d	Urinary incontinence
6e	Fecal incontinence
7a	Speech now limited to six or so words per day
7b	Speech now limited to one word per day
7c	Can no longer walk without assistance
7d	Can no longer sit up without assistance
7e	Can no longer smile
7f	Can no longer hold up head

In neurological exams, there were similarly precise inverse relationships in EEG activity, brain glucose metabolism, and neurologic reflexes. The only possible conclusion Reisberg could draw was that, like the winding and unwinding of a giant ball of string, Alzheimer's unravels the brain almost exactly in the reverse order as it develops from birth. Clearly, the phenomenon warranted more formal study, and a name. Reisberg called it "retrogenesis"—*back to birth*.

Retrogenesis is not a perfect reversal, of course—not literally the unwiring of the brain, neuron by neuron, according to some bizarre genetic instruction booklet. But the deconstruction is remarkably similar to the construction. What researchers realized in delving further into this comparison was that Alzheimer's degeneration followed the opposite pattern of brain *myelinization*—the insulation of nerve axons with a white myelin sheath in order to boost the strength of their signals.

Imagine a house thoroughly wired for electricity and phone use, but without any wire insulation—all the unprotected copper wires wrapped up together and touching one another. Infants are born with billions of neurons but almost no myelin insulation protecting these neurons, rendering them virtually useless. As neurons in various regions of the brain become insulated during child development, generating the famous "white matter" of the brain, these regions are *brought online*, made effective.

We know much about child brain development, thanks to J. L. Conel, a Boston neuropathologist who in 1939 began painstakingly dissecting the brains of deceased children. Over nearly thirty years, he examined the cerebral cortex from brains aged one month, three months, six months, fifteen months, two years, four years, and six years.

What he discovered comported with every parent's experience of their growing child: The first neurons to gain myelin insulation are in the primary motor area, enabling gross movements of the hands, arms, upper trunk, and legs. Next come the primary sensory area neurons in the parietal lobe, bringing gross touch sensations online. After that comes some development of the occipital lobe for visual acuity, followed by the temporal lobe for auditory processing. Gradually, the association areas are then formed, allowing the brain to make more and more sense of the perceptions being registered. Symbolic processing areas then begin to develop slowly, enabling language. Eventually the frontal cortex matures, enabling concentration, abstract thought, and the ability to plan.

One of the very last structures in the brain to be covered in protective myelin is the hippocampus, making it one of the last places to work effectively. This is why children generally don't have any permanent memories prior to age three (although the amygdala can store some very early emotional memories).

The reverse myelinization process of Alzheimer's begins with the most recent and least-myelinated brain region—the hippocampus. From there it moves to the next least-myelinated, and so on. In this one respect, at least, the disease process makes sense. It has its own logic.

For better or worse, the strange notion of reverse childhood turns out to be the best map we have to understand the terrain of Alzheimer's. Think of a teenager you know today and try to imagine her rapid development suddenly halting and beginning to reverse course at roughly the same developmental pace. Over the next twelve years or so, she loses everything she has gained, slowly and steadily.

First, she begins to lose her sense of humor and fashion sense. Now, watch her ambitions become less and less pronounced; then begin to peel away what she has learned from school and parents and peers and television over the last couple of years. Her sense of the world and her place in it fades away. Week by week she becomes not more but less articulate, less independent. She loses her Dairy Queen job because she has forgotten what "ice cream" and "cone" mean, and cannot add very well. As time ticks forward but seems to be going backward, she is now having a hard time picking out her own clothes; most of what she is saying you can no longer understand, and vice versa.

Further imagine your backwards teenager traversing her way back to infancy, to her very first day of birth, her first breath, and you have a surprisingly good grasp of the unraveling of mind, soul, and body that Alzheimer's inflicts on a person. Every skill, feeling, and fact that the patient has learned slowly, satisfyingly, is being steadily erased as if by some sort of cosmic punishment.

The child analogy understandably rankles many caregivers. They are deeply offended at the suggestion that their mother or father or husband or wife is now to be regarded as a mere child. It feels like the ultimate insult one could inflict on someone. Not yet fully formed, children are regarded as incomplete persons. We love them, of course, and recognize them as human beings, but we do not fully trust them. We assume a certain responsibility and even moral superiority over them. To assume this same posture toward a parent or grandparent who has stood for a lifetime in a position of moral authority is a sad and sour thing. It is tragic and demoralizing to suddenly strip our esteemed elders of their authority and reposition them as untrustworthy and intellectually inferior.

But the comparison is a valid, and even necessary, one to make. Here is an instance where scientists fighting disease and caregivers trying to make peace with a human tragedy can come to some common ground: the science of retrogenesis can help caregivers forge a new understanding and appreciation of what their loved ones are going through. Caregivers like Daisy from Raceland find the prism of second childhood helps ease both their chores and psychological strain. By viewing their loved ones as reverting back to childhood abilities and mentalities, caregivers can establish a more humane formula for their care. Whether or not it feels demeaning, retrogenesis can be *instructive*.

As reverse childhood came to seem more and more medically relevant, Alzheimer's researchers in the 1990s began dredging up everything known about developmental biology and psychology to test it for the possible application to their field. Colleagues of Reisberg, for instance, decided to test on severely demented patients a specially modified version of the Ordinal Scales of Psychological Development (OSPD), a test originally designed for infants and toddlers and based on Jean Piaget's theories of development.

This kind of ultra-basic testing had never been done before on Alzheimer's victims. The testers stripped down the OSPD so that it required no vocal abilities at all. They designed it to measure five rudimentary skills:

1. *Visual pursuit and object permanence.* Can the patient keep track of an object moving through an arc of 180 degrees?

2. *Means-ends.* Can the patient reach out for an object, causing an event to occur?

3. *Causality.* Does the patient react to a spectacle with an expression of understanding, such as a smile or frown?

4. *Spatial relations.* Can the patient adjust her vision between two objects?

5. *Schemes.* Can the patient visually inspect an object in her hands?

The experiment worked beautifully. Using criteria initially crafted to measure infant development, the researchers found what they called "residual cognitive capacities" in advanced-stage Alzheimer's patients who had previously been considered untestable.

The implications of this discovery are enormous for the development of caregiving strategies for middle and late-stage Alzheimer's patients. With new layers of understanding what patients are capable of and what they are no longer capable of at any specific stage of the disease, caregivers can be much more *prepared*. They can train themselves, in effect, to be competent reverse parents—not a skill that comes naturally.

If an Alzheimer's sufferer, for example, has progressed to the point where he is trying to put on an undershirt over a sweater, it now could be easily discerned that he has slipped into stage 6a of Alzheimer's, which, via retrogenesis, can be reasonably correlated to age four. Knowing that, one can also infer that the patient has now slid into what Piaget called the "Preoperational" stage. He is still able to represent reality through symbols (to count on his fingers, for example), but he is no longer able to rely on a solid foundation of logic (to understand the importance of going to bed early if he has to get up early the next day). He is also on the cusp of losing the sense that his point of view is distinct from that of others.

Properly utilized, the lens of retrogenesis can allow caregivers to enter the world of Alzheimer's disease with a broad new understanding. Caregivers can hone a sense that something coherent is happening, rather than what looks to the uninitiated like a random and unintelligible breakdown. Anyone who understands childhood can grasp the basic concept of reverting to that state, of developing in reverse. It helps make Alzheimer's caregiving a more human endeavor.

In *Max's New Suit*, Rosemary Wells's popular children's book, Max the young rabbit bumbles through the task of dressing himself. His older sister Ruby tries to teach him, but Max still puts his pants on over his head and his shirt on his legs. It is written about, and for, a very young child, but will work just as well in any nursing home (where between 60 and 80 percent of the patients are suffering from dementia). The world of children's literature turns out to be highly relevant to Alzheimer's. In Barbara M. Joosse's book, *Mama, Do You Love Me?*, to give another example, a little girl asks, "What if I ran away?"

"Then I would be worried," her mother answers.

"What if I stayed away and sang with the wolves and slept in a cave?"

"Then, Dear One, I would be very sad. But still, I would love you."

". . . What if I turned into a polar bear, and I was the meanest bear you ever saw and I had sharp, shiny teeth, and I chased you into your tent and you cried?"

"Then I would be very surprised and very scared. But still, inside the bear, you would be you, and I would love you."

The book is about a child exploring the boundaries of unconditional love. But in a home tainted by Alzheimer's disease, it also comes off as a perfect parable for the anxieties of both sufferer and caregiver. The sufferer wants to know, *What will happen when I become a real burden?* The caregiver wonders how bad the wandering, stubbornness, irritability, and bursts of snarling anger will become. As the illness progresses, she will struggle to look through the *disease* and recognize the *person* inside.

Not surprisingly, caregivers report that Alzheimer's patients in the middle and later stages find a tremendous comfort in children's books and music. They also like stuffed animals and dolls. The child's world—nurturing, safe, colorful, full of soft edges and sweet treats—is what middle-stage patients crave. "Mom enjoys car rides," says Pam from Baton Rouge, Louisiana. "It doesn't matter where we go or if we go anywhere other than drive around. She likes to look at the trees and anything green. . . . She got to the point where being in the store didn't work out too well. Now we still go but not to accomplish anything. We walk the mall and window-shop. If we go in a store it's like the Disney Store or a toy store to look at the stuffed animals. We look at the plants and decorations. We get ice cream."

The daughter has become the mother, the mother the daughter. Catastrophic disease often alters roles, but only Alzheimer's disease can fully reverse them.

Some days are so normal, I am guilty of thinking, "Well maybe he really isn't . . . ?" Then, to bring me back to reality, he wraps all my Tupperware in masking tape. Today, he went out to his workshop to "fix" an old LP record player, got side-tracked and ended up in the yard with a pair of clippers where he decimated my carefully cultivated rosemary bushes.

He was so proud of what he had done. Got rid of those weeds! Oh, well, the air was redolent with the aroma of rosemary. Rosemary is supposed to be the herb for remembrance. Maybe I should rub it in his hair.

—M.V.
Ft. Pierce, Florida

Chapter 9

NATIONAL INSTITUTE OF ALZHEIMER'S

∾

In the 1960s, public officials in industrialized democracies around the world began to notice something: There were more old people than ever, and they voted. The portion of the population living to eighty-five or beyond had tripled since 1900, and the elderly were becoming conspicuous for the first time in human history. In the U.S., a new lobbying organization, the American Association of Retired Persons (AARP), founded in 1958, was on its way to making senior citizens the most powerful interest group in American politics. In 1965, the U.S. government established Medicare, a sweeping federal program designed to protect every citizen "against the ravages of illness in his old age."

Around the same time, researchers were finally uncovering the true significance of one of those illnesses. At the Albert Einstein College of Medicine in New York, neuropathologists Robert Terry and Robert Katzman were shocked to see plaques and tangles turning up in so many brain samples. "We found Alzheimer's cases coming out of the woodwork," said Terry. "It was very common, and that surprised us. We didn't know that Alzheimer's was so common. Everybody thought that senile dementia was due to small artery disease."

After Katzman's sixty-four-year-old mother-in-law was diagnosed with Alzheimer's, he finally realized the larger hidden problem—the very problem that Meta Neumann had tried to expose two decades earlier. "It became obvious to me that Alzheimer's disease was a single entity regardless of age of onset," he said. "When I did simple multiplication, it became evident that this was a very important public health problem."

According to Katzman's calculations, Alzheimer's was already one of the leading causes of death in the United States, probably already killing 100,000 people per year in the U.S. alone. Those numbers would only get larger as the population aged even more.

The world had ignored Meta Neumann in 1953, but now people were ready to listen. Katzman's speeches and editorials in the early 1970s struck a chord with the medical community, which finally seemed open to the idea of senile dementia being a *disease*. As society aged, mores were shifting. So many people were living so long that senility didn't feel so normal or acceptable anymore. A critical mass of doctors began to *prefer* to see senility as a disease. The medical establishment was now ready to take on the moral challenge of Alzheimer's, to make a commitment to intervention.

But how? Researchers didn't know much more about Alzheimer's in the 1960s than they had in 1910. Robert Terry used an electron microscope to observe plaques and tangles at magnifications of up to one hundred times greater than Alois Alzheimer's original view, enabling him to begin to map out a cellular "ultra-structure" of the disease. But his extreme close-ups still did not reveal a cause, or even indicate whether plaques or tangles were closer to the root of the problem. Further progress would require a major new investment in the science of aging and the biology of Alzheimer's. In the early 1970s, health experts called on Congress to establish a National Institute on Aging.

The National Institute of Health (NIH) was established by Congress in 1930, but it wasn't until the late 1940s that two Washington activists began to transform it into the world's foremost center for medical research. Florence Mahoney was a former newspaper reporter and the wealthy widow of the publisher of the *Miami Herald;* Mary Lasker was cofounder of the prestigious Albert Lasker Medical Research Awards, the recipients of which commonly go on to win the Nobel Prize. Together, the two women devised a lobbying technique known as "the politics of anguish," coaxing friends in government and the media into focusing on the ravages of particular diseases rather than general scientific research.

This disease-by-disease approach converted dispassionate intellectual curiosity into a series of personal crusades. Politicians effortlessly gravitated to a war on cancer. They found it easy to convince their constituents that everyone's grandchildren should be spared from polio. Between 1950 and 1960, thanks to Mahoney and Lasker, the NIH budget grew from $46.3 million to $400 million—and became the National Institutes of Health.

Questions about aging research, though, caused a rift between the activist duo. In the early 1970s, Mahoney became convinced that the NIH needed a distinct institute to focus exclusively on the problems of the fastest growing part of the population. Lasker disagreed. She felt that the best way to deal with the problems of aging was to continue the fight against heart disease and cancer. Mahoney went ahead on her own, helping to push the Research on Aging Act of 1972 through Congress. It was vetoed that year by Richard Nixon.

Congress did not have the votes to override Nixon's veto, but two years later it unexpectedly had a different sort of leverage. In 1973, the Nixon White House began to fall under the siege of the Watergate investigation. By 1974, impeachment seemed a very real possibility, giving Congress the upper hand on Nixon. When the Research on Aging Act of 1972 was passed essentially unchanged by Congress as the Research on Aging Act of 1974, Nixon—desperate not to provoke the representatives controlling his fate—signed it. It became law on May 31, 1974, less than two months before he left office.

Robert Butler, the first director of the new National Institute on Aging (NIA), immediately signaled that he intended to make Alzheimer's a top priority. He hired the neurobiologist Zaven Khachaturian to wage war on Alzheimer's.

Khachaturian had been interested in the biology of memory since his days as an undergraduate at Yale in the late 1950s. Later, at the University of Pittsburgh's psychiatric department, he had started to focus on the physiology of forgetting and dementia. Along the way, he also felt the personal sting of the disease: His mother suffered from a progressive memory loss that he later came to suspect was Alzheimer's. "She was increasingly unable to remember the names of people she had just met," he recalled. "She repeated the same questions again and again, as though they had just popped into her head for the first time." Her forgetting progressed slowly; for many years before she died (from heart disease), she was lucid enough to question her son about his memory research—and yet unable to remember much of what he said.

As his mother drifted away, Khachaturian fashioned himself as the brigadier general of the modern war on Alzheimer's. Over two decades, he recruited top researchers, designed research paradigms, collaborated on funding proposals and translated the science to Congress and the public. "I started a crystal growing in all of the major areas—a group on neurochemistry, a group on protein chemistry, one on the infection hypothesis, and one on genetics. I tried to get all the major ideas started because I had no idea which one was going to pay off.

"I also purposefully tried to recruit people who had opposing points of view. There were royal battles. But since I was doling out the money on behalf of the government, my attitude was that I was going to get all these folks started on a level playing field."

The organic crystal quickly grew into a research palace. In the first five years, NIA research funding rose from $19.3 million to $70 million. By 1985, the NIA had established ten federally funded Alzheimer's disease research centers—a brainchild of Khachaturian—to coordinate clinical, behavioral, and laboratory research. The battle was on.

The public also started to learn about Alzheimer's for the first time in the late 1970s, from doctors and the media. In the U.S. Rita Hayworth was diagnosed in 1980. That same year, the syndicated columnist Abigail Van Buren printed an aching letter about Alzheimer's in her "Dear Abby" column. In 1982, President Reagan conferred the first of his two giant spotlights on the disease by proclaiming November "National Alzheimer's Month."

George Glenner, chief of molecular pathology at NIH and one of Zaven Khachaturian's star recruits to Alzheimer's research, was invited to the White House for the proclamation. As one of the few Alzheimer's experts present, Glenner was given the task of explaining the little-known disease to Reagan.

"The President looked at me and asked, 'What is Alzheimer's disease?' " Glenner recalled. "I explained that it was tangles and plaques that form in gray matter that keep neuronal cells from being nourished. Well, he looked at me and smiled.

" 'All I know is that my mother died in a nursing home and she didn't recognize me at the end,' he said."

Turning Alzheimer's into a household word was an official part of the political research strategy—using the "politics of anguish" as a tool to raise as much public interest and as many public dollars as possible. But there was a fallout from educating masses of people about a haunting and incurable disease. While scientists regarded Alzheimer's as a great new frontier, an exciting challenge, the public was left merely bewildered and anxious.

The new message was oppressive and hopeless: Old people did not sometimes gently "go senile." Rather, they were afflicted with a disease. No one was immune from this disease. The cause was unknown. There was no foreseeable treatment or cure.

The longer one lived, the greater one's chance would be of getting this disease.

Inadvertently, health officials had created two new problems: a new disease and a new cultural demon. The public needed more. To exist alongside the frightening unknown is often simply intolerable. In order to cope, we all need some comprehensible grasp of events outside our control, whether or not the interim explanations turn out to be true.

Senility had been frightening enough to people before it was called Alzheimer's disease, of course, and people had always sought comforting explanations for it. One ancient Roman superstition held that old people lost their memories as a result of reading epitaphs on tombstones. A tenth-century Arabic medical text blamed senility on cold, tenacious phlegm in the brain. Then, in the seventeenth century, the suspicion shifted to an excess of internal humidity—followed by a counter-theory that the real culprit was excessive dryness.

In 1984, amidst the surge in popular interest, the Nobel laureate Torsten Wiesel offered an irresistible, if accidental, explanation for senile dementia at a New York City cocktail party. In casual conversation, Wiesel made a vague reference to a possible link between aluminum and Alzheimer's disease.

Immediately, ears around Wiesel perked up. *What's this? A plain explanation for Alzheimer's disease?* The remark spread like a virus, and mutated. Word got out, incorrectly, that Wiesel was about to publish a paper proving that aluminum causes Alzheimer's disease.

Even (perhaps especially) in our modern age dominated by science and reason, people need to fill the void of ignorance with something; Wiesel's suggestion clicked, for many, with their intuitive suspicion of modern life. *Of course* we are killing ourselves with the invisible residue of progress—radioactivity, pollution, trace molecules from the plastics and metals that define the contours of our daily existence. *Alzheimer's from aluminum:* a new disease for an advanced civilization. People may not have understood the link exactly, but somehow it made perfect sense. A powerful myth was born.

Suddenly, in New York and spreading elsewhere, people began to toss out their aluminum cookware, their aluminum-laden antiperspirants, and their aluminum-based antacids. The Aluminum Association went on the defensive, insisting to reporters that its foils and saucepans were safe. But the image of aluminum-as-brain-toxin stuck. The link between aluminum and dementia became the one "fact" about Alzheimer's disease that every literate adult seemed to know.

The truth was less captivating than the buzz. Aluminum wasn't a cause of Alzheimer's disease, but an effect. High concentrations of aluminum had indeed been found in victims' brains during autopsy; this meant, though, that something had gone wrong with the filter system, called the "blood-brain barrier," that was supposed to keep such elements out of the brain. Everyone ingests significant amounts of aluminum and other metals from the water, air, and many natural foods. In healthy individuals, these complex elements are safely kept out of the brain, where they would do serious damage.

Researchers couldn't figure out why the blood-brain barrier was being compromised, but it was clear enough that avoiding aluminum pots in order to escape Alzheimer's disease was like refusing to drink out of glass containers because someone might come along and break one over your head: The hazard has nothing whatever to do with ordinary use.

It turned out that Wiesel was not even working on Alzheimer's disease, let alone writing a paper on the dangers of aluminum. When reached for comment by a *Washington Post* reporter, he quickly corrected the misimpression and laughed nervously about the unintentional power of his offhand remark, vowing to be more careful.

What of the people, though, who would not make such a vow?

> INTERVIEWER: So you're saying [Alzheimer's] is not just a brain problem?
>
> DR. RICHARD SCHULZE: Oh, no, not at all. [One patient of mine] came out of it by cleansing his bowel. . . . Some people are there because they are toxically poisoned from the outside. Some people are toxically poisoned from the [inside]. Or it's from emotional strain they couldn't deal with. Some from metal poisonings like aluminum. I've met people who were just overdosed with aluminum from the fluorides to the antacids to aluminum pots and pans. So I think you have to take each case individually. . . . There's no such thing as Alzheimer's disease, that's what I've discovered. Every person has a different story, from mothballs to aluminum, to "I couldn't handle my life because my husband was cheating on me."
>
> —from *The Last Chance Health Report,* edited by Sam Biser

A popular figure in the world of alternative healing, Dr. Schulze is not a medical doctor. Among other credentials, he has a doctorate in herbology from the School of Natural Healing, an unaccredited correspondence school based in Orem, Utah. He sells books, audiotapes, videotapes, and several "original" herbal formulas to combat a wide variety of diseases. He offers a special tea for dementia patients:

15 parts ginkgo leaf

1 part gotu kola herb

1 part galamus root

1 part rosemary flowers

1 part kola nut

1 part cayenne pepper, the hottest you can get

One teaspoon of herbs to a cup of tea. Six cups per day.

Schulze is not alone, of course, in supplying the wishful world with simple explanations and cures for Alzheimer's. Others have blamed fluoride in the drinking water, amalgam tooth fillings, pasteurized milk, green tea, refined flour, polished rice, gallstones, and tiny parasites in the colon. Among the alleged cures: unrefined sea salt, flaxseed oil, lemonade (in the morning), miso, mistletoe, red grapes, turmeric, essiac tea, chlorela algae, barley grass, shark cartilage, olive leaf extract, acupuncture, electromagnetic pulse therapy, hyperbaric oxygen therapy, ultraviolet blood irradiation, and—another Richard Schulze suggestion—deep, painful massage of the feet.

A 1995 survey indicated that more than half of Alzheimer's sufferers have tried at least one of these therapies. Twenty percent have tried three or more of them. The impulse is certainly understandable. A relentless, degenerative disease eats away at a person's cognition while most well-meaning doctors throw up their hands and declare that there is virtually nothing to be done. Legitimate suspicions arise: These doctors are Western—what about thousands of years of Eastern wisdom? What about substances that the famously slow U.S. Food and Drug Administration hasn't yet approved? On the Internet, there is excited talk about drugs available only in Europe or Asia. With seemingly little to lose, sufferers and caregivers may grasp for anything that glitters.

Buyers should beware, though. Conventional science, indeed, does not have all the answers; any serious Alzheimer's researcher would be the first to acknowledge that. But how do the explanations of others hold up under scrutiny?

Few of Schulze's claims are upheld by medically supported fact. Alzheimer's *is* a recognizable disease, with a predictable set of symptoms and recognizable pathology. No single case of Alzheimer's disease has ever been cured by a bowel cleansing, or psychotherapy, or any other treatment. The cause of Alzheimer's is not yet known, but there is considerable evidence that it is caused by a combination of genetic and environmental factors.

Schulze's specific list of environmental culprits—though terrifying to the layman—is not confirmed by any serious scholarship. Reputable studies of fluoride, amalgam tooth fillings, aluminum, and other popularly suspected substances have so far come up empty.

In the end, though, Schulze's supreme confidence is the best clue to his illegitimacy; genuine scientists speak in more tentative terms, always careful not to overstep the bounds of what has been proven. Much is known about Alzheimer's, but the many unanswered questions and its incurability demand humility, not the pretension of certainty.

As for Schulze's tea: While heavy doses of gingko have been shown to have some very mild effects in ameliorating some of the symptoms of dementia, the effects always appear to be temporary and do not appear to slow its progress. The final ingredient in Schulze's dementia tea, moreover, should raise eyebrows. No reputable medical studies show that cayenne powder has a demonstrable effect on the brain, and the quantity he is prescribing will make any beverage fiery hot. Imagine the effect of slipping a copious amount of red-hot pepper into the drink of an unsuspecting patient who is only half-lucid and has no powers of communication left. Now imagine doing that six times a day.

A year after George Glenner helped explain Alzheimer's to Ronald Reagan at the White House, he delivered the first major combat victory in Zaven Khachaturian's war on Alzheimer's. In 1983, he unlocked the molecular structure of *beta-amyloid,* the main component of plaques.

Laboratory science had improved considerably since the day of Alois Alzheimer. In 1906, the forefront of brain research was the ability to view cells and their components at a magnification of several hundred times. Alzheimer could see the outlines of the plaques and tangles; he could draw them, count them, describe them, stand in awe of them. But he could not learn much about them. He could not get inside of them and see what they were made of, or understand how they were altering the surrounding tissue.

By the time Glenner came to the subject, the view of plaques and tangles through a light microscope was akin to looking at New York City from the Goodyear blimp: a vivid scene, intriguing, but not very enlightening. What interested modern researchers was the street-level view, and the scene behind closed doors—the nearly hidden molecular and chemical processes cooking inside. From the blimp, plaques were large, dense, menacing-looking clouds of foreign matter. Up close, Glenner could see that tiny strips of *beta-amyloid*, a sticky, insoluble protein fragment, were sticking to one another like wisps of used packing tape torn from a package as it was opened in haste. The tape strips spilled onto the floor, stuck to dust, to hair, to each other. After a while, they started to gum up the whole room.

Glenner decoded the molecular composition of the starchlike beta-amyloid (from *amylum*, the Latin word for starch), which in turn enabled other researchers to find its source. This was the foot in the door that many other researchers had been waiting for. "George came along and sequenced the protein," recalled Zaven Khachaturian, "and, oh my God, it was like the floodgates opened." The story of how plaques become plaques was finally unraveled.

Plaques were caused by a chemical accident, the defective breakdown of a benign substance called amyloid precursor protein (APP) that lives throughout the body—in the brain, heart, kidneys, lungs, spleen, and intestines—and has some still-unknown role in cellular function. As a part of routine function, APP regularly gets broken down into much smaller soluble components and washed away with other decomposed tissue and chemicals. But under some mysterious conditions, the breaking-apart doesn't work right, and out come sticky shards of beta-amyloid. As they stick to each other and attract other detritus—fragments of dead and dying neurons—they slowly form into dense, misshapen clumps: plaques.

Three years later, in 1986, the tangles were also decoded. Researchers discovered that they were made up of another contaminated protein called *tau*, which normally serves as railroad ties for a tracklike structure that transports nutrients and other important molecules throughout the cell body of every neuron. The tangled tau had somehow become hyperphosphorylated—corrupted by several extra molecules of phosphorus. Without the railroad ties, the tracks had no integrity. They got bent into a twisted mess.

Imagine some metal-chewing gremlin working its way down railroad tracks, chewing up the steel ties (the tau). Then, under the weight of the train (the nutrients being transported), the tracks buckle. The damage is compounded as the train continues to speed along, causing a mass of twisted wreckage all along the tracks.

Inside the neuron, the twisted debris gets worse and worse, as the filaments keep twisting around one another. Communication and cell nourishment are at first compromised, and then drop off to nothing; the neuron cannot sustain itself in any way and begins to wither. The cell membranes collapse, and every part of the neuron—the long axon that is responsible for sending out signals to other neurons, the short, branchlike dendrites responsible for receiving signals from other neurons, and everything else—disintegrates. The thousands of synapses, each representing a fragment of a memory, vanish like a plane flying over the Bermuda Triangle. At the end, there is no trace that the neuron itself ever existed—except for one thing. All that's left, if a pathologist stains the tissue just right, is a small clump of what neuropathologists call "ghost tangles." There, a neuron once stood.

A decade after Khachaturian had gone hunting for new Alzheimer's researchers, here were the first big payoffs. It was suddenly a very exciting time to be in the field. The modern race to understand Alzheimer's and defeat it had begun in earnest. But many more hazards lay ahead.

George Glenner fell mysteriously ill about ten years after his important breakthrough with beta-amyloid. He had shortness of breath and fatigue, and when doctors started doing tests, none of the obvious possibilities checked out.

When they finally discovered what it was, the entire Alzheimer's research community took a shudder: Glenner had somehow contracted a very rare disease called systemic senile amyloidosis—the unexplained proliferation of amyloid proteins throughout the body, clogging up his heart and other organs. It was, in a sense, Alzheimer's disease of the body.

"How I got this? We don't know," Glenner serenely said to a reporter shortly before he died. "It's just one of those mysteries." Whatever the ultimate explanation, it looked like more than a coincidence. It certainly seemed that he was inadvertently sacrificing his own body for the sake of scientific discovery.

Just before he died in 1995, Glenner was asked if he thought there would be a cure for Alzheimer's.

"Of course," he said.

I have really struggled with the honesty issue. What do you say to someone who sits on her bed and says that she has never stayed out overnight without letting her parents know where she is? What do you say to someone who thinks she is a teacher and if she doesn't get home and into her classroom there will be a whole class of children left unattended? What do you say to someone who thinks she has no money to pay bills and will lose everything she owns if she doesn't get home to a job that you know she has been retired from for years? I couldn't find any reason for telling her over and over that she has a horrible terrible degenerating disease that was making her feel the way she does.

I found that she became less anxious if I just listened to what she was saying and feeling. Sometimes saying nothing was better than anything I could say. Telling her that I would take care of some of these things put her a bit more at ease. It may feel better for me to verbalize the facts, but what she needs is comfort and security—not the truth. The truth won't change anything.

—N.B.
Merrimack, New Hampshire

Chapter 10

TEN THOUSAND FEET,
AT TEN O'CLOCK AT NIGHT

∽

Taos

Dusk settled in on the first night of the Molecular Mechanisms conference. Two hundred scientists, weary from travel but rejuvenated by the cold, pure mountain air, fell into their chairs to listen to Stanley Prusiner's keynote address. Perhaps he couldn't compete with Monica Lewinsky's pitiful tale, but he had prepared some drama of his own.

Prusiner had swept-back white hair, and an arched brow that conveyed authority when he spoke. He also had a surprisingly bitter tone in his voice, as though someone had taken something from him that he knew he would never get back. Though he was world-famous for his discovery of "prions"—the previously unknown infectious proteins that cause Creutzfeldt-Jakob disease in humans and bovine spongiform encephalopathy (a.k.a. "mad cow disease") in cows—the accomplishment seemed to have left an emotional scar.

For many years Prusiner had been a pariah in the scientific community, openly ridiculed for a theory many regarded as off the wall. It seemed preposterous that mere proteins could be infectious, since they weren't really alive.

Gradually, though, the evidence accrued and Prusiner was vindicated. The prion notion was so distinct from the rest of science that the distinguished American physician Lewis Thomas called it "the strangest thing in all biology." In contrast to a virus, which injects its own DNA into the host's nucleus, using the cell machinery to make copies, infectious prions require no genetic manipulation to spread. These oddly shaped proteins destabilize other nearby proteins simply by rubbing up against them, converting the neighbors into the same malignant shape. One prion transforms the next which transforms the next, creating a chain reaction that leads to what Prusiner calls a "sticky sheet" of clumpy protein. As the immune system responds by attempting to remove all the unwelcome particles, the host brain becomes a spongy mass.

As far as anyone could tell, Alzheimer's is not an infectious prion disease (though George Glenner's death from amyloidosis had caused concern). But there were enough common elements to interest Prusiner. He also seemed interested in being here in a moral capacity, as a successful fellow researcher from a nearby disease who perhaps had some lessons to share with his research cousins.

The message was embedded in his tone of resentment. As he delivered a detailed overview of his work on an overhead projector, Prusiner also retaliated against his past tormenters. He repeatedly displayed a cartoon image of a younger Stanley Prusiner (with dark hair) being squashed by a giant thumb. The thumb represented mainstream science, which kept him down because of his unconventional ideas. Prusiner finished his talk with an acrid quote from Winston Churchill:

> Men occasionally stumble across the truth, but most of them pick themselves up and hurry off as if nothing had happened.

A fitting statement from a man of politics and war, perhaps, but not a very uplifting note from a champion of scientific inquiry. Prusiner was a sore winner; it was not very becoming. But he was a winner, nonetheless, and his tale of triumph over adversity conveyed the intended message to these elite researchers: *Don't be afraid to buck the conventional wisdom; that's how scientific progress is made.*

Seventy-two of the world's most coveted ski runs were about a ten-minute drive away from the conference. Free shuttle buses waited out front on Civic Plaza Drive, with their doors wide open; eleven hundred skiable acres under a sun that famously shines 323 days a year. But with the high stakes in mind, almost everyone quietly declined, on account of what they would have had to miss; sessions were running from 8:00 A.M. to 10:00 P.M. each day, with breaks for coffee and meals.

There was so much ground to cover, including the entire human genome, with its 30,000 genes and three billion nucleotide base pairs. In the early 1990s, much of the work had shifted to molecular genetics, as researchers began to uncover genetic links to Alzheimer's all over the human genome: Chromosomes 1, 14, 19, and 21, they discovered, each have genes that can help cause Alzheimer's.

They learned that only 5 percent of Alzheimer's cases—most of them involving onset in middle age—are caused directly by a single gene. In this small minority, the disease is inherited as simply as detached earlobes or brown eyes, from just one parent's dominant gene. Anyone carrying this gene will get the disease, if they live long enough; statistically, the victims will pass the gene and the disease on to 50 percent of their children.

The cause or causes of the other 95 percent of cases were not so clear. Much emerging evidence supported a theory that the disease is "multifactorial"—caused by an unfortunate accumulation of genes and environmental factors. According to this analysis, initiating Alzheimer's disease is like pushing a school bus over a small hill: No single individual can possibly do it alone, but the right group of players coming together at the right time can make it look easy.

Making sense of such a complex landscape required an unprecedented amount of cooperation. Scientific discovery has always depended on an ever-growing scaffold of ideas and observations. But this brand of sped-up science, where data can be retrieved, analyzed quickly, and shared instantly over the Internet, required an unimaginably intricate network. The presentations in Taos—e.g., ". . . working from data on presenilin mutations published by Karen Duff in New York and Gerard Schellenberg in Seattle, and using transgenic mice supplied by Karen Hsiao in Minneapolis, we set out to . . ."—conjured up a histopathological ballet. Teams of researchers scattered around the world, constantly aware of and reacting to the movements of everyone else, were creating an improvisational dance with a startling number of graceful interchanges.

But there was also awkwardness, and discord. At the end of the first complete day, devoted almost exclusively to understanding the building blocks of the amyloid plaques, and to whether it is not the plaques but perhaps the free-floating beta-amyloid that actually does the damage, the Mayo Clinic's John Hardy, a warm and irreverent Brit with droopy eyes and an easy smile, rose to speak. He emphasized from the outset that he wasn't promising much. "Just sort of a potpourri, bits and bobs to finish off the evening.

"I've always wanted to give a talk at ten thousand feet at ten o'clock at night with four gin-and-tonics in me," he quipped to the tired group. "We'll see how it goes."

Before he got into the meat of his talk, though, he couldn't resist a poke at an absent rival. "Allen Roses isn't here, in case you haven't noticed," he said with a grin, "so I thought I'd show this slide."

The slide, entitled "Diseases Are Processes," was a wry allusion to a long-standing dispute. For several years, Hardy had been one of the leading proponents of the "amyloid cascade hypothesis," which suggested that plaques are closer to the root of Alzheimer's than tangles. According to this theory, the disease is preceded by a buildup over time of beta-amyloid, which eventually reaches a critical mass and triggers other unwanted events, including the formation of tangles. Most Alzheimer's researchers—probably some 80 percent—had come to embrace this line of thinking and had dedicated their research to some aspect of it.

Roses, director of genetics research at the pharmaceutical giant Glaxo Wellcome, dissented. He dismissed plaques as "tombstones" and "scar tissue" that are largely irrelevant to the underlying mechanisms of the disease. The "amyloid establishment," he complained, was drawing far more resources than it merited. Roses's research had led him to believe that tau—tangles—are closer to the root of the problem. In 1992, as director of the Alzheimer's program at Duke, he had made probably the most important genetic discovery to date: a variant of a gene called ApoE, located on chromosome 19 (a human cell has 46 chromosomes), that appeared to increase the risk of developing Alzheimer's by a factor of twenty. Seven years later, it was still the only verified genetic discovery related to the more common form of the disease.

Roses had felt ignored after his discovery. No one seemed interested in following up on his breakthrough research. He saw it as a classic case of herd-mentality science. The spectacular popularity of the amyloid hypothesis, he said with his famously unvarnished candor, was simply a matter of "good scientists not being able to look objectively at science, being so subjectively involved in being right and organizing posses to make sure that other people are kept from [getting the grants]—'hang these guys so they're not in the way of what we're doing.'

"It happens in this field, and I think it has really slowed therapy. The reason I say that is because these guys don't make drugs. Drug companies make drugs. And when drug companies want to start an Alzheimer's program, what do they do? They go for what's popular, for what's in the press. They say, 'Oh, here's something in *Nature*.' And if in fact 85 percent of what you see is [amyloid research], well, some drug exec without a scientific background is going to say, 'I don't know about this crazy guy Roses, who everybody says is wrong. We'll invest in amyloid.' So what happens is that the drug companies' Alzheimer's programs are actually amyloid programs, and it feeds upon itself."

Scientists can vehemently disagree and still be close friends, of course. But not John Hardy and Allen Roses. In 1991, when Hardy was still stationed in Britain, the two got into a transcontinental telephone screaming match over a paper that Hardy was about to publish.

It was not a small event. Hardy had established a link between a rare, early-onset form of the disease and a mutation on chromosome 21. The paper would be the first genetic linkage to be associated with Alzheimer's (this was before Roses's big discovery), and it included some of Roses's data as part of the proof. On the advice of a patent lawyer and because Roses had made it clear that he didn't really believe in such a link, Hardy had decided not to show the paper to Roses or offer him coauthor credit.

But then someone leaked the paper to Roses in an anonymous fax from London's Paddington Station. "I went berserk," Roses said. The imbroglio that ensued left the Alzheimer's research community polarized.

Things had simmered down somewhat since then, but the Hardy-Roses rivalry endured. "John and Allen are civil to each other," someone close to Hardy told me in Taos, "but there's no good feeling between the two." Roses was, in fact, supposed to speak at this conference, but he bowed out at the last minute. In an E-mail correspondence, Roses dismissed the Taos conference. "Most of that is academic rehash that some of our [company] people will filter," he said. "We are advancing other technologies toward a treatment. Universities do not make drugs. Governments do not make drugs. Pharmaceutical companies make drugs."

So here, at ten thousand feet, at ten o'clock at night, Hardy was poking at Roses in his absence. "Diseases are processes" was Hardy's cagey depiction of their essential disagreement: From

Hardy's point of view, Roses didn't think of Alzheimer's as an aggregation of materials and sequence of events so much as a switch turned on by a gene.

On the third night of the conference, the "tauists" got their chance. This was the stalwart minority of researchers exploring the possibility that tangles, not the plaques, were the real key to understanding Alzheimer's.

The tau (tangle) vs. amyloid (plaque) rivalry had become intense over the previous decade. "The battle is raging like the religious wars of medieval times," observed Zaven Khachaturian. "But it's good for everyone. I like to sit on the fifty-yard line and cheer."

In her talk, Virginia Lee, half of an award-winning husband-wife team from the University of Pennsylvania, playfully jabbed the predominantly amyloid crowd. "I'll give some background info for those few of you who don't understand a lot about tau," she said. Her rivals laughed.

But it was Lee's colleague Khalid Iqbal who launched the direct assault. "The amyloid cascade hypothesis has been around for almost ten years," he said, "and some of the best scientists have been working on it. But this relationship is still not understood.

"Tonight I will propose to you that we also consider an alternative hypothesis—that Alzheimer's is fundamentally a metabolic disorder. Like hypertension and coronary heart disease, Alzheimer's is a metabolic disorder of mid to old age which requires a genetic predisposition and one or more environmental factors."

Iqbal pointed out that of all the genetic mutations and environmental factors found to correspond with Alzheimer's, none are causative—none cause Alzheimer's every time. It's also important to note, he said, that the disease can arise outside of the presence of all known risk factors.

In other words, we don't know all the causes and may never know them. The causes are so many and so complex that they aren't even what matter. What matters is the common *pathway* that the disease takes after it has started. The challenge of researchers is not to stop the train just as all the cars are being assembled and put onto a track. Rather, it is to block that track after the train gets rolling but long before it gets to its destination.

The likely pathway of this disease that ends in the death of neurons, Iqbal said, is not the formation of beta-amyloid but the hyperphosphorylation of tau—the creation of tangles.

Then Iqbal delivered the sharpest blow, suggesting that amyloid may not only *not* be the problem—it may actually be a part of the solution. Amyloid, he said, seems to be not a destructive protein but a *repair* protein. Amyloid levels, he noted, go up every time there is some harm to the brain.

This was tantamount to marching into a meeting of the Federal Reserve Board and saying, "Tonight I will propose to you that inflation is not our enemy but our ally." Iqbal was lobbing grenades here. He had not come to Taos to make new friends. Prusiner, wherever he was in that large dark room, no doubt wore a narrow grin of satisfaction. Here, clearly, was a scientist not following the pack.

It all came back to Prusiner, then, and his Churchillian taunt: "Men occasionally stumble across the truth, but most of them . . ."

Was the amyloid bandwagon a classic example of "herd science," as Allen Roses and Ruth Itzhaki charged, or was it the legitimate outcome of sober investigation? This, and not any strict question of biology, was the unspoken theme of the conference. The amyloid camp seemed to have infected nearly everyone with optimism. But was that optimism sound?

The future of Alzheimer's disease would rest on the answer.

From a distance, scientific research can seem sterile, all test tubes and assays and peptides and risk factors. The Latin terminology and white lab coats create an impression of scientists as geek technicians, anti-people people who, for reasons of extreme shyness, prefer to wallow in details, crunch numbers, and deal only with objective truth. The stereotype: Scientists are smarter than the rest of us, are uncomfortable in their extreme intelligence, and find it hard to deal with others.

But close up, the view is entirely different, much more textured and colorful. The better I came to know this elite scientific group of Alzheimer's researchers, the more I understood how profoundly human their shared endeavor really was. Not far below the surface talk of microtubules and missense mutations was a culture steeped in ambition, loyalty, secrecy, warm companionship, resentment, and greed. There were real, lasting friendships here, and career-threatening antagonisms. Science turns out to be more similar to statehouse or boardroom politics than an outsider would suspect.

As I was taking it all in, one scientist at the conference quietly reminded me that there was a lot going on beneath the surface of these talks. "An important subtext of these battles," he whispered in the middle of a presentation, "is that all of these scientists have patents on their discoveries. There's a lot of money at stake."

Not just research money, but Lear Jet and beach house money. A sweeping change in U.S. law in 1980 allowed American universities and researchers to begin applying for their own patents on discoveries made with federal research dollars. Scientists were also permitted to create for-profit corporations on the side, while maintaining their publicly sponsored university research positions. "An entrepreneurial atmosphere has begun to alter the ethos of science," is how the Tufts University ethicist Sheldon Krimsky puts it. "Norms of behavior within the academic community are being modified to accommodate closer corporate ties."

For this reason, even though the scientists traveled from all around the world to speak to one another, there was also clearly much *not* being said. While this seemed to be in direct contravention of the historically open-air philosophy of all scientific inquiry, it was also conceivable that market incentives were just what ambitious researchers needed to drive themselves even harder to win this critical race.

Just before the weekend ended, I caught a telling glimpse of this invisible layer of information. One of the last to speak was Ivan Lieberburg, not a director of a university lab but head of research and development for Elan Pharmaceuticals, based in San Francisco. *Universities do not make drugs . . . pharmaceutical companies make drugs.* Lieberburg discussed, in very general terms, all the possible treatment possibilities, and then hinted at a few areas that his company is now focusing on. He apologized to the group for having to restrict his talk; for proprietary reasons, he said, there was much he could not say. But he did drop a few hints. "We're really on the threshold of a new age," he said. "I think we're coming very close to the goal line now, thanks to what many of you have done." The tone was beyond hopeful—it was celebratory.

Afterwards, as he packed up his slides, Lieberburg turned to me and said, "This was one of the most frustrating experiences I've ever had in my life, to speak to a group like this and not tell them what I know." Stay tuned, he said. Something big is coming this summer. Something very big.

Mom hasn't been feeling good the last couple days,
I wonder if her medication has something to do with it.
She takes:

Propulsid 20 milligrams, twice a day
K-Dur 20meq SA TAB, once a day
Synthroid 0.025 milligrams, once a day
Imdur 30 milligrams, once a day
Procardia XL 60 milligrams, once a day
Prilosec 20 milligrams, once a day
Aspirin 325 milligrams, once a day
Betagan eye drops, two drops for each eye, twice a day
Trinsicon/Ferocon, once a day
Paxil 30 milligrams, once a day
Neurontin 100 milligrams, once a day
Nizoral (cream), once a day
Ditropan/Oxybutynin chloride 5 milligrams, twice a day
Extra-Strength Tylenol, once a day

After sleeping for just a little bit last night, she woke up crying. She wanted us to take her to the bank. We told her it was the middle of the night— the bank was closed. She threw a fit. We told her we have cash here in the house in case she needs it. It was futile. Everything we said made no sense to her, and she made no sense to us. She went back to bed and cried. We let her cry herself to sleep.

This morning when I went to wake her for breakfast I found her pajama bottoms "hung up to dry" and she had no Depends on. It could be that she needs a change in mood medications.

—C.J.
Toledo, Ohio

Chapter 11

A WORLD OF STRULDBRUGGS

~

Alois Alzheimer did not get to pursue his namesake disease for very long. In 1912, just a year after publishing his first substantial paper on Alzheimer's disease and only two years after it was named for him, he accepted a new job as head of psychiatry at the University of Breslau. On the train to assume his new post, he collapsed; a case of infectious tonsillitis had developed into rheumatic fever, spreading to the kidneys, joints, and the lining of the heart. He was taken directly from the Breslau train station to the hospital. Though he eventually gained enough strength to leave the hospital, he never fully recovered. "At the conference of German Psychiatrists in 1913 I saw him," Kraepelin later recalled. "Although outwardly he appeared sprightly/active, his mood was dejected and depressed; he looked into the future with bleak foreboding. . . . In the effort to complete his duties to the full, Alzheimer did not understand how to protect himself."

Alzheimer grew weaker and weaker and finally died in 1915. He was fifty-one—the same age that his famous patient Auguste D. had been when she first experienced symptoms of forgetfulness.

For someone born in the mid–nineteenth century, fifty-one years was not brief: Life expectancy for Alzheimer's generation in Germany was somewhere in the low forties. Alois Alzheimer's boss in Frankfurt, Emil Sioli, lived to be seventy; the legendary cellular pathologist Rudolf Virchow lived to be eighty-one; but these were the exceptions. "Although historical records indicate that older people have always existed in human societies," says University of Chicago epidemiologist S. Jay Olshansky, "survival beyond age fifty for most members of a population was a rare event until the twentieth century."

Today, endurance is the norm. One in eight Americans is over sixty-five. Ninety percent of all babies born today in the developed world will live past sixty-five.

Such a dramatic expansion of life's quantity begs the question: Can we hope to match it with comparable gains in quality?

Because there were relatively few elderly at the time, it would have been impossible for Alzheimer to imagine the implications of his work. He had identified a disease that would become a serious epidemiological problem only as human populations achieved much longer life spans. Neither he nor any of the extraordinary minds in his circle could have foreseen that "this Alzheimer's disease" would in the next century emerge as *the* central public health epidemic of the industrialized world.

Perhaps it is not so bad that they couldn't see clearly into the future. If doctors in 1910 could somehow have envisioned the appalling side effects of medical progress, the agony of neurodegeneration and other diseases of deterioration experienced mostly by people who live into their seventies and beyond, they would have found this very difficult to reconcile with their work. "Modern health care permits growing numbers of people to live to advanced age under circumstances that call into question the meaning of survival," concludes Hunter College's Harry Moody.

Olshansky echoes this sentiment. "Our society is experiencing unprecedented rates of survival into older ages," he writes, "but this success has also been accompanied by a rise in frailty and disability in the general population. This is a consequence that neither the medical community nor society was prepared for."

A 1997 "State of World Health" report by the World Health Organization began this way: "Dramatic increases in life expectancy, combined with profound changes in lifestyles, will lead to global epidemics of cancer and other chronic diseases in the next two decades. The main result will be a huge increase in human suffering and disability."

Epidemiologists call this extension of frailty time a "prolongation of morbidity." It is the paradox that the extension of life inevitably yields new suffering. Alzheimer's is perhaps the perfectly poignant emblem of this medical quandary: As we defeat disease, we also create disease. Any particular illness may be conquered, but mortality is unavoidable.

Evolutionary biologists are also fascinated by the rapid increase in longevity and its unintended consequences. From their perspective, the central concept here is one of *hidden diseases*—disorders that have always existed for human beings in a potential state, but that have never been fully realized until recently.

Hidden diseases only emerge after inordinate wear and tear. A serious cyclist buying a state-of-the-art touring bicycle, for example, can expect to repair and replace many parts on a fairly predictable schedule: tires, inner tubes, and brake pads will all wear down; the bike's chain and ball bearings in the wheels' hubs will require constant lubrication, and even then they will seriously fatigue after several thousand miles. For these parts and others, replacement is common, expected, necessary.

It will take some extreme use, though—imagine crisscrossing the United States several hundred times—to wear out a set of handlebars or the bicycle's frame. There are weaknesses hidden somewhere in those durable parts that are impossible to predict and not even relevant until an extremely advanced age of use.

The long-term frailties are there somewhere, but they cannot be seen. For some fifty thousand years, as the vast majority of human beings died under the age of fifty, disorders like hearing loss, prostate cancer, osteoarthritis, breast cancer, colon cancer, amyotrophic lateral sclerosis, and Alzheimer's disease were mere diseases-in-waiting. Only in the last fifty to one hundred years have they started to come into view.

Given this, perhaps the most remarkable thing about the history of senile dementia is that it has been so conspicuous. In practical terms, it was a hidden disease with very few victims before the twentieth century, and yet references to senility are strangely ubiquitous throughout recorded history—not just in medical records, but also in legal, political, and cultural texts. Sometime around 500 B.C. the Greek legislator Solon mentioned that impaired thinking due to old age could invalidate a last will and testament. A reference to dotage is included in the "Story of the Larrikin and the Cook," one of the tales from the fifteenth-century *The Thousand and One Nights*. The *Florentine Codex*, a history of Aztec culture in Mesoamerica compiled by the Franciscan monk Bernardino de Sahagún in the sixteenth century, mentions the "childish" grandfather and other "foolish" old people. Other earlier chroniclers of senility include Euripides, Chaucer, Montaigne, Chekhov, Balzac, Carlyle, Hugo, Trollope, Conan Doyle, Bernard Shaw, Joyce, Melville, Conrad, Tocqueville, Wharton, Darwin, Cooper, Poe, Hawthorne, Sinclair Lewis, O. Henry, Sir Walter Scott, Dickens, and Thoreau. In *War and Peace,* Tolstoy wrote:

> The prince had aged very much that year. He showed marked signs of senility by a tendency to fall asleep, forgetfulness of quite recent events, remembrance of remote ones, and the childish vanity with which he accepted the role of head of the Moscow opposition.

The question is, *Why* was senile dementia such a popular topic when the sufferers were so few and its practical impact on society minimal?

In myth and fable, senility often intersects with immortality. In the Greek myth "Eos and Tithonus," Eos, goddess of the dawn, asks Zeus to grant immortality to her mortal lover Tithonus. Acting like a vindictive schoolmaster intent on teaching a lesson about linguistic precision, Zeus complies in letter but not in spirit; he bestows onto Tithonus immortality—but not eternal youth. Tithonus does live on and on, but in time becomes decrepit and senile. Eos, instead of being blessed with an endless life of passion and companionship, is consigned to the role of everlasting caregiver. Unwilling to bear the endless burden, she eventually shuts Tithonus up in a box, where he remains forever, paralyzed and babbling.

In *Gulliver's Travels,* Jonathan Swift amplified this ancient tale into the grisly spectacle of the Struldbruggs, a subrace of immortal beings born at random among the mortal Luggnaggians. When first told that these rare immortals exist—some eleven hundred of them, including fifty in the city he is currently visiting—the foreign traveler Lemuel Gulliver is gleeful. A society with immortals in its midst, he presumes, is virtually guaranteed to be enlightened—"Happy People who enjoy so many living Examples of ancient Virtue, and have Masters ready to instruct them in the Wisdom of all former Ages!" The immortal elites, he reasons, will provide the best possible insurance against the repeating of past mistakes. With a living history as its guide, civilization will inevitably become smarter and stronger.

But Gulliver has gotten it all wrong. After much laughter at his expense, the Luggnaggians politely explain that immortality, far from being a blessing, is in fact the worst imaginable curse. The actual lives of the Struldbruggs fell into this pattern:

> They commonly acted like Mortals till about Thirty Years old, after which by Degrees they grew melancholy and dejected. . . . When they came to Fourscore Years, which is reckoned the Extremity of living in this Country, they had not only all the Follies and Infirmities of other old Men, but many more which rose from the dreadful Prospect of never dying. They were not only opinionative, peevish, covetous, morose, vain, talkative; but uncapable of Friendship, and dead to all natural Affection, which never descended below their Grandchil-

dren. . . . They have no Remembrance of any thing but what they learned and observed in their Youth and middle Age, and even that is very imperfect. . . . In talking they forget the common Appellation of Things, and the Names of Persons, even of those who are their nearest Friends and Relations. For the same Reason they never can amuse themselves with reading, because their Memory will not serve to carry them from the Beginning of a Sentence to the End.

Gulliver's Travels was completed in 1725, when Swift was fifty-eight. He had long since established himself as a powerful intellect, able to wield his severe wit as a weapon against religious and political adversaries. For all of his success, though, Swift had also long exhibited a deep personal fear—a near-obsession—with the idea that his mind would slowly fade away. As a boy, he had watched in horror as his uncle Godwin withered under the forces of senility, and Swift never seemed to let go of the dark certainty that he would follow the same course. In his middle years, on a walk with the poet-clergyman Edward Young and other friends, Swift dramatically pointed to a diseased elm tree and declared, "I shall be like that tree; I shall die first at the top." He frequently complained in letters to friends about the quality and future of his memory. Swift's close friend John Boyle, the fifth Earl of Orrery, later recalled that he "heard him often lament the particular misfortune to human nature, of an utter deprivation of the senses many years before a deprivation of life." He arranged that most of his estate be devoted to the creation of a new psychiatric hospital. (Swift also complained of dizziness, nausea, and hardness of hearing all of his life, which in hindsight has been identified with some confidence as Ménière's disease, a disorder of the inner ear. Ménière's disease does not lead to memory loss or dementia.)

As he headed into his early sixties Swift's prodigious intellect was still clearly intact, but written and spoken complaints of memory loss increased. In "Verses on the Death of Dr. Swift," an autobiographical caricature written in 1731 (at age 64) about his own future demise, Swift proclaimed:

> Poor gentleman, he droops apace:
> You plainly find it in his face.
> That old vertigo in his head
> Will never leave him till he's dead.
> Besides, his memory decays;
> He recollects not what he says;
> He cannot call his friends to mind;
> Forgets the place where last he dined. . . .

Finally, as Swift approached the age of seventy, his worst fears were realized. Little by little, he began to lose his memory. Aphasia also slowly set in. He complained in one letter, "I neither read nor write, nor remember, nor converse," and in another that he could "hardly write ten lines without blunders, as you will see by the numbers of scratchings and blots before this letter is done. Into the bargain I have not one rag of memory." He became dependent on his generous cousin Martha Whiteaway as a full-time caregiver. Friends began to address their letters directly to her, and she would respond on his behalf.

Swift's decline was clearly a steady and progressive one, chiefly centered on memory. It was not, as later claimed by William Makepeace Thackeray, Samuel Johnson, and other Swift detractors, the emergence of a full-fledged, violent "lunacy" that had always been lurking in his personality. Like Cordell Annesley's oldest sister, Thackeray and Johnson sought to misappropriate the symptoms of dementia for their own purposes—in their case to diminish Swift's literary stature. History reveals their cynicism, and connects them morally with every other soul who lazily and/or greedily contorts a case of senility into some general impugning of the victim's character.

The unraveling continued. By 1740, when Swift was seventy-three, Mrs. Whiteaway reported to friends that his memory had gotten so bad he could no longer finish or correct any of his written work. Swift himself wrote in a short note to her, "I hardly understand one word that I write." Two years after that, he no longer recognized Mrs. Whiteaway and became violently abusive of her. Even with all her affection for Swift, it was more than she could take. A housekeeper and a servant were left to care for him. A commission of friends and local officials concluded in a report in 1742 (when Swift was seventy-five) that he was "of such unsound mind and memory that he is incapable of transacting any business, or managing, conducting, or taking care either of his estate or person." In other words, he had apparently reached the middle stages of senile dementia.

It was in June of that same year that a violent and controversial episode with a local rector, Dr. Francis Wilson, marked the end of Swift's social interactions. There are differing accounts as to exactly what happened during the afternoon Swift spent with Wilson, a friend who was at that time seeking a high position at Dublin's St. Patrick's Cathedral, where Swift was dean. It is clear that Wilson came to visit Swift and persuaded him to leave his home and dine with him without the usual accompaniment of Swift's housekeeper/aide. It is also clear that Swift drank a good deal of wine and spirits at the meal and afterward—perhaps at the strong urging of Wilson. Whatever happened between the two, whether or not Wilson was loading Swift up with liquor in order to gain his endorsement for the new post, the evening ended badly.

On the way home in a carriage, Swift became enraged with Wilson and struck him. According to Wilson's account, Swift had suddenly and without provocation flown into "a most astonishing rage," cried out that Wilson was the devil, hit him, scratched him, and tried to poke his eyes out. Swift's arm was later very badly bruised. Wilson then ordered a stop to the carriage and cursed his companion. "You are a stupid old blockhead," he yelled at the severely demented Swift as he fled, "and an old rascal." Swift was taken back to his home.

By the time he got there, though, he had apparently forgotten the entire event. "Where is Dr. Wilson?" he asked his servant. "Ought not the doctor to be here this afternoon?" He could not recall even having seen him that day.

The clear intent of Swift's Struldbrugg morality play was to illustrate the same paradox that demographers would stumble onto two centuries later: *By extending our lives, we achieve suffering.* Of this Swift was certain. He also seemed to know somehow that his own demise would embody this theme. The combination of his progressive dementia and a series of unrelated and excruciating physical setbacks rendered him an almost perfect icon of wretched aging. As things got worse and worse, Lord Orrery wrote to Martha Whiteaway. "I am sorry to hear his appetite is good," he offered. ". . . The man I wished to live the longest, I [now] wish the soonest dead. It is the only blessing than can now befall him."

Orrery's ambivalence is now ours. It is estimated that one in nine baby boomers could live to be one hundred years old. For their grandparents' generation that figure was one in five hundred. We are in essence creating a world full of Struldbruggs, people living *en masse* into very old age and paying the consequences for it— the "rise in frailty" and prolongation of morbidity that will inevitably accompany increasing age.

Still, we pursue longevity, as individuals and as a species, and we do so without apology. It is our natural instinct to want to live, or perhaps more accurately to desperately want not to die, and to want our friends and relatives also not to die.

How will we face this new abundance of frailty: By merely trying to conquer it all, crying out in frustration whenever we fail? Or by also seeking to reconcile with the inevitable, to decline with grace, to establish a calm acceptance of our mortality? "It is time to be old/To take in sail," Emerson wrote in "Terminus." ". . . 'The port, well worth the cruise, is near/And every wave is charmed.' " In his diminished vista, he set out to live a life of peace and acceptance, a slow and happy fade.

In order for us to make intelligent choices about how we decline, it is important to understand why death exists in the first place. Why, indeed, are we not immortal? Is there some social or biological utility to death? Most everything in the physical world seems to have a rational basis if we look closely enough. So what is the point of dying?

In 1825, a British actuary named Benjamin Gompertz noticed

something peculiar in his mortality tables. Plotted on a graph, ages of death formed a graceful U. The probability of dying, he noticed, was very high at birth; it declined rapidly during the first year of life, and continued to decline up to the age of sexual maturity. From there it increased rapidly, exponentially even, until very old age. In sum, the older you got after birth, the less of a chance you had of dying—up until puberty, that is, at which point the older you got, the *more* of a chance you had of dying. Gompertz theorized that he had detected a hidden Law of Mortality, some sort of natural order of living and dying.

He had. Over the following two centuries, evolutionary biologists and population geneticists helped refine this law, which helped them understand the purpose of death—or, rather, its purposelessness.

Death, they came to realize, is not a part of the plan. It is not programmed into the code of life in the same way that, say, a firecracker is designed to explode. Death is also not nature's way of clearing space for future generations. Nor is it a genetic guarantee that miscreants will not be able to make trouble into eternity. Death is not nature's way of rationing energy so that the maximum number of individuals get a chance to live.

Rather, death is an unwanted but unavoidable by-product of life in the same way that a wood fire leaves us with a pile of carbon residue. The fundamental design of all life, according to the law of natural selection, is the continual adaptation of a species, *through reproduction,* to maximize long-term survival. Adaptation happens through a natural genetic variation; those variants best suited to the environment will survive the longest.

There is no particular requirement that all of these genetic variants have a built-in death spiral. It just happens that, so far, *all* of the best possible designs for a successful reproductive organism result in a structure that is highly vulnerable to deterioration sometime *after* the reproductive period. Think of a light bulb that is designed to burn very brightly; its essential purpose is its intensity, and a by-product of that intensity is that it will burn out.

A more precise analogy, one suggested by the University of Chicago's Olshansky, is the Indianapolis 500 race car, a machine designed with one very specific goal—to get to the end of that five-hundredth mile with as much speed as possible. What happens to the car in the 501st mile and every mile thereafter is of no particular concern to the designer. Every detail of design must be aimed toward the first five hundred miles. "From an evolutionary perspective," says Olshansky, "the race is to reproduction, which includes a time for the production of offspring, a possible child-rearing period, and for some species (for instance, human beings) a grandparenting period where parental contributions can be made to the reproductive success of their own offspring."

The point of the analogy is that, in designing a vehicle to go a precise distance at top speed, specific choices have to be made that favor those priorities. Those choices seem to inevitably result in long-term weaknesses that will prevent the car from lasting as long as it might have. "It is important to realize," says Olshansky, "that the cars are not intentionally engineered to fall apart—they are simply not designed to run indefinitely beyond the end of the race."

Hence Benjamin Gompertz's U-shaped mortality curve. The Law of Mortality dictates that every living organism makes reproduction a priority *at the expense of longevity.* If an individual survives the harrowing process of being born, it has a built-in maximized chance of making it to sexual potency. After that, the forces of deterioration start to overcome the forces of life.

Epidemiologists refer to the postreproductive period of life as the "genetic dustbin," because any genetic expression that occurs only in late life is simply beyond the reach of natural selection. A gene that causes a man to be very short in stature *might* help or hurt his chances to adapt to the environment and to procreate. But a gene that causes a woman's hair to turn gray when she is seventy will have no effect at all. Her genes are already passed on or not passed on, without any regard to whether that trait was a desirable one.

So-called hidden diseases, then, are hidden not just in the sense of not being visible to pre-twentieth-century human beings. More importantly, they are hidden from the forces of natural selection.

In 1998, Olshansky and his colleagues were surprised to discover something new about the Law of Mortality: that medical science had been able to *alter* it. Sorting through mortality data from mice, beagles, and humans who had died of natural causes, they were able to chart Gompertz U-shaped mortality curves in order to reveal each animal's genetic schedule of mortality—what they called their "mortality signatures." The human mortality signature turned out to be eighty-three. This means that if all of the external threats to the human body were removed, the point at which it would be most likely to simply give out averages around the age of eighty-three.

What they didn't expect, though, was a U-shaped mortality curve with a different *shape* for humans than for the other animals.

This meant that modern medicine has not only reduced external threats, but has also somehow overcome internal rhythms. "The change in rates," reported Olshansky, "indicates that the intrinsic mortality signature of human beings, something that we once thought was intractable, is being *modified.*"

We're pushing our bodies past their own innate limits. Due to extraordinary medical interventions in cancer, heart disease, and other conditions, humankind is now living longer than our genes would ordinarily allow. We are outliving our own mortality signature, living on what epidemiologists call "manufactured time." It is the cushion of extra life that we are creating for ourselves with our ingenuity and our tools.

The real challenge, of course, is to insure that this new time is something we are happy to have.

This was the second day of nearly total confusion for Ed. He was back pretending to drive the locomotives and imagining that I was one of the crew. I was asked to call the dispatcher and find out how to get back to Walla Walla.

Periodically, he asked me what Arda was doing and if I'd heard from her and telling me what a special person she is to him. (Arda is me.)

This afternoon we went for a ride, then stopped for a bite to eat. Our bill was $13.11, which Ed insisted on paying. He pulled two fifty-dollar bills out of his wallet. I told him I had the right change so I took the bill and paid it.

When we pulled up under the carport at home he said, "I'll wait here. What are we stopping here for?" He is at least cheerful and relaxed, much like a little child waiting to be told what to do. It could be worse.

—A.B.
Walla Walla, Washington

Chapter 12

HUMANIZE THE MOUSE

❧

In the 1980s, as researchers began to contemplate the possibility of trying to defeat Alzheimer's disease, the search for a fitting animal model became paramount. No one could develop a successful Alzheimer's drug without first testing it, and refining it, on animals. In order to save human lives, many thousands of nonhuman lives would first be forfeited to science. These animals would be bred according to certain desirable characteristics, kept in strictly controlled environments, examined for changes in behavior and intelligence, and ultimately sacrificed. Their brains would be taken apart, fixed in solution, sliced thinly, and examined under a microscope; or their brains would be spun in a centrifuge and analyzed chemically; or their brains would be placed in a petri dish with a variety of toxins. Collectively, these brains would serve as the proverbial drawing board onto which researchers would sketch all possible ideas for a cure.

The trouble was that, as far as anyone could tell, no other creature naturally suffers from Alzheimer's. It is a disease of sophistica-
tion. In much the same way that a bicycle cannot acquire muffler
problems, animals with much less developed brains cannot experience the same sort of progressive memory loss and insidious cognitive decline as human beings.

So researchers looked for the best possible substitute, indications
of a less elaborate senile dementia in lesser-developed mammals. At
ten or eleven years of age, they noted, some dogs start to have sleeping trouble, pacing around at night and getting lost in familiar sur-
roundings. When researchers took a look at their brains under the
microscope, they found amyloid plaques similar to those in human
Alzheimer's victims—but no tangles. They also discovered the same
tangle-less pathology in cats, bears, squirrel monkeys, and lemurs.

In aging polar bears and sheep, they saw just the reverse—tangles but no plaques. No one could find a single animal, aside from
humans, that had them both.

But that wasn't the biggest impediment. Ultimately, what
made each of these animals unsuitable for Alzheimer's research was
their longevity. Few researchers can afford to spend a decade or
more waiting for a lab animal to be old enough for study.

Mice, by contrast, age quickly. They rarely live longer than two
years. Mice are also easy to breed and to handle. They are by far
the most popular animals for lab research. But to Alzheimer's researchers, mice were virtually useless. Very old mice displayed
some slight cognitive impairment, but nothing that could be clas-
sified as dementia. Their brains accrued neither plaques nor tangles. So researchers set out to "humanize" mice—to somehow trick
their bodies into acquiring a disease that evolution had spared
them.

Humanizing mice was an outlandish scientific scheme. It was one thing to try to understand an animal's biology in great detail, and quite another to try and fundamentally change it—not after it was formed but during assembly. Engineers could make a car more like a train by putting it on tracks. But how could biologists change the construction of a mouse so as to make it more like a human being?

There was no way, prior to the 1980s. But then came a new technology that made humanizing not only possible but almost routine. It was called *transgenics*—the transfer of genes from one species to another.

The science of genetics dates back to the Austrian monk Gregor Mendel who, in the 1850s and 1860s, conducted hundreds of controlled breeding experiments with the garden pea *(Pisum sativum)* that proved the existence of genes. Heredity was not, Mendel demonstrated, a process of indiscriminate blending in which the traits of the parents were simply mixed together in a metaphoric vat. Rather, it was a composite of the parents' distinct genes, a mosaic of sorts.

But Mendel's work wasn't publicly recognized until 1900, sixteen years after his death. In the meantime, Charles Darwin, in 1859, introduced the broader concepts of evolution and natural selection, which were immediately catapulted into worldwide prominence. For a while, Darwin's lofty ideas levitated in the culture without essential infrastructural support, without a grounded explanation for how genetics actually works. What scientists at the time failed to realize was how volatile such intellectual instability can be. Without the nitty-gritty Mendelian details, Darwinism was left vulnerable to misunderstanding and manipulation.

One extremely dangerous misconception was the notion of "degeneration," introduced by psychiatrist and theology student Augustin Morel. Morel reasoned that if evolution helped the fittest rise to the top, it must also actively push the least fit to the bottom. Undesirable traits would not merely be passed over; they would grow less and less desirable with each successive generation. The hook nose of the parent would become more hooked in the child, the cleft palate more cleft, the low intelligence even lower. Character traits and morals would be passed on and amplified in the same way. Morel wrote:

> This deviation even if, at the outset, it was ever so slight, contained transmissible elements of such a nature that [the patient] becomes more and more incapable of fulfilling his functions in the world; and mental progress, already checked in his own person, finds itself menaced also in his descendants.

The traits from one generation would get worse in the next; the entire family line would *degenerate.* In effect, Morel proposed that undesirable genetic traits—and their human carriers—were themselves diseases. The health of human society depended on the eradication of these diseased genes.

It was a perverse, wrongheaded proposal, made in ignorance and with the hubris that science could serve humanity by destroying many humans. But in the pre-Mendelian vacuum, many scientists found degeneration theory irresistible. All over Europe, doctors rushed to create lists of physical and mental deformities that indicated a degenerative spiral in a particular family or group.

In Germany, the Society for Racial Hygiene was formed in 1905 as a way of defending civilization against genetic impurities. Emil Kraepelin and Alois Alzheimer both joined. Though not overtly racist in its conception, degeneration theory helped to nudge German society down a slippery slope toward ethnic bias and xenophobia of all nonconforming individuals and groups.

At the bottom of that slope: Hitler's Final Solution, the systematic extermination of Jews, Gypsies, homosexuals, the handicapped, the mentally ill, and others considered degenerate. "We may—and we must—rely on the healthy instincts of the best of our people," zoologist Konrad Lorenz wrote in 1940 to support Nazi aims, "for the extermination of elements of the population loaded with dregs. Otherwise, these deleterious mutations will permeate the body of the people like the cells of a cancer."

Alois Alzheimer, whose wife came from a prominent Jewish family, was not a proto-fascist. Though he was receptive to the notion of degeneration, he was also wary of its social implications. "Perhaps the future," he wrote, "will let us see more clearly here and then show other principles to advantage; today we would go on interminably, if we were to see ourselves as justified in placing into the balance the inferiority of the descendants of the mentally ill, when we have to decide whether a termination of pregnancy is appropriate or not." In a 1999 biography of Alzheimer, Konrad Maurer wrote, "With that [remark], Alzheimer distinguished himself very clearly, and very early on from his colleagues [Alfred Friedrich] Hoche and [Ernst] Ruedin, who would later provide the weaponry for a terrible development."

Science as weaponry: the metaphor is a reminder of scientists' awesome power. The naming of diseases is a powerful social act that in turn can dictate social behavior. It therefore behooves the public to keep a close watch over the definition of diseases, of the power of doctors to decide what is and is not a part of healthy human society. Like the military, the scientific establishment should ultimately be under the watch of civilians ensuring the public will.

In 1953, James Watson and Francis Crick proposed the double-helix model as the structure of DNA, a spiral-shaped chain of deoxyribonucleic acid molecules that contained programming information for the function of all living organisms. In the following decades researchers began to construct a crude map associating particular genes with specific functions and diseases. By the 1980s, scientists could not only analyze the sequence of DNA strands but, incredibly, could also chemically remove—"knock out"—a tiny snippet and insert a replacement. When they had honed the technique enough to do this inside a just-fertilized mouse egg, the first humanized mouse was born. So-called knock-out mice became a powerful new tool for researchers all across the disease spectrum.

Nature may favor survival of the fittest, but with their startling new power, geneticists often found themselves working in the other direction—toward a degeneration of their own making. Commonly, knock-out technology was used to proliferate flawed genes—what Konrad Lorenz called the *dregs*—for closer study. Instead of building a "better mousetrap," as the business cliché goes, they created worse mice: artificially obese mice, diabetic mice, deaf mice, muscular dystrophy mice, Huntington's disease mice, asthmatic mice, cystic fibrosis mice, cancer mice, heart disease mice, and—in 1996—Alzheimer's mice.

Or at least the first reasonably close approximation. By splicing in a human gene that causes harmless APP to disintegrate into sticky beta-amyloid, the University of Minnesota's Karen Hsiao created the first mouse with plaques. The descendants of this humanized mouse appeared normal at birth. But at nine or ten months, they started having considerable memory trouble. In a pool of water, they would lose the ability to learn and remember the location of a platform. In dry mazes, they kept forgetting where the exits were. It was about as close to Alzheimer's disease as researchers could imagine in a mouse. When Hsiao opened up their brains, she saw that they were filled with amyloid plaques. It was a major breakthrough.

Of course, not everyone liked the idea of inflicting human diseases on animals. In 1999, animal rights activists broke into several University of Minnesota labs. They took forty-eight mice—including several of Hsiao's—along with thirty-six rats, twenty-seven pigeons, and five salamanders, and destroyed lab equipment worth several million dollars. They also spray-painted walls with slogans such as "No More Torture" and complained of electrodes being attached to animals' heads.

Five of the "liberated" animals were found dead the next day in a nearby field. Meanwhile, university scientists effectively refuted the activists' claims: The electrodes were not a part of some shock treatments, but harmless measurement devices, the same as those used to measure brain waves on humans. By no means were these animals being "tortured." To the contrary, lab animals all across the country were now protected by an elaborate legal and ethical regimen that guaranteed them a hygienic, nutritious, and pain-free environment. For reasons of liability, personal conscience, and good science, modern researchers generally treated their animals well and sacrificed only as many as were necessary.

Still, lab animals were being held against their will, drugged, and killed. The relatively humane treatment of the animals did not address the most basic charge of animal rights activists: that it is immoral to sacrifice animals merely to improve the health of human beings. To their credit, many modern researchers seem ready to address the issue head-on. "I am sure that we do have such duties to behave kindly and with respect to other animals, with the minimum of violence and cruelty, not to damage or take their lives insofar as it can be avoided," writes British neurobiologist Steven Rose. ". . . [B]ut all such duties to nonhuman animals are limited by an overriding duty to other humans." If sacrificing these animals can reduce human suffering, most researchers strongly believe, it is morally necessary. Their duty is not to the preservation of life in general, but human life in particular.

Despite protests, overall public sentiment and market economics strongly supported transgenics, and it flourished. By 1998, more than 500,000 transgenic mice were being used annually in experiments across the research spectrum. The technology was a critical breakthrough for Alzheimer's research in particular, finally giving scientists a reliable animal model. Dozens of variant strains followed from the original Hsiao knock-out Alzheimer's mouse and became the basis of many important Alzheimer's breakthroughs in the late 1990s.

The marketplace not only encouraged the creation of these

mice; it also insisted on their commodification. Not long after the Taos conference, Elan Pharmaceuticals—the company promising a dramatic development "very soon"—instead slammed the community with litigation. The company filed suit against the nonprofit Mayo Foundation for selling a strain of Hsiao mice on which Elan claimed to hold a patent.

The lawsuit hit the field like a cluster bomb, with subpoenas hitting other researchers all over who were working with knock-out mice created on the Hsiao model. Elan demanded to see the contents of their lab notebooks. "It's outrageous," remarked Karen Duff of the Nathan Kline Institute. Johns Hopkins microbiologist David Borchelt insisted that he would go to jail before turning his notebooks over to Elan.

The Mayo Clinic's Steven Younkin lashed out at Elan by contrasting the company's ethic with that of the mouse's original "inventor," Karen Hsiao. "Karen decided on Day One that she was giving her mouse to any academic researcher who asked for it," he said. "I think [Elan's] strategy is, 'Let's make sure we make all the money we possibly can, and if it slows down research, that's too bad. We've got our shareholders to worry about.' "

The notion of scientists fighting in court for the exclusive right to create a defective mouse was grotesque. But the new genetics lent itself to such absurdity, since it gave humans the power to alter the basic building blocks of life. In pursuit of their own interests, corporate managers saw little choice but to reduce transgenic creations to matters of contract and property law. The irony of the effort to "humanize" these mice, then, was that they were also simultaneously pushed in a very different direction—out of the realm of living beings entirely. It is as though the mice, now that they were programmable, were nothing more than machinery.

A California judge dismissed the Elan lawsuit, ruling that the company's patent was invalid. Officials from Elan declined to make any public comment on the case, other than to say that it was "Elan's policy to enforce its intellectual property rights," and that in the wake of the court dismissal the company was continuing to examine its legal options. Its litigiousness reflected the changing climate in science, a lurch toward the free market that gave primacy to making money rather than sharing information. Since 1980, when Congress significantly loosened restrictions on the interaction between public and private research efforts, many academic researchers had taken personal investment stakes in their own research. A 1996 survey of articles in leading U.S. biomedical journals revealed that close to one-third of the lead authors had some significant financial interest in the issues discussed in their published report.

Overall, the community was ambivalent about the new opportunities to benefit financially from their own research. "It brings out the worst in some people," said Glaxo Wellcome's Allen Roses. "And there is no field as bad as Alzheimer's. I've been in several fields including muscular dystrophy and human genetics, which is known to be bad because things can be so easily stolen, but Alzheimer's disease is the epitome of this because there's so much money at stake."

But Roses also had much to say in favor of the marketization of science. From where he sat, it was clearly faster and more efficient. Just two years after leaving Duke University for his new corporate post, he had already pioneered the use of a new technology called "SNP mapping." SNP, pronounced "snip," stands for single nucleotide polymorphisms, single-molecule variations in human DNA that determine whether someone is susceptible to a certain disease or would be responsive to a certain drug. SNP mapping helps to narrow substantially the search for disease genes by reducing the amount of information that needs to be analyzed—the equivalent of telling a researcher at the Library of Congress that instead of having to search randomly through the open stacks for a particular book by Kurt Vonnegut, he can instead check the card catalogue file under "Von." "In diabetes," Roses cited as an example, "we can go from 50 million base pairs down to ten thousand."

Because his discovery was privately funded, Roses openly bragged, he was not bound to share anything about it until after the money is in the bank. "One of the things we want to do before we release it," he said about one SNP development, "is get the functional genomic mice we need ready to go. That way, we're way far ahead and it's very expensive for anybody to try and catch up— like when Duke is ahead of its opponent and the students turn their back and scream, 'It simply doesn't matter.' " He laughed.

This was the new scientific ethic, as dictated by corporate managers: *Get products to market*. In his former academic life, Roses had spent decades applying for government grants, publishing in prestigious journals, and attending a whirlwind of academic conferences. He no longer did any of this—not just because he didn't have to, he said, but also because he was convinced that academic science had become permanently corrupted by money, and that he had found a new and much better way. As an academic, Roses said, he merely fought over ideas. As a corporate pharmacogeneticist, he was actually working to conquer diseases.

"I was in a situation where I was spending 50 to 60 percent of my time writing grants that never got funded," he said of the contrast. "We argued for three years about whether ApoE is inside neurons or not. It is in the neurons. We went to every meeting. They said, 'It's not in the neurons.' We would write a grant proposal. 'Oh, you can't do that—it isn't in neurons.' No grant. So what we have now done is say, 'Piss off. We're just going to do it. We're going to do it right and objectively, on the basis of the data.' I can tell you, we have found differences in the brain metabolism in these mice where the only difference is ApoE3 versus ApoE4. What they are and how we target them—I don't have to publish that. I don't have to take the time or the people it would involve to publish it.

"Am I keeping anything from my fellow researchers around the world in Alzheimer's disease? Hell no! All they ever did when I ever said anything was to say, 'No, no, no.' We would just argue it at all these scientific meetings. Now we debate in the context of very critical, highly skilled scientists who know that our viability as a team, our viability as a company, and our jobs depend on it—not whether we get it first into publication."

In fact, Roses *was* withholding information, as he acknowledged. His point seemed obvious. He was arguing that, in the new context of market science, withholding information was more efficient. The ends justified the means. The market would sort things out.

❧

Mother has for some time referred to herself in the third person. Usually this happens when we have been talking about her for a little while. She will ask a question that fits right in to the conversation, but begins, "Does she . . ." If I ask to whom she is referring, she'll answer, "That woman we have been talking about."

There are also lots of double people here. My husband is "the boys." My daughter's friend, who came over so I could go to a support group, was just one person when she walked out the door, but within fifteen minutes was two! I am a different person in the morning, afternoon, and night, which is logical considering that she thinks she's living (and working) in an institution. She was a nurse, so three shifts, right? Sometimes I'm different within the hour: "I can't go to the store with you because that other girl is taking me somewhere else."

—M.A.J.
Nampa, Idaho

❧

Chapter 13

WE HOPE TO RADIO BACK TO EARTH
IMAGES OF BEAUTY NEVER SEEN

·~·

In a short story by Jorge Luis Borges, a group of elite mapmakers are given an inherently unrealizable task: to create a map of the empire that is on the same scale as the empire—a map as big as its subject matter. Analogous is the challenge Morris Friedell took upon himself after receiving his Alzheimer's diagnosis. He wanted to unravel the mystery of a brain disease just as this disease was unraveling *him*. He wanted to study his own undoing.

In a sense, he'd been preparing for this project for most of his life. His college courses focused on human dignity and what he called the "social psychology of affliction." Now, in his unexpected new role among the afflicted, he could test the practicality of his ideas.

Shortly after his diagnosis he wrote a short essay entitled "Introduction to Myself and My Plight." The essay concluded:

I hope to be able to contribute to existential philosophy from a unique perspective. Perhaps, as my selfhood diminishes, I can add to the general human understanding of matters such as "self" and "time" and "nothingness." With this orientation I can perhaps make my slow dying a final intellectual and esthetic adventure.

When I was in my early teens in the 1950s I avidly read science fiction by Robert Heinlein and Arthur C. Clarke. I fantasized being an "astrogator." We collide with an asteroid, there is not enough fuel to get back to earth. We turn the ship straight away from the sun, we voyage out beyond the orbit of Pluto. We know we will perish in the interstellar void, yet we hope to radio back to earth images of beauty never seen as well as valuable information. . . . On August 19, 1998, my neurologist told me [Alzheimer's] is what the PET scan indicated. And here I am on that spaceship.

It wasn't long before he sent back his first dispatch, about a surprising advantage he discovered in forgetting. With less of a grip on what happened two hours or ten minutes ago, Morris reported feeling dramatically more involved in the present. "I find myself more visually sensitive," he said. "Everything seems richer: lines, planes, contrast. It is a wonderful compensation. . . . We [who have Alzheimer's disease] can appreciate clouds, leaves, flowers as we never did before. . . . as the poet Theodore Roethke put it, 'In a dark time the eye begins to see.'

"So many of us go through life like tourists with a camera always between our eyes and the world," Morris observed. Alzheimer's won't allow that sort of detachment. Like H.M. from the 1950s, the short-circuiting of memory forces every Alzheimer's sufferer to be always in the Now. This is widely regarded as one of the horrors of the disease. But from his firsthand experience, Morris argued that being perpetually in the Now has an upside. It leads to an actual *heightening* of consciousness. "I can watch kittens playing in a way I couldn't before," he said.

How could a neurological disease enrich awareness?

All of waking life is a stew of familiar and unfamiliar experiences; it is the brain's job to turn the unfamiliar into the familiar. Familiar sights, sounds, and ideas don't demand as much energy or attention, and can elicit quicker and more graceful responses. Thanks to familiarity, a person can do many things at once, and even process relatively complex ideas almost completely in the background, without having to bother the conscious mind.

New experiences, by contrast, demand conscious attention, so that they may be examined, understood, contextualized, reacted to, memorized, *learned.* Think of learning to play the piano or to ride a bike; think of the first time you went to a baseball game or ate sushi. The unfamiliar demands focus, greedily occupies consciousness. Confronting the new is a captivating, exhausting experience.

Alzheimer's keeps things new. After onset, the unfamiliar can never become familiar. The Alzheimer's mind is constantly flooded with new stimuli; everything is always in the moment, a rich, resonant, overwhelming feeling. "I've noticed that I have a large amount of appreciation for whatever I'm focused on," commented fellow Alzheimer's sufferer Laura S. in response to Morris's declaration. "It is very clear and real. Look away and it is gone. Look back and it is fresh and new. I am checking this out with a red geranium blossom right now. When I look away, 'red' no longer exists except as an abstract term. No blossom image remains. . . . But I can look again."

Ever-freshness, then, may be considered an Alzheimer's consolation prize. This may be a particularly difficult idea for caregivers to swallow because their own experience is often precisely the opposite. As their forgetful loved ones repeatedly stumble over the same tasks and information, caregivers must suffer through the oppressive repetition. They repeat the same mind-numbing instructions over and over again. Life threatens to become less and less fresh in the way that a tour guide quickly loses any real enthusiasm and interest in the material that she must repeat twelve times a day, five days a week. In the often deadening, disheartening world of Alzheimer's care, caregivers wake up thousands of days in a row facing the same tourist wanting to take exactly the same tour.

Still, caregivers must try to understand both the frustrations and the unexpected benefits of having an unraveling mind. What they may at first presume to be a uniformly awful experience for the victims can sometimes perhaps be peculiarly satisfying and even enriching—"a final intellectual and esthetic adventure."

In the late 1970s, close friends of the master Abstract Expressionist painter Willem de Kooning began to notice that he was having trouble remembering names and recent events, and following the thread of conversations. At the time, de Kooning was trying to escape from a decades-long dependence on alcohol, and the memory problems were assumed to be acute side effects of his difficult recovery.

It turned out that the forgetting was not the end of his alcoholism; it was the beginning of his Alzheimer's disease. He recovered his strength and, with the aid of friends, family, and a drug called Antabuse—which nauseated him every time he tasted alcohol—managed to stay on the wagon. But his forgetfulness grew steadily worse. Slowly, over nearly two decades, he unraveled entirely. His estranged wife, Elaine, who came back into his life in 1978 and became the chief architect of his recovery from alcoholism, eerily predicted the course of his later years in a frank lecture she gave him that same year.

"Bill," she said. "Your genes are sensational. Your mother lived to be ninety-two and was strong as a rock. Your father lived to eighty-nine, your grandmother to ninety-five. So your body's going to last, but your brain is going to go. You will be a vegetable."

"You're scaring me," de Kooning replied.

"Good," said his wife.

By 1983, five years later, he was forgetting so much that he started to experience moments of genuine confusion. On a transatlantic flight from New York to Amsterdam that year, de Kooning turned to Elaine in the middle of the in-flight movie and said, "This is a lousy film. Let's get out of here."

When his wife gently reminded him they were not in a New York cinema but on a plane to Europe, de Kooning revealed an even deeper confusion. "This is terrible," he said. "They'll find out I left the U.S., and they'll never let me back in again." De Kooning had originally come to the U.S. as a stowaway in 1926, and had not become an American citizen until 1961. Now, on the plane to Amsterdam in 1983, he was stuck in an old awareness, a sense of himself that had long since expired.

Such a time regression is common for Alzheimer's sufferers in the confusional stages; quite often, they find themselves jerked back so forcefully to earlier memories that they expect spouses to be young and parents to still be alive. They might also think of themselves as younger looking, failing to recognize their own faces in the mirror. All of this happens because relatively fragile memories from recent years have dissolved, leaving only much older, more durable memories. While a memory formed forty years ago is not inherently more resilient than one formed four years ago, older memories of childhood playhouses and wedding vows have become more durable through thousands of recollections in the intervening years. Since the act of remembering itself creates a brand-new memory of that memory, the most powerful images from childhood and early adulthood get replayed over and over again in a person's mind and thus become virtually indestructible by the time a person reaches his seventies. Those seasoned memories are as durable as limestone, while the more recent are still relative impressions in sand.

De Kooning, remarkably, kept painting. In fact, as he recovered from his drinking problem, he commenced in 1981 what would turn out to be one of the most productive, if also controversial, periods of his career. De Kooning not only produced an extraordinary 341 paintings over a ten-year period, but created work that has since received high critical praise—even given the general awareness of his dementia.

The paintings from the 1980s are, in many respects, very different from his earlier work. They are more melodious, graceful, and far less dense. Overall, they seem happier, far less angst-ridden, than his more famous creations. In contrast to his previously complex color palette, premixed with great care, de Kooning came to rely heavily on primary colors pulled straight out of the tube. In contrast to his thickly layered paintings from before, these late works have a lot less texture. The strokes are less animated, more relaxed; the dominant form is a bright, ribbonlike weave vaguely suggesting human curves and natural landscapes. Blank space takes a more prominent role in these late paintings—"like a blank mind picturing itself," observed art journalist Kay Larson.

"There is no question in my mind that it's an extraordinary body of work," San Francisco Museum of Modern Art curator Gary Garrels told Larson in 1994 as he organized a major exhibition of the eighties work. "There is intense concentration and consciousness in these paintings. They are not just someone spreading paint around. This is definitely an artist in control." Garrels went on further to say that many of de Kooning's works from this period are "among the most beautiful, sensual, and exuberant abstract works by any modern painter."

Critics took special notice of the 1995 Garrels exhibition because they had, by 1980, more or less written de Kooning's artistic obituary—one which included an especially unflattering final chapter. "Anyone who remembers the [1983] Whitney [retrospective] exhibition knows there are acres of sloppy, slack, fizzled paintings from the sixties and seventies," wrote Larson. "Nobody had a reason to think the eighties would be different."

But this new work, everyone agreed, *was* very different from previous periods. "The effect they gave was one of lightness and joy," Curtis Bill Pepper wrote in the *New York Times* after seeing a collection of de Kooning's latest paintings in the early 1980s. "It was an old man's lyrical elegy distilled from the turbulent recesses of the self."

Pepper did not mention that a metabolic process in de Kooning's cerebral cortex was radically redefining his "self." What was taking place in that Long Island studio was much more than a personal resurgence; de Kooning was documenting on canvas his own progressive forgetting.

Was he really a happier man? It's entirely possible. Alzheimer's can be severely frustrating to patients at certain periods, but can also leave its victims extraordinarily serene. The patient loses the awareness of what he has lost. He has fewer thoughts, fewer worries. Life is not as complex or demanding. In this sense, Emerson was speaking hopefully on behalf of all Alzheimer's sufferers when he said, "Things that go wrong . . . don't disturb me," and "I have lost my mental faculties but am perfectly well."

When, in the 1990s, the art community finally got to see the eighties work as a whole, now very aware of de Kooning's slide into dementia, there was a flood of interest in the paintings and curiosity about what they meant. Inevitably, a debate ensued about their artistry, their importance, and their connection to the artist's previous work. Ultimately, these were subjective judgments, of course, but it was only natural to wonder if de Kooning had maintained his greatness throughout illness. Were his late works genuinely a part of the *oeuvre* of one of the most important painters in the twentieth century, or should they instead be thought of as works by a once-great artist now "on autopilot," without any fresh ideas or even any ideas at all?

This was not just an academic question. Millions of dollars and the reputations of many collectors, curators, gallery owners, and critics were riding on the answer. The stakes were so high that in 1995 the San Francisco MOMA's Garrels assembled a panel that included the painter Jasper Johns and directors of several major modern art museums. (De Kooning was in the final stages of his illness at the time, no longer painting; he died in 1997.) Over two days, they reviewed and discussed scores of the late paintings, and considered some fundamental questions:

Should current works be judged as a group or individually?

Should they be judged purely on their own merits or in comparison to prior work? If the latter, how much familiarity with de Kooning's past was necessary to make sound appraisals of this work?

Should the viewer's own expectations play a role?

Should de Kooning's intentions be taken into account? If so, how could one best discern his intentions?

These were all formal and polite ways of poking at a very uncomfortable question: Could this new direction of work legitimately be seen as an extension of de Kooning's provocative career, or had he lost his artistic spark along with his functioning hippocampus? It is an impossible question to answer fully, of course, but still one well worth asking. The insidious creep of Alzheimer's erases the self in such tiny increments that trying to determine any sort of distinct cutoff point approaches the paradoxical quality of a Zen koan. What is the sound of fewer neurons firing?

One factor in sizing up the effect of Alzheimer's on the artistic process is the distinction between *mind memory* and *muscle memory*. Mind memories are formed in association between the hippocampus and the cerebral cortex, stored in the cortex, and are highly vulnerable to suggestion, to the vagaries of time, and to the plaques and tangles of Alzheimer's disease.

Muscle memory, also called *procedural memory*, exists as an entirely separate neural network in different regions of the brain. These are the unconscious, but exquisitely detailed, movements that a person makes when walking down the stairs, riding a bike, playing the piano, typing, clapping, painting, kissing. Muscle memories are much harder to lay down than mind memories—they take practice, practice, practice. But once ingrained, they are also far more difficult to erase. Notice that even victims of extreme amnesia do not "forget" how to walk. It takes a stroke or some other traumatic brain injury for muscle memories to be disrupted. Doctors were interested to discover that H.M., whose ability to form new mind memories was immediately and forever removed along with his hippocampus, could in fact develop new coordination skills—even though he was never actually aware of the new skills he had.

In the same way as H.M., Alzheimer's sufferers generally retain complete muscle memories until the very late stages of the disease, when the plaques and tangles finally creep into virtually every area of the brain. This steady erosion of intellectual capacity without noticeable physical disruption is what sparks public fascination with the disease in the first place, and haunts even the most seasoned observers. Even for people who spend years immersed in the culture of the disease, it is positively ghostly to be in the presence of a man who for several years has not recognized his wife but who can still walk or sing or even dance a waltz.

Or paint. We know, both from firsthand reports of de Kooning's studio assistants and from the closely studied patterns of Alzheimer's disease, that de Kooning's signature brushstroke did not erode at the same time that he had trouble remembering what he had eaten for breakfast. His muscle memory remained intact for a long while, and the act of painting remained important to him. People who spent time with him during his long period of forgetting say that his sagging posture and lethargic manner abruptly shifted into an erect, energetic, passionate professionalism whenever he walked from his kitchen to his adjacent studio.

What was ebbing slowly in de Kooning's brain was a refined cognition and a capacity for lucid discourse. He could no longer manage his practical affairs, engage in sophisticated conversation, or socialize on any significant level. Many years before he was forced to stop painting, he became effectively cut off from the world around him, losing the ability to discuss his work intelligently or consider it in the larger context of society and art history.

From a certain creative standpoint, such forfeitures might not be considered a liability. After all, artists are not analysts. To the contrary: Every creator knows that thinking can disrupt creativity. "Art . . . is not cognitive," Israel Scheffler wrote in his book *Symbolic Worlds,* "but rather emotive in its import. Its function is to stimulate, express, or vent emotions rather than describe reality."

Throughout his long career, de Kooning had not relied on elaborate conceptualization in the same way, for example, that Andy Warhol had to create his Campbell Soup silk screens or Georges Seurat had to create his painstaking pointillist *Sunday Afternoon on the Island of La Grande Jatte.* "De Kooning was never a very intellectual painter," wrote Kay Larson. "Even in the beginning, in the *Women* [series], in *Excavation,* his talents emerged from the moment—from the thrust and parry of the brush, from the 'excavation' of his emotional state."

One essential component of self that Alzheimer's patients do *not* come untethered from early on is their own emotional reservoir. From this vantage, it almost seems as though de Kooning contracted just the right disease, the one neurological disorder that would spare his ability to create as it ate away at most of the rest of his abilities.

Perhaps, then, Alzheimer's did not dim de Kooning's art, at least not until much later in the disease. Perhaps Alzheimer's *enhanced* his art. Morris Friedell's observation about the heightening of consciousness in the early stages of Alzheimer's would seem to apply perfectly to de Kooning and other abstract artists. If Abstract Expressionism exists predominantly as an emotional response to the world, the new freshness of consciousness forced upon early-stage Alzheimer patients could presumably serve as a creative impulse.

De Kooning himself had complained in the mid-seventies (pre-Alzheimer's) that his way of working had become "almost a habit," and critics seemed to agree wholeheartedly. It seems more than a mere coincidence that his art was rejuvenated at precisely the same time he began to succumb to the disease—to lose his ability to follow habits. One reasonable analysis is that the disruption of memories fortuitously dissolved chronic work patterns that had become such a burden. In this way, the disease may have, if only temporarily, *rescued* de Kooning's career, granting him an extra few years of creative energy by releasing him from a tired routine.

"Collectively, the pictures . . . seem to glow with an inner light," the *San Francisco Examiner*'s David Bonetti wrote of de Kooning's late work. ". . . They remind you that even during bleak times, art can offer emotional and spiritual solace like nothing else." Kay Larson, writing in the *Village Voice*, pared the rejuvenation theory down to its perfect reductionist epithet: De Kooning, she wrote, rounded out his career in a fertile period of "Alzheimer's Expressionism."

One does not, of course, want to exaggerate the advantages of a slide toward oblivion. Many important faculties are, in fact, adversely affected early on in Alzheimer's: constructional abilities, spatial relations, orientation, perspective, and concentration. So even as an abstractionist, de Kooning would have had a somewhat reduced command of his craft after the onset of Alzheimer's. His ability to execute a desired stroke would in certain ways have been compromised.

Another important consideration is the impairment of so-called executive function skills, including goal-setting and self-evaluation. A person's introspection begins to wither away from near the beginning of Alzheimer's—the constant "How-am-I-doing?" inner dialogue that people with functioning brains take for granted. When introspection begins to break down, so does will-fulness—"Here's-what-I-should-do-next." As the plaques and tangles proliferate and the brain begins to shrink, a psychic barrier arises between the victim and the outside world. The Alzheimer's sufferer becomes an island.

In that isolation, argue some, de Kooning's art in particular vanished completely. "Art, in the way that de Kooning conceived it, is something that is produced in a conscious dialogue with the rest of art history and culture," argues art historian András Szántó. "De Kooning is an excellent example of what we call the 'professional artist,' one who worked strictly within the context of other art. His was actually a very conceptual, aesthetic agenda, turning the art world upside down, demolishing certain assumptions that were in place up to the 1960s.

"If, later on in life, we end up with someone who is merely doing things in his head, then de Kooning's art, as he understood it, is gone. Once the dialogue with the rest of the world is severed, it is impossible to speak of this as art with a capital 'A.'"

Amidst stark disagreements about the quality of de Kooning's eighties paintings, the 1995 panel did not manage to come to a real consensus. "No single point of view predominated," Garrels politely reported, except for the agreement that the works produced after 1989 could not be counted as "fully realized works of art." Some panel members felt that the work had lost its essential structure in the mid-1980s—which is roughly when de Kooning passed into the middle stages of the disease. But others agreed with Garrels and MOMA curator Robert Storr that the work up to 1989 stands on its own.

A year after the panel deliberated, the neurologist Carlos Hugo Espinel published an essay about de Kooning in the British medical journal *Lancet.* "These paintings [are] not merely the product of someone who had simply retained colour perception and the motor strength to copy," Espinel wrote. "Even if at times he confused his wife with his sister . . . De Kooning went on to create. His resurgence is a testimony to the potential of the human mind, evidence for hope."

And there *was* hope—not that de Kooning might somehow recover from his forgetting, but that he could live serenely within it; that we could all live in harmony with the specter of senile dementia.

De Kooning was, after all, speaking for all of us, and to us. He had spent his long life producing abstract emotional pastiches, painting images from his psyche in the same way that radio announcers would depict a boxing match: in quick, emotional bursts that said something very personal about the artist and, often, also something profound about the human condition. "I am always in the picture somewhere," he said in 1950. "... I seem to move around in it, and there seems to be a time when I lose sight of what I wanted to do, and then I am out of it. If the picture has a countenance, I keep it. If it hasn't, I throw it away."

In these late paintings, de Kooning was presenting one final series of communiqués to his public, messages of tranquillity and transcendence in decline. It was a message that Emerson, Shakespeare, Erasmus, and others had sent: Senility, while devastating, is also a part of life.

In his essay, Espinel also briefly alluded to a feature in the late-period de Koonings that every other observer had missed: the unmistakable resemblance between the wispy strokes on his canvases and the neurofibrillary tangles in his brain.

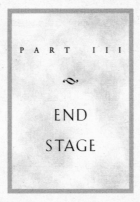

PART III

❧

END
STAGE

Chapter 14

BREAKTHROUGH?

◇

San Francisco, California: July 1999

In July, with patents filed and publication pending, Elan Pharmaceuticals finally broke their long silence: They had a new drug that had *eliminated* plaques in mice. In the next few months they would begin testing it in humans.

The news caught researchers completely by surprise.

"It's wild and amazing," said Sangram Sisodia, chairman of neurobiology at the University of Chicago.

"This is a major step forward," said the National Institute on Aging's Marcelle Morrison-Bogorad.

Even officials from the famously cautious Alzheimer's Association gushed. "It's a fascinating finding with immense potential," offered Vice President Bill Thies. This was the first time in the organization's twenty-year history that it had issued an unqualified statement of optimism about a potential treatment.

The most surprising part of the news was the type of drug: a simple antibody vaccine, no different in principle from the vaccines for polio, measles, mumps, and diphtheria. Those vaccines work by injecting weakened bits of live virus into the bloodstream, stimulating the immune system to develop specific antibodies that quickly recognize and remove any future virus to come along.

Antibodies are not limited to virus removal; they can theoretically be programmed to tag and remove any foreign object— beta-amyloid, for instance, the main component of plaques. Beta-amyloid is just as foreign to the human body as any virus. Elan's new approach was to inject bits of beta-amyloid into the bloodstream the same way that Albert Sabin injected weakened polio virus.

It seemed like one of those ideas that was too simple to work, so much so that when lead researcher Dale Schenk had first mentioned the concept to coworkers in a brainstorming session a few years earlier, he said, "Everyone looked at me like I was crazy." The notion seemed dead on utterance; as a demonstration of its apparent absurdity, one of Schenk's colleagues pinned it to an office bulletin board of outrageous comments.

Now, other Alzheimer's researchers were admitting they would have had the same reaction. "If someone had suggested that experiment to me," said the Mayo Clinic's John Hardy after the breakthrough announcement, "I would have told them not to waste their time."

Chicago's Sisodia said: "I wouldn't have imagined it could ever work. We haven't even *thought* about a vaccine for Alzheimer's."

But to Schenk, his self-described "nutty idea" was the natural outcome of tracing what he already knew about plaques through a number of logical steps. "The absolute levels of production of beta-amyloid in the brain tissue seem to be a critical factor in whether or not you get amyloid plaques," he explained. "So I was thinking about that one day, and I thought, 'If there was only a way to tie up that beta-amyloid in the brain, to keep it occupied.' Then I thought, 'Well, maybe if we had antibodies there, that would work. It's too bad that there are no good ways to get antibodies into the brain. You could inject them straight into the brain, but that's not a good idea. . . .'

"And then it suddenly hit me like a stone: Actually, we could put antibodies into the *bloodstream,* and a small amount would likely leak into the brain. Furthermore, why don't we just immunize with beta-amyloid? Then the body would be constantly making a ton of antibodies and over time a small amount of that antibody would get in and change the equilibrium."

To most scientists, the idea would immediately have seemed like a nonstarter because of the famous blood-brain barrier, the protective mechanism that keeps carbohydrates, proteins, metals, and other impurities out of the brain. While the rest of the body's organs can easily tolerate a rich and coarse blood flow, the brain's fine vasculature cannot. Brain arteries are a delicate silk web as compared to the body's rope artery hammock, and would easily clog and burst under the pressure of such bulky particles.

The brain does need fresh blood, though, which delivers a constant infusion of oxygen and glucose in order for it to survive. So it relies on a fine mesh filter system—the blood-brain barrier. Schenk was very familiar with the barrier through some recent research he had done—so familiar that he was mindful of something that most other neuroscientists seemed not to be: The blood-brain barrier *is not perfect.* For whatever reason, it has a tiny built-in leak—about three out of every thousand unwanted particles get in.

Schenk's epiphany was that a body constantly manufacturing its own supply of beta-amyloid antibody would produce so much of it that three parts per thousand would be plenty.

Like so many other breakthroughs in history, his eureka moment capped off years of hard work. Schenk and his colleagues had been researching Alzheimer's aggressively on several fronts since 1987. With no expectation of near-term profit, they'd invested tens of millions of dollars. "For years, we've had a major, major, major commitment to Alzheimer's research, far more than any single university center," Schenk boasted. "It has been a giant effort. At one point, we had sixty people working on it at once, and that doesn't count the labs of our collaborators. It's not by chance that we came up with the vaccine. It really isn't chance."

For the vaccine experiment, Schenk cordoned off three groups of mice genetically designed to develop plaque-filled brains. The first batch, the control group, received no vaccine. The second group received a series of injections of vaccine beginning at six weeks of age (young adulthood). The third group started getting injections at twelve months (old age)—only after they had started to accumulate plaques.

After about a year, mice from groups one and two were sacrificed and dissected: Brains from the control group were, as expected, riddled with plaques. Of the nine mice in the group receiving the vaccine from early on, though, seven had virtually no plaques; the remaining two had significantly fewer than the control mice. The results were so dramatic, Schenk says, that when they first looked at the tissue slides, "we thought maybe the animals had been mixed up."

They had not. To an extent beyond the Elan team's wildest expectations, the injected bits of beta-amyloid had evidently stimulated the immune system to attack and dissolve the plaque deposits as they were being formed. It is a two-step process. First, the injected beta-amyloid prompted the immune system to tag all beta-amyloid in the brain for removal. Then white blood cells and another class of cells called microglia, acting as the body's garbage collectors, swept through and picked up everything that had been tagged. The result: no more plaques. Individual strands of beta-amyloid floating free were nabbed before they could glom on to a plaque.

Eighteen months after the experiment began, they got even better news. When they sacrificed the third group of mice—those who received the vaccine only as elderly mice—they again saw fewer plaques compared to the control group at that same age. The vaccine not only prevented plaques from forming, but also disassembled and removed plaques already in the brain. It was a true plaque-buster—not just a shield but also an antidote.

This new drug, temporarily named AN 1792, was not by any means a certain cure for Alzheimer's disease. First, the company would have to see if it was safe in humans. There was a serious worry among some neuroscientists that the injected beta-amyloid could stimulate a troublesome (possibly even lethal) autoimmune response, wherein the immune system behaves as though the body's own cells are a foreign enemy needing to be destroyed. (Other autoimmune disorders include psoriasis, rheumatoid arthritis, lupus, diabetes mellitus, and multiple sclerosis.)

Another possible scenario was that the vaccine could prove safe but ineffective. It might not clear away human plaques as effectively as mouse plaques.

Finally, of course, the vaccine might work brilliantly but not end the disease. No one could say for sure that clearing away the plaques would be enough to beat Alzheimer's.

These were serious hurdles, but all the same, Elan's announcement seemed to have inaugurated a new era in Alzheimer's research: *the beginning of the end.* This particular drug might not be the cure, but at least it was the first contender.

Yesterday when I visited my mother at the new home, she had taken her outer garments off and was taking a nap in someone else's bed (alone). Her personal teddy bear was in someone else's room. This is one of her best friends, and she used to constantly carry it around and talk to it. I rescued it and put it in her arms as she slept. I realize that residents take things from others' rooms, but feel bad that her teddy bear was not close by her.

　　The old house had five to eight residents. This new one has sixteen. She has sixteen closets to hide in. The staff is cautious when opening closets, because Mother will jump out and "boo" them.

—J.T.
Cross Plains, Wisconsin

Chapter 15

ONE THOUSAND SUBTRACTIONS

❧

The late years of Ralph Waldo Emerson's senile dementia were probably about as peaceful as anyone could have hoped. "He suffered very little," wrote his son Edward, "took his nourishment well, but had great annoyance from his inability to find the words which he wished for. . . . He went to his study and tried to work, accomplished less and less, but did not notice it." Emerson became intermittently confused about where he was, lost his ability to write letters and to understand what he was reading and much of what was said to him, and lost grasp entirely of many important figures in his life. Within a week of Henry Wadsworth Longfellow's death, in the spring of 1882, Emerson could not be made to understand *who* his old friend was. The entity of "Longfellow" in Emerson's mind had comprised a broad constellation of synapses, and that particular constellation was now inaccessible. Did it still exist? Only as cellular residue.

By far the most vivid account of Emerson's late-stage dementia comes to us via the efforts of an industrious and conniving young man named Edward Bok. A Dutch immigrant who settled in New York City with his family in 1870, when he was seven, Bok quickly became smitten by the unrelenting American can-do spirit, and particularly seduced by the allure of celebrity. By his early teens, as an office boy at Western Union Telegraph and a budding freelance reporter, he developed an ambition to meet and interact (however superficially) with the most popular public figures of the time. Emerson was near the top of Bok's wish list.

After easily engaging former President Ulysses S. Grant and then-President Rutherford B. Hayes, Bok traveled to Boston to make more famous "friends" and collect their autographs. Just eighteen, he was already savvy enough to understand how one association could lead to another, and planned his visits accordingly. Over the course of just a few days in November 1881, Bok parlayed a meeting with Oliver Wendell Holmes into one with Longfellow; the Longfellow interaction begat an audience with the Episcopal bishop Phillips Brooks (composer of "O Little Town of Bethlehem"). Brooks, in turn, advised Bok on how to see Emerson. "I don't know whether you will see him at his *best,*" he warned the young man in polite understatement. Bok had no idea what he was talking about.

The next day Bok went to Concord, where he managed to enchant *Little Women* author Louisa May Alcott. Now nearly fifty, Alcott had grown up with Emerson as a neighbor and uncle figure. "Our best and greatest American," she called him in her journal, ". . . and the man who has helped me most by his life, his books, his society." Alcott agreed to make an introduction for Bok, while also warning him that Emerson was not the man he once had been.

When they arrived at the house, though, Ellen Emerson politely declined to show them in. "Father sees no one now," she said, "and I fear it might not be a pleasure if you did see him." Bok was prepared for this contingency. At just the right moment, he expertly dropped in a line from his previous day's conversation with Phillips Brooks, and once again a door opened.

The vacant ghost of Emerson was sitting quietly at the desk in his study. "Father," said Ellen, gently alerting Emerson to his uninvited guests. He looked up at them and smiled, but said nothing. Then, slowly rising from his desk, he offered his hand and gestured vaguely toward some empty chairs. But as soon as he had turned away for just a moment, something very unsettling happened: Emerson wandered away from his visitors and toward the window. There, he stood for a while, apparently oblivious to any other presence in the room. In a split instant, he seemed to have forgotten entirely about the others.

Ellen, who had been slowly losing her father for more than a dozen years, started to cry and left the room, but Louisa and Edward stayed on quietly. After a few minutes, Emerson headed back to his desk, noticing them along the way. Again, he bowed a silent greeting, then sat down at the desk; once more, out of sight, out of mind.

What no doctor in 1881 could have known was that Emerson was by now operating with a virtually obliterated hippocampus, occasioning a virtually perfect case of anterograde amnesia—the loss of ability to create any new memories. If his was an Alzheimer's pathology, plaques and tangles germinating in the hippocampal formation had first started to create a noticeable disturbance in Emerson's functioning almost fifteen years earlier. Since that time, as the unwelcome particles spread to other regions of the brain, they also continued to proliferate in their original nest. Slowly, steadily, a critical mass of neurons and connections between neurons had been hacked apart; probably no more than half of the original healthy cells now remained. In this state, not only was the hippocampus completely incapable of consolidating short-term into long-term memories; it could not even establish "working memories" of a duration of minutes.

All that was left, then, was a limited capacity for "immediate memory" of mere seconds. Emerson was still conscious, and somewhat sentient. He could still coalesce different fields of information—verbal, visual, auditory—into a cogent sense of the present tense, a working (if constricted) consciousness. He was still, in some sense, *there*.

But how much of the great mind remained was an open question. Gently probing that consciousness for its eroding boundary, his old friend Louisa now spoke up in a nervous attempt to end the dreadful silence in the room.

"Have you read this new book by Ruskin yet?" she asked.

The voice didn't register. Emerson rose slowly and looked up at Louisa. "Did you speak to me, madam?" he asked. At the moment, he had no apparent recognition of a friend of nearly half a century—the realization of which sent Louisa into tears. As she retreated to the other side of the room, Bok, now left alone with Emerson, saw his opportunity and blurted out his long-planned request.

"I thought, perhaps, Mr. Emerson, that you might be able to favor me with a letter from Carlyle."

"Carlyle? Did you say Carlyle?"

"Yes," repeated Bok. "Thomas Carlyle."

"Yes, to be sure. Carlyle. Yes, he was here this morning. He will be here again tomorrow morning." In fact, as even Bok knew, Carlyle lived in England. The two had not seen each other for many years.

There was a pause, into which Emerson lost his train of thought. Emerson looked at the boy for a cue. "You were saying?"

Bok repeated his request. Could Emerson give him one of the original Carlyle letters?

"Oh, I think so, I think so. Let me see. Yes, here in this drawer I have many letters from Carlyle." He ruffled through some papers in his desk drawer and then again lost himself. More quiet moments passed. Finally, Bok, sensing correctly that his visit was about to come to an end, pared down his request. He asked for a simple autograph.

"Mr. Emerson," Bok said, "will you be so good as to write your name in this book for me?"

"Name?" said a puzzled Emerson.

"Yes, please. Your name: Ralph Waldo Emerson."

"Please write out the name you want, and I will copy it for you if I can."

Bok, stunned, wrote out "R. Waldo Emerson, Concord, November 22, 1881," on a slip of paper and handed it to Emerson along with the book. Emerson then copied Bok's dictation, very slowly copying letter by letter:

R. Waldo Emerson
Conocord
November 22, 1881

(Notice the extra "o" in Concord. In his fog, Emerson had misspelled the town which he himself had made world-famous.)

After the autograph came the most chilling occurrence yet. Emerson forgot about signing his name just as soon as he had done so. A few moments after Bok placed the autograph book back in his pocket, Emerson caught sight of the slip with Bok's handwriting on his desk and fell into a wide smile.

"You wish me to write my name?" he said. "With pleasure. Have you a book with you?"

Bok, now "overcome with astonishment," again handed him the autograph book. And so it was that Emerson autographed Bok's book not once but twice, bestowing on the young man two separate handwritten pieces of evidence of having met the great Transcendentalist in person—when, as a matter of both neurobiology and humanity, he had arguably never met Emerson at all.

Two weeks later, Emerson was dead, of pneumonia.

If Emerson was, as it appears in medical hindsight, afflicted with a reasonably straightforward case of what we now call Alzheimer's disease, it is also clear that he was mercifully released from the scripted drama before its dismal finale. In the end, for those Alzheimer's sufferers who do not die of something else along the way—pneumonia, stroke, heart failure, cancer, etc.—speech dissolves completely, incontinence sets in, muscles become stiff, walking becomes impossible; the face loses all elasticity, breathing becomes labored, swallowing ceases. All of this happens slowly, incrementally, insidiously, over months or even years.

In the brain, the pathway of the disease is the steady continuation of retrogenesis completing its relentless undoing on the way back to birth, the plaques and tangles moving into those regions that control gross motor function and are the very first to become myelinated in an infant.

Stage

7c	Can no longer walk without assistance
7d	Can no longer sit up without assistance
7e	Can no longer smile
7f	Can no longer hold up head

After the motor skills begin to collapse, limiting the patient to a wheelchair and then to a bed; after the eyes lose their ability to focus, something happens that is chilling even for this disease: the return of the infant reflexes.

In normal development, infants younger than six months will, when the soles of their feet are stimulated, raise their big toe up and spread their other toes outward. This is called the Babinski sign, after the French neurologist Joseph François Félix Babinski, who first described the phenomenon in 1903. The Babinski sign disappears after approximately six months of age; from then on the toes reflex downward in response to the same stimulus. Alzheimer's patients reclaim the Babinski sign (also now called the plantar response) in the very late stages, along with the other well-known infant reflexes: rooting, sucking, grasping. They all come back. If you scratch the palm of a late-stage patient, you might notice a twitch of the chin muscle on the same side. If you put your finger in the palm of his hand, you'll feel an instant, familiar grab.

After much of the cortex has been decimated, and thinking and mobility are all but at an end, the tangles launch their final assault on the brain in its most primitive and evolutionarily oldest region: the brainstem, at the base of the brain, just above the spinal cord. The brainstem controls involuntary, hard-wired functions such as breathing, blinking, blood pressure, heart rate, and sleeping cycles. It regulates the lungs, intestines, liver, kidneys, pancreas, and other organs, freeing up the cortex to worry about sensations, movements, and ideas. A person with extensive cortical damage but an intact brainstem can live for years in a "persistent vegetative state" with feeding tubes and meticulous care. But Alzheimer's does not let that happen. It finishes the job by slowly destroying the brainstem just as it has destroyed the hippocampus and the other regions of the brain along the way.

No matter how long the end has been anticipated by friends and family, no one knows quite what to expect. On the Alzheimer List, Stephanie Zeman, a nurse specializing in dementia care, counseled her listmates about the final path toward death. "The last few days of life for most people with dementia," she said, "go something like this: The person will stop taking anything by mouth. They may sleep a lot. At this point families worry about the discomfort of hunger or thirst. Studies indicate that at this stage the person does not experience discomfort from either hunger or thirst because the body is literally shutting down. This is a natural process. The digestive system and kidneys can no longer process nutrients or eliminate waste normally. Loading the system with IV fluids often puts the person into congestive heart failure and their lungs may become congested because the heart is also beginning to fail and cannot pump the larger blood volume any more.

"The hands and feet will begin to feel cold and may develop what is called mottling, a blotchy look, because now some of the tissues are not getting a normal level of oxygen. The person is now fairly unresponsive and their breathing becomes shallower and may sound noisy from an accumulation of fluids in their throat. At this point the head can be elevated slightly and turned to the side to help with this. This stage may last a day or more. Hands and feet are now very cold. Family may want to put blankets on the person but in fact, as the body shuts down, it conserves all of its resources for the trunk and brain so the core body temperature is not sub-normal but may in fact, be elevated. A light sheet is usually all that is needed.

"The end of life is usually very quiet and the person just slips away. Families at the bedside may suddenly realize the person is not breathing any more. Within a few minutes the heart stops and the person is truly at rest."

Life passes, and the caregiver can no longer give care. Into the void rushes a powerful sea of emotion, with uneven waves of relief, regret, guilt, anger, emptiness, and renewed purpose. On the surface, the caregiver is finally cut loose from an extraordinary burden, and is relieved. The long decline is over.

Under any circumstances, mourning a lost life is a complex emotional event. With Alzheimer's, though, it is particularly torturous because in this long disease there have already been so many expirations along the way. In *Man's Search for Meaning*, Viktor Frankl raised the specter of "emotional death," the death of the spirit occurring well before the death of the actual body. Alzheimer's specializes in such split-level death. The final passing from Alzheimer's is really just the last in a long series of deaths. It is death not by a thousand cuts but by a thousand subtractions.

This understanding of Alzheimer's death, in turn, suggests

something important about death in general that ordinarily goes unnoticed. The truth is that, no matter the cause, death is *never* a single end but a collection of ends that are ordinarily so tightly bound together that they appear to be one entity. In the same way that visible light usually appears to be a single colorless article, death usually looks like a single experience. One moment the person is there, alive, and the next moment—*flick*—the light switches off and the person is gone. Here, then not here. The doctor looks over at the clock on the wall and quietly says, "Time of death, 11:19."

But the reality of death is not so crisp. Even when the dying is instantaneous, as from a catastrophic collision, death is not just the squelching of the heart, not just the end of oxygen to the brain, not just the cessation of energy in the body. It is the smothering of a veritable universe of living fibers, the death of billions of individual cells and trillions of connections among those cells. A constellation of memories is dissolved, as are habits, feelings, cravings, annoyances. Not just a body, but its constituent parts: ten long fingers and ten knobby toes, a playful mouth, eyes that can be piercing or despondent.

Why are so many people fascinated by Alzheimer's disease? Because it is not only a disease, but also a prism through which we can view life in ways not normally available to us. Through the Alzheimer's prism, we can experience life's constituent parts and understand better its resonances and quirks. And as the disease relentlessly progresses toward the final dimming of the sufferer, it forces us to experience death in a way it is rarely otherwise experienced. What is usually a quick flicker we see in super slow motion, over years. It is more painful than many people can even imagine, but it is also perhaps the most poignant of all reminders of why and how human life is so extraordinary. It is our best lens on the meaning of loss.

Like Emerson, Jonathan Swift did not live long enough with his progressive dementia to unravel completely. He did, though, die quite a few deaths along the way to his final passing. His late stages were marked by intensive walking, sometimes up to ten hours a day. He gradually lost access to nearly all his words and would rarely speak. Once, near the end, a servant picked up Swift's watch to find out the time. Curious, Swift managed to utter "Bring it here" and stared at the watch for some time. He also once reached for a knife; when it was taken away, he shrugged his shoulders and said, "I am what I am. I am what I am."

His last recorded words were spoken to his servant. He couldn't find the words that he wanted, and finally settled for "I am a fool." Swift died mourning the death of his own intellect. He died grieving for himself.

I had a dream three nights after Dad died: The telephone rang and I answered. Turning around I saw my father—no longer emaciated and ill with cancer, but round, rosy, and healthy. He put his arms around me and said, "I just want you to know that everything's all right."

Strange, but I had no such dream about Mother returning after her death. Alzheimer's had taken so much from her and from us that she, literally, didn't seem to linger here on earth. As my daughter said, "It's almost like Grandma said, 'I'm outta here!'" Who can blame her?

However, shortly after her death my father returned in a dream, wearing an absolutely terrible red plaid jacket. (Only mother could have gotten him to wear that thing! She loved red plaid.) He said that Mother had sent him to tell me they were together and all was well.

I learned to not be afraid to hurt. I learned to get all the help I needed in order to heal. As a result I'm beginning to remember the happier side of Mother.

—S.P.
Denver, Colorado

Chapter 16

THINGS TO AVOID

❧

Doctors cannot yet cure Alzheimer's, or prevent it, or even mask its symptoms for very long. But hundreds of studies have begun to produce a pointillist portrait of how people can help themselves— things to do for the body, mind, and spirit that *might* reduce the risk of getting the disease, or at least delay its onset:

Avoid head injuries.

Avoid fatty foods.

Avoid high blood pressure.

Eat foods rich in antioxidants, which eliminate damaging free-radical molecules. Eat, specifically: prunes, raisins, blueberries, blackberries, kale, strawberries, spinach, raspberries, brussels sprouts, plums, alfalfa sprouts, broccoli, beets, oranges, red grapes, red peppers, and cherries. (Foods listed according to their antioxidant content, in descending order.)

Eat foods rich in folic acid, and in vitamins B6, B12, C, and E.

Eat tuna, salmon, and other foods rich in fatty acids.

Don't drink too much alcohol. (A moderate amount might be slightly beneficial.)

Don't skimp on sleep. (Sleep is rejuvenating to the brain and the body; sleep seems to play a very important role in long-term memory formation.)

Exercise.

Maintain a high level of social contact (and consider marriage—one study shows fewer married people getting Alzheimer's).

If you are a woman past menopause, consider estrogen replacement therapy. (Some studies suggest it may reduce Alzheimer's incidence by as much as half.)

If you like to chew gum, continue chewing gum. (This is very tentative. One study suggests a mysterious connection between chewing and the health of hippocampal cells.)

If you regularly take nonsteroidal anti-inflammatory drugs such as ibuprofen for another reason, continue. (Some studies show a benefit.)

Get a thorough education.

Keep your mind active. Read, discuss, debate, create, play word games, do crossword puzzles, meet new people, learn new languages. Studies show that people with very high levels of education, while not immune from Alzheimer's, do tend to get the disease later than others.

Ancients in Greece and Rome did not have to be goaded into keeping their minds limber. They had no choice. By necessity, they relied on mind and memory to an extent that people today would find hard to believe. The men that Emerson admired in his journal—"L. Scipio knew the name of every man in Rome. . . . Seneca could say two thousand words in one hearing"—had no convenient alternative. There was no printing press, no pen and ink; the cumbersome wax tablet was the best external device they had. So the mind was always the default notebook of choice.

To put it to the most efficient use possible, the Greeks invented *mnemonics*—a technique to assist memory. The art of mnemonics was built around the observation that while the human capacity to remember ideas, language, and numbers seems frightfully limited, visual memory is nearly infallible. The hackneyed phrase "I never forget a face" turns out to be a literal fact of human biology; in tests running into the thousands of faces, there seems to be no limit to powers of recognition. By contrast, remembering a string of fifteen to twenty numbers is a strenuous chore.

The strange disparity between visual memory and word/number memory impressed Greek intellectuals somewhere around the fourth century B.C. The legend is that mnemonics was first demonstrated by the poet Simonides of Ceos (556–468 B.C.), the sole survivor in the collapse of a large banquet hall. Simonides had just stepped outside the hall to receive a message when the roof caved in and crushed everyone inside. To his surprise, the poet found that he was able to reel off a flawless list of the victims, and to identify each crushed body. He did this by recalling where each person had been sitting in the banquet hall. It was as if he had a tiny map of the banquet hall imprinted somewhere in his brain.

We all do. Neuroscientists would later discover that a particular region of the hippocampus is filled with "place cells" programmed to create cellular landscape maps from visual perception. While not photographically flawless in their registration of detail, these place cells help us recall the position of an object in relation to the position of other objects. Recall that in the very early stages of Ronald Reagan's illness, he turned to his wife and said, "Well, I've got to wait a minute. I'm not quite sure where I am." The early destruction of hippocampal place cells in Alzheimer's disease is the reason for sudden "Where-am-I?" moments. Much like a brittle old road map in the closet, the spatial map in Reagan's brain was disintegrating.

With only an intuitive understanding of place cells, the Greeks went on to develop a series of mnemonic devices rooted in the power of visual memory. Many were based on the architectural model that Simonides had inspired—a visualization of rooms in a home, for example, into which the mnemonist would "deposit" pieces of information: one name on a dining room table, another name in the fireplace, yet another in the hallway, and so on. Over time, people found that, with the right devices, the brain could be turned into a startlingly reliable reference tool.

Mnemonics proved to be a critical tool in the long human struggle toward enlightenment. So-called memory palaces and memory theaters were a dominant feature of the intellectual landscape for more than a thousand years, well through the Renaissance. The historian Frances Yates suggests that Shakespeare's Globe Theater was actually based on the model of a memory theater. "I come to the fields and vast palaces of memory," Saint Augustine wrote in *Confessions*. "Hidden there is whatever . . . has been deposited and placed on reserve and has not been swallowed up and buried in oblivion. When I am in this storehouse, I ask that it produce what

I want to recall, and immediately certain things come out; some things require a longer search, and have to be drawn out as it were from more recondite receptacles."

Today, we treat the brain differently. Even those who think for a living don't rely on it as a data storehouse. In place of the vast internal memory palace, we have Post-it Notes, steno notebooks, Palm Pilots, libraries, and the Internet. We are awash in external memory, upon which we have built edifying worlds of art, literature, science, law, and philosophy. The modern brain is saved primarily for synthesis of ideas, emotional impressions, rhetorical flair, and amusement.

In the transformation, we have surrendered some of memory's importance. In 2001, I do not need to remember a long list of names (I write them down), or the full text of a speech (I use note cards or a TelePrompTer), or every bone and blood vessel in the body (I can refer to a textbook). I do not need to know how to calculate a circumference (calculator), or even how to spell "calculator" (spell checker). I just need to know that these information resources exist, and how to use them. This is one of the essential truths of the post-Gutenberg age: We live in a world of shared information and understanding—the challenge is not to know it all, but to know how to know. "Our age is retrospective," Emerson wrote in *Nature*. "It builds the sepulchres of the fathers. It writes biographies, histories, and criticism. The foregoing generations beheld God and nature face-to-face; we, through their eyes."

Shared understanding and memory is an obvious step forward in human civilization, but it is not without its trade-offs. Emerson's chief worry was that the flood of knowledge from others would cut us off from the wisdom of personal experience. But he was also very concerned by the steady loss of life-affirming skills due to the gradual adoption of more and more labor-saving and thought-saving conveniences. "The civilized man has built a coach," he said, "but has lost the use of his feet. He is supported on crutches, but lacks so much support of muscle. He has a fine Geneva watch, but he fails of the skill to tell the hour by the sun. . . . His notebooks impair his memory; his libraries overload his wit . . . and it may be a question whether machinery does not encumber; whether we have not lost by refinement some energy . . . some vigor of wild virtue."

It was not a new warning, even then. Plato had cautioned two thousand years before that the new tool of writing was "a recipe not for memory, but for reminder." He prophesied a world with more external knowledge and less internal proficiency: "If men learn this, it will implant forgetfulness in their souls: they will cease to exercise memory because they rely on that which is written."

The lesser-used mind does, almost inevitably, become a somewhat weaker instrument. Is it possible, in our superior modern world, with terabytes of instantly accessible knowledge and machines that practically think for us, that even healthy brains are in something of an insidious decline? We know that labor-saving devices like cars and washing machines have led to couch-potato lifestyles and a steady rise in obesity. What we don't recognize quite so readily is a corresponding link between the rise of external memory and a decrease in brain exertion. Not doing the mental work means not building those internal connections between neurons.

We use our brains to build great tools that make our lives safer, cleaner, longer, easier. But these same tools also dull our minds.

Not surprisingly, modern science has already risen to treat this emerging problem. The start of the twenty-first century saw neuroscientists classifying mild memory loss as a new disease: mild cognitive impairment (MCI). Society seems eager for this, already flocking to herbal tonics like adrafinil, deprenyl, gingko biloba, and piracetam as potential medical solutions to cognitive frustration.

It is intrinsically human to want to better ourselves with tools. But there may also be a price paid in the quest. Of all the quantitative perks acquired through technological progress—convenience, efficiency, longevity, the thrill of electronic contact—none add a whit to the one true qualitative pursuit: to make life more meaningful. To the contrary, the manic chase of material improvements can easily crowd out the pursuit of meaning.

If material gains are spiritually empty, the obverse is also true: hardship or loss can offer a window to spiritual transcendence. "The helpless victim of a hopeless situation," Viktor Frankl says, "facing a fate he cannot change, may rise above himself, may grow beyond himself, and by so doing, change himself."

Finding meaning through loss: it is an observation that anyone who has flunked a test, skinned a knee, or lost a friend can easily relate to. Meaning through loss is one of life's chief—and most reliable and universal—paradoxes.

While it is perfectly understandable, then, to want to *overcome* loss—and we all yearn to, and always will—it's equally important to remember loss's utility. If Alzheimer's is, as I have already argued, one of our best lenses on life and the meaning of loss, then the medical war on Alzheimer's presents two substantial dangers:

1. We may get so distracted by the goal of defeating Alzheimer's that we lose sight of the disease's essential humanity.

2. In winning the war, should we be so fortunate, we will also be eliminating the lens that has served humanity so well for thousands of years. Defeating Alzheimer's will be like defeating winter. Once it is gone, we'll face less hardship, but we'll also have lost one of life's reliable touchstones.

The same lesson applies to other scientific ambitions. Since we now have the power to overcome nature—to tinker with our own genetics—it is crucial to try to realize what we'll be giving up as we overcome our limitations. The burden ultimately rests with nonscientists to insist on a full exploration of these issues, since very few scientists will stop to explore them on their own accord.

One scientific movement that presses ahead without a full consideration of the ramifications is called *posthumanism*. "We are at the point of remaking human biology," Gregory Stock, director of the Science, Technology and Society program at UCLA, wrote in 1998. Stock, author of *Metaman: The Merging of Humans and Machines into a Global Superorganism,* was talking about the virtues of germline engineering—the creation of *knock-out people* by adding and subtracting traits as we see fit. Posthumanists ask: What qualities in particular would you like your next child to have? They want to take the design process away from natural selection and put it in the hands of individual human beings.

Now that we have transgenic mice with muscular dystrophy and asthma, it is no great stretch of the imagination to think about scientists manipulating human genes to enhance the prowess of the brain. Is the power of memory a gene-based trait? The man with the perfect memory, A. R. Luria's remarkable human subject S., would have said so. Both his parents also had otherworldly memories, as did a cousin. In 1995, Tim Tully, a scientist at Cold Spring Harbor on Long Island, kicked off the brain-enhancement era with an insect counterpart to S., a transgenic fly that forms scent memories much faster than ordinary flies and keeps them forever. He called it the fly with photographic memory.

Advocates of germline engineering imagine a world not too far away that will be populated by "posthumans." Our post-human children, they predict, will have faster, more reliable brains, germ-resistant bodies, and other adaptations that make us clearly better. The apotheosis of posthumanism is the death of death: the "manufacturing" of an unlimited amount of time for humans to enjoy life. "I am now working on immortality," University of California at Irvine evolutionary biologist Michael Rose told *Wired* magazine for its January 2000 issue. Rose is not the only serious scientist aiming to obliterate life's ultimate boundary. The Silicon Valley genetic engineering firm Geron is trying to unlock the secrets of telomerase, an enzyme found in sperm cells and cancer cells that seems to be the key to keeping such cells youthful. Another corporate stem-cell researcher, William Haseltine, founder of Human Genome Sciences, predicted that this research arc will lead to what he called a "transubstantiated future" for human beings within seventy years—meaning that the generation born in the late twentieth century could be the last to face death as an inevitability.

The number of obstacles to immortality make it impossible to guess seriously about whether it will ever happen. But its plausibility demands that we begin to ask: *Do we want this?* Do we want perfect memories and endless lives?

In *Gulliver's Travels,* Gulliver changes his mind about the glories of immortality after he sees that it is fraught with problems. But what about a *clean* immortality, one that would actually work well? What if, short of eternity, we could live four hundred relatively healthy years instead of seventy-five? Imagine being able to stick around and see your children's children's children's children's children's children's children's children's children's children's children's children's children's children's children's children's children's children. If we could do so in sound mind and relatively sound body, without being too much of a burden on our families or our communities, we could indeed live out the original aspirations of Gulliver—to first acquire great material wealth and a formidable education and then spend subsequent lifetimes putting those resources to great use, pursuing modernization, universal health care, and other high-minded humanistic pursuits.

It sounds wonderful, and perhaps would be in many ways. But it would also be a fundamental challenge to how we understand ourselves, and it is almost impossible to imagine the ramifications—good and bad—for humanity.

To be human as we know it today is to experience the cycles of life, to experience great loss and pain—not just the pain of tragedy but the pain of inevitability. The essential joy of life is embedded in our mortality, and in our forgetting. How we would be changing ourselves if we decide to cross the Rubicon to posthumanity is impossible to tell. Life as we know it is an incalculably complicated web of interdependence. Species rely on other species for survival, and abilities and capacities are balanced out by other abilities or inabilities. But more important than the unintended consequences of manipulating DNA is the essential loss of humanity that happens as soon as we begin doing so. As Plato, Nietzsche, Emerson, and others have argued, humanity is something we should savor for all of its frailties as well as its abilities. The only true wisdom, said Joseph Campbell in a paraphrase of the Caribou Eskimo Shaman Igjugarjuk, "lives far from mankind, out in the great loneliness, and can be reached only through suffering. Privation and suffering alone open the mind to all that is hidden to others."

One cannot appreciate life's majesty without experiencing its hardships. In the Wim Wenders film *Wings of Desire,* angels abandon a perfect but colorless heaven for a life on earth with all of its Technicolor problems. Perfection is boring and lifeless; reality, with its grit and loss, is fulfilling.

Perhaps no human being has experienced this hard truth as completely as S., the man with the perfect memory. Recall that although he remembered everything he ever came into contact with, S. could make sense of almost nothing. Simple stories baffled him, and even people's faces were difficult for him to place because he recorded so much information about each moment's expression. S. spent his entire life looking at everything with a magnifying glass, taking in so many details that he could never pull back far enough to make sense of the patterns. He saw the trees but not the forest. "The big question for him, and the most troublesome," wrote Luria, "was how he could learn to forget. . . . there were numerous details in the text, each of which gave rise to new images that led him far afield, until his mind was a virtual chaos. How could he avoid these images, prevent himself from seeing details which kept him from understanding a simple story? . . . The problem of forgetting . . . became a torment for him."

S. tried everything he could think of to forget. He tried writing things down, reasoning that if he wrote something down he wouldn't need to remember it, would be free to forget it. "But I got nowhere," he reported. "For in my mind, I continued to see what I'd written." Even when he tried writing everything down on the same sort of paper with the same pencil, the information would not blur together as he'd hoped. He kept seeing it all distinctly in his mind's eye.

So he tried burning it, literally. He would record information on paper, set it afire and then watch the paper burn into a charred scrap. But that didn't work either. In his mind, he still saw the information under the black char.

The image of a man literally burning information in his struggle to forget is perhaps the most poignant way to marvel at memory and its gorgeous fragility. Our limitations *are* our strengths. Perhaps it is true that with very slight modifications our brains and bodies could be made virtually invulnerable. But in escaping loss we would also be escaping life.

❦

We are like the dead in Thornton Wilder's Our Town. *As we drift away from life, no longer fearing to die nor craving and striving for our place in the sun, we can look back on the world that was, and see it as a whole.*

—Morris Friedell

❦

Chapter 17

THE MICE ARE SMARTER

✥

Washington Hilton, Washington, D.C.: July 2000

Near the entrance to this hotel nineteen years ago, John Hinckley crouched to his knees and opened fire on Ronald Reagan and his staff, as the President left the building following a speech to labor union delegates.

Now Reagan's daughter Maureen returned to this place of dreadful memory to address another assembly, the World Alzheimer Congress. It was the largest-ever professional gathering on the disease.

Her father was in the final stages. He had stopped talking, and was having some trouble walking. Maureen, meanwhile, had emerged as a powerful voice in the crusade against Alzheimer's, skillfully using her family's public tragedy to raise awareness and to campaign for more government research funding. In the Hilton's expansive basement conference center, she joined physicians, nurses, counselors, and more than three thousand researchers for a broad review of the latest scientific developments and caregiving techniques.

There was also a pack of journalists. Everyone wanted to hear the bulletin about Dale Schenk's vaccine—about how the knock-out mice were getting *smarter*.

The vaccine really seemed to be working, at least in animals. A number of labs around the world had replicated Schenk's results, and one had gone further. At the University of South Florida, researchers gave vaccine injections to the knock-out mice and then months later tested their memories. They found just what they'd hoped: In water mazes, the mice did not bumble about the way they had been genetically designed to; instead, they learned how to navigate the maze just like normal mice. They were normal now, apparently. For these humanized mice, at least, Alzheimer's disease was now preventable.

This has to be taken in context, of course: Mice don't really get Alzheimer's, so they can't really be cured of it. The mice whose brains had been artificially contaminated with plaques had now been artificially cleansed of them; it *seemed* like a step in the right direction, but one had to remember that a disease that only exists in humans can only be cured in humans.

In a small room crowded with microphones and cables, Schenk and his boss Ivan Lieberburg gave a briefing to an international press corps, sharing even better news: Phase I safety trials had ended with no observable side effects of the vaccine on humans. Phase II multidose human trials would therefore soon commence, this time to test the drug's effectiveness. They could have the first results in as few as eighteen months—at the end of 2001. That's when the world would first get an inkling of whether or not this was going to be a useful treatment for Alzheimer's, or a cure, or nothing at all.

That same morning, Schenk shared the fine points with fellow researchers in the hotel's underground ballroom. Reviewing the data from follow-up studies on mice, guinea pigs, rabbits, and monkeys, he said it was now clear that the vaccine was working exactly as they predicted: The injected beta-amyloid was prompting the immune systems to produce targeted antibodies, a small portion of which were crossing the blood-brain barrier and binding directly with beta-amyloid in the brain. Then the offending substances were effortlessly being cleared away as cellular trash.

Even though most of these scientists had known something about the vaccine for almost a year, many still seemed startled to hear Schenk's presentation. Just a few years earlier, no one could have even imagined that anyone would be talking about a potential cure so soon. It was as if President Kennedy had called for a moon landing within a decade and NASA soon reported back that they were about to land men on Mars.

After the talk, as everyone filed out of the large ballroom to head for the smaller specialized sessions of the day, one researcher turned to another and asked, "So if this thing works, is the game over?"

On the surface, of course, that was the big question: Will clearing the plaques abolish this disease? Going deeper, though, there was a more fundamental question raised by this vaccine's sudden emergence: Why had Dale Schenk been the only person on earth to think of it? And why had he been laughed out of the room when he first shared his thought?

It was a variation on the recurring theme of outcast scientists. Why was Stanley Prusiner vilified for years over his unusual—but as it turned out, correct—idea about infectious prions? Why was Allen Roses denied grants for follow-up research to his important ApoE discovery? Why was Ruth Itzhaki ignored in her pursuit of herpes simplex virus 1? Why was Meta Neumann ignored? Alois Alzheimer? Why does the culture of science seem to so often punish the most inventive?

Science is ultimately a human endeavor. Its language is uniform, its methods are strict, but the questions posed and the analysis applied are as idiosyncratic as love affairs and operas and football games. There is, thus, an organic incongruity. Scientific discovery is, and always will be, an inherently clumsy matter as scientists attempt to fit the round peg of humanity into the square hole of objectivity.

The most adventuresome of these scientists, pushing against the limits of comprehension, are inevitably bruised by the friction. They are threatening existing power structures and, perhaps more dangerously, jeopardizing people's basic understanding of the world around them. They are casting doubt on "truths" on top of which people have built their careers, and around which they have oriented their lives. If a scientist named Galileo suggests in the early seventeenth century that the earth revolves around the sun, the veracity of that statement does not matter nearly as much to his peers as how its consideration may immediately affect their lives. So Galileo is forced to recant. That particular truth will have to wait.

The persistent challenge of science, and all edification, is to minimize the friction: to encourage the pursuit of new ideas while helping to sustain the integrity of people's lives.

Other enticing developments were revealed at the July 2000 conference. Researchers from the Mayo Clinic had just produced the first knock-out mouse with both plaques *and* tangles. Several drug companies had isolated the brain enzyme that seems to convert harmless APP into malicious beta-amyloid; perhaps a drug could arrest that process. "There's a smell of success in the air," said the NIA's Marcelle Morrison-Bogorad.

Hundreds of more mundane, if still important, presentations were also taking place. In the Jefferson Room, New York University's Yaakov Stern was comparing the hippocampal memory network with the prefrontal memory network; in the Monroe Room the University of Texas's Rachel Doody was reviewing the limited success of Aricept and other similar drugs.

The real heart of the conference, though, was in the free-for-all poster sessions at midday. In a vast, low-ceilinged room, the entire community of researchers came together every day at noon to eat bland sandwiches and browse the hundreds of large bulletin board presentations lined up in long rows. These were novel bits of research from experiments, many of which were still in progress. It was old-fashioned science, with data open for review and critique. Charts were pinned next to graphs, were pinned next to microscopic photographs, were pinned next to project summaries, were pinned next to tentative conclusions, were pinned next to contact information. Gerontologists from Sweden huddled in front of one poster, right next to a group of microbiologists from New Orleans. There was barely enough room to squeeze through.

The variety of material was fierce.

Poster #40, presented by Tohru Hasegawa, discussed the potential preventative effect of Japanese green tea.

Poster #96, presented by R. Distl & V. Meske, revealed that microdensitofluorometrically determined free cholesterol is higher in tangle-bearing neurons than in tangle-free neurons.

Poster #168, presented by Jennifer W. Catania *et al*, reviewed the genetics of Alzheimer's disease in the Caribbean Hispanic population.

The paradox of these poster sessions, and of the entire scientific portion of the conference, was that amidst all the data and ideas the *disease* was nowhere to be found. Science had fragmented it into almost unrecognizable shards—cholinergic transmitters, vascular risk factors, nicotinic receptors, aspartyl proteases, synaptic plasticity in mice, and on and on. The crowd had the patina of a large cohesive community, but was really a collection of superbly focused specialists—most of whom barely knew how to talk to anyone outside their constricted microfield. In the name of science, good science, they were far too close to the trees to see the forest.

It would take a trailblazer to try to show them the panoramic view. On the last day of the conference, in the last row of the poster session bazaar, the very final display stood out from the others. It had an entirely different flavor:

#1231

POTENTIAL FOR REHABILITATION IN ALZHEIMER'S

Standing beside #1231 was a man in a brown tweed coat and a graying beard: Morris Friedell, the college professor from Santa Barbara. Struggling to maintain his dignity and his wits as Alzheimer's slowly advanced, he had made the long journey from out west to present his ideas to the community of scientists. Until now, conversations about his ambitious ideas had mostly been limited to fellow victims, caregivers, friends, and family. His dream was to share them with professionals. He thought he might be onto something important. From his poster:

Central hypothesis:
The typical qualitative symptoms of mild to moderate Alzheimer's, gross forgetfulness, disorientation, and loss of abstraction and judgment, stem from quantitative decrements in processing capacity underlying these functions. Since patients retain substantial strength in procedural memory and memory for emotionally significant events, there is major potential for rehabilitation through relearning activities using a greater number of simpler steps.

The complex presentation contained fragments of neurobiology, sports psychology, and spirituality. There were quotes from Frankl, Thoreau, and Lao-tzu ("In the pursuit of learning, every day something is acquired. In the pursuit of Tao, every day something is dropped.") There were poems from victims, a color copy of a de Kooning from 1984, and a diagram from the psychologist A. R. Luria demonstrating rehabilitation of a brain-damaged patient. Morris's own PET scan report was also pinned up on display. Appended to the conclusion was a note: "I welcome feedback and discussion. I'm staying at——. Phone is——. E-mail is——."

But his poster drew almost no interest. Researchers peered at it for a second and moved on. They didn't know what to make of this unorthodox exhibit, and seemed anxious to find something more technical and less ambiguous—something closer to their own specialty. There was, of course, no one at this conference—or any conference—who specialized in rehabilitating Alzheimer's patients. That's just why Morris was there.

He gently looked around at the sea of researchers passing him by. "I feel like I'm living a dual life right now," he said quietly. "On the one hand, I feel like a kid at a science fair. But I also feel like a kind of a ghost, hovering here as an afterthought."

Selfishly, I was happy that he was there. It was our first face-to-face exchange ever, after about a year of long-distance interaction. We had corresponded via E-mail mostly, except for the one day several months before when Morris called to talk. On the phone, we had spoken for a while about his disease and my book. I had thanked him for his many insights, for introducing me to Viktor Frankl and tipping me off to Emerson's dementia. He seemed interested in my aim to write a biography of the disease, and eager to help. We agreed to stay in touch, to keep exchanging ideas.

Now I was eager to continue our discussion. The poster scene, though, was a little too chaotic for a real conversation. We agreed to meet the next day for lunch.

Over sandwiches and coffee at a grill across town, we climbed back into some of our shared curiosities, starting with rehabilitation. He was of course not talking literally about beating this disease with brain exercises, but about minimizing and slowing the cognitive loss by adapting to it.

Why shouldn't Alzheimer's patients get as much conditioning as stroke victims, for example? The disease's ultimate mortality should not automatically annul patients' expectations of living the fullest possible life for the longest possible time.

Alzheimer's is a very slow disease, and there was no particular reason to settle for a passive approach of managing loss—which was often tantamount to hospice care in slow motion. If drugs like Aricept could lead to marginal improvements, it was tantalizing to imagine what a professional rehabilitation program could do. Intensive rehab, in the spirit of what knee and hip surgery patients go through routinely, had just never been considered before in Alzheimer's disease. In the new era of people discovering their disease very early on, the idea made abundant sense.

Morris's proposal was not a first draft. "My previous approach to rehabilitation," he said, "was to substitute intense meaning and emotional organization for [cold analysis], refining your sense of what's important to compensate for your inability to deal with everything.

"I've revised that. If a person has a block in problem solving and it gets too emotional then their memories can get *more* scattered.

"Most of the focus on brain injury has to do with the frontal lobes—auto accidents with younger people and such. People with mild Alzheimer's still have frontal lobes that are functioning very well. They know what they want to do, but they are not able to learn anything from the attempts. There is some work with the Montessori approach to problem solving with people with dementia that's been encouraging. Rather than relearning to pay attention to the problem, I suggest a reeducation vaguely inspired by

Montessori: Do something that's extremely simple, just to get into a confidence mind-set—stringing one or two beads, or something like that. And gradually learn to solve problems in new, simpler ways.

"The spirit of *feng shui* is interesting. I tell other early-stage patients, 'The practical application of my theory is to start getting rid of your clutter,' and this strikes a chord in the way that my other ideas haven't. Eliminate physical clutter as a path to get rid of mental clutter. I'm saying, 'simplify, simplify, simplify'—just like Thoreau."

We talked for two hours. Some of his ideas I understood, some I did not, entirely. Morris sometimes paused for a while, and had to occasionally struggle to stay on track. There was no question that he was slowly succumbing to the disease. Mostly, though, I was left with the impression that he was onto something important, that he *did* understand his own unraveling in a way I would not have ever imagined possible when I first started to learn about this disease. Throughout our lunch, I repeatedly encountered a *frisson* of realization that in several years of research, the most thought-provoking discussions I'd had about Alzheimer's were with one of its victims.

I realized that, in a peculiar way, Morris had rehabilitated *me*—and my understanding of Alzheimer's. When I started my research, I conceived of a book that might, on the one hand, catalogue the horrors of Alzheimer's, and on the other, relay the hopeful story of the race to cure the disease.

I still respected that dichotomy, still feared the disease, and still hoped for a cure, of course—as did Morris. But I also now realized that the story of Alzheimer's is in some ways exactly the opposite of my original premise: It is a condition specific to humans and as old as humanity that, like nothing else, acquaints us with life's richness by ever so gradually drawing down the curtains. Only through modern science has this poignancy been reduced to a plain horror, an utterly unhuman circumstance.

It wouldn't be fair to say that I had transcended the disease in the same way that Morris obviously had, or in the way that Emerson and de Kooning admirably had. After all, I was still only an observer. But it's worth noting that, personally, I migrated over several years' time from morbid fascination and dread of Alzheimer's to a new kind of peace and reconciliation.

As this realization unfolded, I thought of another presentation at the conference, given by the social worker and author Lisa Snyder. In the Indonesian island of Bali, she reported, there is a powerful myth of life cycles that centers on memory:

Babies are born with no memory. They gather memories as they grow. As they get old they lose these memories so that they can be reborn again in a void.

All of these things I was thinking about as I drove Morris back to his hotel room. I told him again how much I appreciated his ideas, and wished him well.

Then, just before I dropped him off, Morris asked me if we'd ever spoken before today.

EPILOGUE

～

*I cannot promise you everlasting life, but I can promise you life
RIGHT NOW.*

—Bruce Springsteen

Two blocks from my home in Brooklyn is the main entrance to
Prospect Park, an arrow-shaped 526-acre retreat from urban intensity. It is a wondrous place, with a mile-long hilly green meadow, a
great lake, and the last surviving natural forest in Brooklyn. There
is a working nineteenth-century carousel, a band shell for concerts,
picnic tables and barbecue pits, a horse trail, plenty of swing sets,
and wild geese. About six million times a year, people come here
to find themselves.

The park was designed by Calvert Vaux and Frederick Law
Olmsted from 1865 to 1873, just after the pair had completed
their work on Central Park in Manhattan. They had planned to

link the two parks with a ten-mile-long, tree-shadowed "parkway," but could not sell that part of their vision. Still, Olmsted considered his Brooklyn park to be a crowning achievement. "I am prouder of it than anything I have had to do with," he remarked on a later visit.

Olmsted was a champion of urban beautification in the mid-to-late nineteenth century and is now considered the founder of American landscape architecture. He is responsible for an astounding number of treasured urban American refuges, including Chicago's Jackson Park, Boston's Emerald Necklace, and Louisville's Cherokee Park. "The further progress of civilization is to depend mainly upon the influences by which men's minds and characters will be affected while living in large towns," Olmsted argued. A city park, he insisted, must help the resident escape "the devouring eagerness and intellectual strife of town life."

He was abundantly influenced by Emerson, whom he read avidly and met with early in his career. His was an unflinchingly Emersonian notion. "What we want to gain," said Olmsted, "is tranquillity and rest to the mind."

A year or so after Olmsted finished his work on Prospect Park, he moved to Washington, D.C., to design the grounds of the U.S. Capitol, which he worked on for fifteen years, up until 1889. Not long after that, as he neared seventy years old, he started to have memory problems, very subtle at first and then, gradually, more disabling. On the way to pivotal meetings, he would ask his sons to remind him of key names and project details. Then, in North Carolina, he was discovered writing virtually the same letter over and over again to his patron George Vanderbilt, his short-term memory apparently obliterated.

In 1895, at age seventy-three, he wrote his son John, his devoted right hand for twenty years: "I see that I ought no longer to be entrusted to carry on important business for the firm alone." Olmsted retreated into seclusion in Maine (in a house designed by Emerson's cousin, William Ralph Emerson). As John attempted to keep his father tangentially involved in the firm's projects, he made a firm, practical suggestion. "It would be well for you," he wrote his father, "to review the letters we have written you since you went to Deer Isle each time before you write your daily letter to us. . . . [you should] constantly bear in mind that your memory for current events is no longer a working basis for your thoughts."

Things became much darker. Olmsted became paranoid, accusing John of executing a "coup." In 1898, at age seventy-six, it got bad enough that he had to be moved into McLean Asylum, in Waverly, Massachusetts, where he would remain confined until his death in 1903.

Alzheimer's is, in itself, a sort of mental confinement—the sufferer is incarcerated within the collapsing neural structures that he has taken a lifetime to build. But Olmsted, through his own work, inadvertently lived out the metaphor in literal terms. He was imprisoned not just within his own collapsing mind, but also in his own design: Olmsted had created the 275-acre grounds for McLean two decades before. At first, he was bitterly aware of the irony. But by the time he died, he had forgotten not only about his design of McLean, but also about landscapes altogether.

We have not forgotten about him. It has been the great triumph of civilization to compensate for the limits of human life and memory, to extend the fruits of one person's intellect beyond its natural life. Olmsted's magnificent creations have lasted a full century since his decline and are set to last many more. Part of the further progress of civilization will be to help care for those who are truly losing themselves—not to overcome their humanity, but to help them find comfort in it. Just to the right of Prospect Park's main entrance is Prospect Park Residence, a large old apartment building that has recently been renovated and transformed into an assisted-living facility. Many of the residents are in one or another stage of progressive dementia. Through the windows of their apartments and especially through their daily walks into the large park, the residents who are forgetting themselves are finding the peace that they so desperately need in their decline. Through Olmsted's natural landscapes, in a way beyond what he had imagined, they have found tranquillity and rest to the mind.

ACKNOWLEDGMENTS

There is a woman whom I have never met, whose name I do not know. Let me acknowledge her first, because it was her forgetting that started all this. Eating lunch alone one day in my neighborhood taqueria, I found myself absorbed by a nearby conversation about this woman with early-onset Alzheimer's who could no longer recognize her own husband. I closed my eyes and tried to imagine myself as that husband, and then stumbled back to my office determined to learn more about this disease.

Listening to public radio in my kitchen, I have heard authors from time to time insist that they didn't really choose their book topics—that it's more like the books chose *them*. This is not the sort of thing I expected would ever happen to me.

I am blessed to have Sloan Harris for a literary agent. This book simply could not have happened without him. Much of Sloan's insight into this project, sadly, came out of firsthand experience with the decline of his own grandmother, Louise Walker, to whom I also want to pay tribute.

Bill Thomas, at Doubleday, provided the perfect nest for the fledgling work, and proved to be a masterful and nurturing editor.

I am indebted to Karen Duff, at the Nathan Kline Institute, for her patient tutorials on the molecular biology of Alzheimer's and the politics of that community.

For help unearthing details of Emerson's decline, thanks to Randall Albright, Howard Callaway, Morris Friedell, Roberto Piccoli, and Joel Porte.

Excavation of the ancient history of senility was facilitated by John Baines, Peter Butrica, Lawrence H. Feldman, Joan Ferry, Carol Fleming-Huskisson, François Hinard, Allen Koenigsberg, Julie Langford-Johnson, Russell A. Johnson, James Lawrence, Gert-Jan Lokhorst, David Lupher, Willard L. Marmelzat, Michael Meckler, Ernest Moncada, Tim Parkin, Elaine Perry, George Pesely, James M. Pfundstein, Gil Renberg, Patrick Rourke, Røy Starling, Juergen Stowasser, and Carl Widstrand.

Steven Johnson and James Ryerson, both of *Feed* magazine, spurred the material on memory molecules and Luria's patient S. András Szántó advanced my understanding of the relationship between identity and the artistic process for the chapter on de Kooning.

Thanks to Jed Levine, Tony Yang Lewis, Julie Rosenberg, Stefanie Roth, Judy Joseph, and Irving Brickman for a gentle introduction to the world of caregiving. I am particularly grateful to Irving for his kindness, conferred even as he faced the cancer that ended his life before the completion of this book.

Carla Flaherty generously shared her journal about her father's decline. Dan Paris, Geri Hall, and dozens of other regulars on the Alzheimer List gave me a better education than I could have hoped for. Thanks also to Julie Miller at the Alzheimer Association.

Heiko Braak and Kelly Del Tredici supplied key neuropathological papers, and Dorothy Rice furnished economic data and estimates. For historical guidance, thanks to Matthias M. Weber. Paulette Michaud and Jeffrey Toward were generous to share their transcripts of interviews with early-stage patients. John Trojanowski and Virginia Lee spent some of their valuable time educating a neophyte.

I am grateful to Neil Levi for sharing his translation-in-progress of a biography of Alois Alzheimer. Michael Strong let me read his fascinating dissertation on James Joyce and neuroscience. Richard Gehr opened the door to Nietzsche.

Bruce Feiler, Gersh Kuntzman, Andrew Shapiro, and Eamon Dolan are cherished confidants and advisers. Richard Shenk gave invaluable support. Thanks to Joanne Cohen and Sidney Cohen and Peggy and David Beers for reading early drafts. I am also very grateful to Teri Steinberg for her powerful encouragement and insight, and to Kendra Harpster for editorial assistance. Thanks to Apple Computer for so quickly replacing my laptop after it mysteriously caught on fire.

For his music, I thank Keith Jarrett.

For help with the manuscript in its late stages, I am indebted to Andrew Hoffman, Linda Steinman, Roy Kreitner, Daniel Radosh, Gina Duclayan, Tom Inck, Ivan Oransky, and Tom Inglesby. Nick Moore, John Holzman, and Jon Shenk served as much-needed compasses in the harrowing final days.

Acknowledgments

Word by word, chapter by chapter, my brother Joshua Wolf Shenk helped me make this a much better book.

As ever, I am grateful to my wife, Alexandra Beers, for her wisdom and friendship. This book was written in the glowing home I share with Alex and the incomparable Lucy Beers Shenk. Lucy: I'm all finished with my chapters now. Let's go play.

RESOURCES FOR PATIENTS AND FAMILIES

✌

For families stranded on the island of Alzheimer's disease, the initial feeling can be one of utter desolation. Many soon discover, though, that there are a host of extraordinary provisions available—medical and social services, support groups, books, and products for safety and security—that can make the long stay somewhat less perplexing and more comfortable. Below is a selected guide to some of these aids. (For more information, including medical research updates and links to the surfeit of online resources, visit www.theforgetting.com on the World Wide Web.)

PHONE HOTLINES
Alzheimer's Society
0845 300 0336
www.alzheimers.org.uk
Provides a full range of information and pointers to local services in England, Wales and Northern Ireland

Alzheimer Scotland - Action on Dementia

freephone helpline 0800 317817 www.alzscot.org

www.alzscot.org

Provides a full range of information and pointers to local services in Scotland

Carers National Association

0207 490 8818

Provides information on all aspects of caring

Age Concern England

0208 679 8000

Provides information and advice for older people, particularly on eligibility for social/health benefits

Alzheimer's Disease International

0207 620 3011

www.alz.co.uk

Provides contact details for Alzheimer Associations throughout the world

BOOKS

General

Alzheimer's at Your Fingertips, by Hary Cayton, Dr. Nori Graham and Dr. James Warner. Class Publishing, 1998

The 36-Hour Day: A Family Guide to Caring for Persons with Alzheimer Disease, Related Dementing Illnesses, and Memory Loss in Later Life, by Nancy L. Mace and Peter V. Rabins. John's Hopkins University Press, 2001.

Introducing Dementia: The Essential Facts and Issues of Care, by David Sutcliffe. Age Concern Books, 2001.

Living with Alzheimer's Disease and Similar Conditions, by Gordon Wilcock. Penguin Books, 1999

For children
What's Wrong With Grandma? A Family's Experience with Alzheimer's, by Margaret Shawer and Jeffrey K. Bagby. Prometheus Books, 1996.

Financial/Legal
Managing Other People's Money, by Penny Letts. Age Concern Books, 1998.

Your Rights 2000-2001: A Guide to Money Benefits for Older People, by Sally West. Age Concern Books, 2000.

Nutrition
Soft Options; For Adults Who Have Difficulty Chewing, by Rita Greer. Souvenir Press, 1998

Memoirs
Iris: A Memoir of Iris Murdoch, by John Bayley. Abacus, 1999.

Remind Me Who I Am Again, by Linda Grant, Granta Books, 1998

SOURCES

◦

By subject, in order of appearance.

Ralph Waldo Emerson

Baker, Carlos. *Emerson Among the Eccentrics: A Group Portrait.* New York: Penguin, 1996.

Bok, Edward. *The Americanization of Edward Bok: An Autobiography.* 1920. Reprint, New York: Pocket Books, 1965.

Cabot, James Elliot. *Memoir of Ralph Waldo Emerson.* 1887. Reprint, New York: AMS Press, 1965.

Emerson, Edward Waldo. *Emerson in Concord: A Memoir.* 1889. Reprint, Detroit: Gale Research Co., 1970.

Emerson, Lydia Jackson. *The Selected Letters of Lydia Jackson Emerson 1802–1892.* Edited by Delores Bird Carpenter. Columbia: University of Missouri Press, 1987.

Emerson, Ralph Waldo. *The Letters of Ralph Waldo Emerson.*

Edited by Eleanor M. Tilton. Vol. 10, *1870–1881*. New York: Columbia University Press, 1995.

———. "Notebook IT." In *The Topical Notebooks of Ralph Waldo Emerson,* edited by Susan Sutton Smith. Columbia: University of Missouri Press, 1990.

———. *Essays: First Series.* 1841. Reprint, Philadelphia: David McKay, 1890.

———. *Natural History of the Intellect.* 1893. Reprint, New York: Solar Press, 1995.

———. *The Journals and Miscellaneous Notebooks of Ralph Waldo Emerson.* Edited by Joel Porte. Cambridge: Harvard University Press, 1982.

———. *The Journals of Ralph Waldo Emerson, 1864–1876.* Edited by Edward Waldo Emerson and Waldo Emerson Forbes. New York: Houghton Mifflin, 1909–1914.

Garnett, Richard. *The Life of Ralph Waldo Emerson.* 1888. Reprint, New York: Haskell House Publishers, 1974.

Gregg, Edith E. W., ed. *The Letters of Ellen Tucker Emerson.* Kent, Ohio: Kent State University Press, 1982.

McAleer, John. *Ralph Waldo Emerson: Days of Encounter.* Boston: Little, Brown, 1984.

Richardson, Robert. *Emerson: The Mind on Fire.* Berkeley: University of California Press, 1995.

Russell, Phillips. *Emerson: The Wisest American.* New York: Brentano's, 1929.

Sealts, Merton M. *Emerson on the Scholar.* Columbia: University of Missouri Press, 1992.

Thayer, James Bradley. *A Western Journey with Mr. Emerson.* 1884. Reprint, Port Washington, N.Y.: Kennikat Press, 1971.

Alois Alzheimer and Emil Kraepelin

Berrios, G. E., and H. L. Freeman. *Alzheimer and the Dementias.* London: Royal Society of Medicine Services Limited, 1991.

Bick, Katherine, *et al. The Early Story of Alzheimer's Disease: Translation of the Historical Papers by Alois Alzheimer, Oskar Fischer, Francesco Bonfiglio, Emil Kraepelin, Gaetano Perusini.* New York: Raven Press, 1987.

Brannon, William L. "Alois Alzheimer (1864–1915) I. Contributions to Neurology and Psychiatry. II. Dementia Before and After Alzheimer: A Brief History." *Journal of the South Carolina Medical Association* 90, no. 9 (September 1994).

Decker, Hannah S. *Freud in Germany.* New York: International Universities Press, 1977.

Lewey, F. H. "Alois Alzheimer." In *The Founders of Neurology.* Springfield, Ill.: Thomas, 1970.

Maurer, Konrad. *A Biography of Alois Alzheimer.* Translated by Neil Levi. New York: Columbia University Press, forthcoming.

——— *et al.* "Auguste D. and Alzheimer's Disease." *Lancet* 349 (24 May 1997).

Weber, Matthias M. "Alois Alzheimer, A Co-worker of Emil Kraepelin." *Journal of Psychiatric Research* 31, no. 6 (1997).

Weindling, Paul. *Health, Race and German Politics Between National Unification and Nazism 1870–1945.* Cambridge: Cambridge University Press, 1989.

Ancient History of Senility

Aristophanes, *The Clouds.* Published as E-text by the Internet Classics Archive, at http://classics.mit.edu/Aristophanes/clouds.html

Berchtold, N. C., and C. W. Cotman. "Evolution in the Conceptualization of Dementia and Alzheimer's Disease: Greco-Roman Period to the 1960s." *Neurobiology of Aging* 19, no. 3 (1998).

Cicero, *Selected Works.* Translated by Michael Grant. New York: Penguin Books, 1960.

Cohen, Gene D. "Historical Views and Evolution of Concepts." In *Alzheimer's Disease,* edited by Barry Reisberg. New York: The Free Press, 1983.

Falkner, Thomas M. and Judith de Luce. *Old Age in Greek and Latin Literature.* Albany: State University of New York Press, 1989.

Finger, Stanley. *Origins of Neuroscience.* New York: Oxford University Press, 1994.

Juvenal. *The Satires of Juvenal.* Translated by C. E. Ramsay. Cambridge, Mass.: Loeb Classical Library/Harvard University Press, 1918.

The New Oxford Annotated Bible. New York: Oxford University Press,

Oxford English Dictionary. Compact Edition. Oxford: Clarendon Press, 1971.

Parkin, Tim. "Out of Sight, Out of Mind: Elderly Members of the Roman Family." In *The Roman Family in Italy,* edited by Beryl Rawson and Paul Weaver. Oxford: Clarendon Press, 1997.

Plato. *Theaetetus.* Published as E-text by Project Gutenberg at www2.cddc.vt.edu/gutenberg/etext99/thtus10.txt

Sahagún, Bernardino de. *General History of the Things of New Spain: Florentine Codex.* Translation. Santa Fe, N.M.: School of American Research and University of Utah, 1950–1982.

The Tale of Sinhue and Other Ancient Egyptian Poems, 1940–1640 B.C. Translated by R. B. Parkinson. Oxford: Oxford University Press, 1997.

Torack, Richard M. "The Early History of Senile Dementia." In *Alzheimer's Disease,* edited by Barry Reisberg. New York: The Free Press, 1983.

Virgil. "Eclogue IX." In *Virgil's Works,* translated by J. W. Mackail. New York: Modern Library, 1950.

Xenophon. *Memorabilia.* Stuttgart: Teubner. 1969.

Ronald Reagan

Altman, Lawrence K. "Reagan's Twilight." *New York Times,* 5 October 1997.

"Maureen Reagan Says She Has Beaten Cancer." Associated Press. 4 May 1998.

Sidey, Hugh. "The Sunset of My Life." *Time,* 14 November 1994.

Strober, Deborah Hart, and Gerald Strober. *Reagan: The Man and His Presidency.* New York: Houghton Mifflin, 1998.

Science of Mind and Memory

Alkon, Daniel L. *Memory's Voice: Deciphering the Mind-Brain Code.* New York: HarperCollins, 1994.

Baddeley, Alan. *Your Memory: A User's Guide.* New York: Macmillan, 1982.

Blakeslee, Dennis. "The Blood-Brain Barrier." Background briefing posted on 5 May 1997 at www.ama-assn.org/special/hiv/newsline/briefing/bbb.htm

Blakeslee, Sandra. "Tests with Rats Offer Clues to Why Memories Change." *Cleveland Plain Dealer,* 25 September 2000.

Bliss, Tim. "The Physiological Basis of Memory." In *From Brains to Consciousness: Essays on the New Sciences of Mind,* edited by Steven Rose. Princeton: Princeton University Press, 1998.

Bolles, Edmund Blair. *Remembering and Forgetting: Inquiries into the Nature of Memory.* New York: Walker and Company, 1988.

Carter, Rita. *Mapping the Mind.* Berkeley: University of California Press, 1998.

Dennett, Daniel C. *Consciousness Explained.* Boston: Little, Brown and Company, 1991.

Goldberg, Stephen. *Clinical Neuroanatomy Made Ridiculously Simple.* Miami: MedMaster, Inc., 1979.

Greenfield, Susan. "How Might the Brain Generate Consciousness." In *From Brains to Consciousness: Essays on the New Sciences of Mind, op. cit.*

Heindel, William C., and Stephen Salloway. "Memory Systems in the Human Brain." *Psychiatric Times,* June 1999.

Johnson, Steven. Interview with Steven Pinker. *Feed* magazine, at www.feedmag.com/re/re181_master.html

Mega, Michael S., *et al.* "The Limbic System: An Anatomic, Phylogenic, and Clinical Perspective." *Journal of Neuropsychiatry* 9 (3): 315–330 (1997).

Meier, Barry. "Industry's Next Growth Sector: Memory Lapses." *New York Times,* 4 April 1999.

Mithen, Steven. *The Prehistory of the Mind: The Cognitive Origins of Art and Science.* London: Thames and Hudson Ltd., 1996.

Noback, Charles R., *et al. The Human Nervous System: Structure and Function.* Philadelphia: Williams and Wilkins, 1996.

Parnavelas, John. "The Human Brain: 100 Billion Connected Cells." In *From Brains to Consciousness: Essays on the New Sciences of Mind, op. cit.*

Pinker, Steven. *How the Mind Works.* New York: W.W. Norton, 1999.

Rhodes, Richard. *Deadly Feasts: The "Prion" Controversy and the Public's Health.* New York: Touchstone, 1998.

Robbins, Trevor. "The Pharmacology of Thought and Emotion." In *From Brains to Consciousness: Essays on the New Sciences of Mind, op. cit.*

Rose, Steven. *The Making of Memory: From Molecules to Mind.* New York: Anchor, 1993.

Rose, Steven P. R. "How Brains Make Memories." In *Memory,* edited by Patricia Fara and Karalyn Patterson. New York: Cambridge University Press, 1998.

Schacter, Daniel L. *Searching for Memory.* New York: Basic Books, 1996.

Scheck, Barry. "Attorney Barry Scheck." *The Connection* (radio program), WBUR, Boston, 16 March 2000.

Sejnowski, Terrence J. "Memory and Neural Networks." In *Memory, op. cit.*

Selkoe, Dennis J. "Alzheimer's Disease: A Central Role for Amyloid." *Journal of Neuropathology and Experimental Neurology* 53, no. 5 (September 1994).

Smith, A. David. "Ageing of the Brain: Is Mental Decline Inevitable?" In *From Brains to Consciousness: Essays on the New Sciences of Mind, op. cit.*

Squire, Larry R. "Memory and Brain Systems." In *From Brains to Consciousness: Essays on the New Sciences of Mind, op. cit.*

Strong, Michael. "When Language Goes on Holiday: *Finnegans Wake,* Neuroscience, and Models of Subjectivity." Dissertation, University of Pennsylvania, forthcoming.

Tanner, J. M. *Fetus into Man: Physical Growth from Conception to Maturity.* Cambridge, Mass.: Harvard University Press, 1990.

Wilson, Barbara A. "When Memory Fails." In *Memory, op. cit.*

S., The Man with the Perfect Memory

Luria, A. R. *The Mind of a Mnemonist: A Little Book About a Vast Memory.* Translated from the Russian by Lynn Solotaroff. Cambridge: Harvard University Press, 1968.

The History of Disease

Aronowitz, Robert A. *Making Sense of Illness: Science, Society, and Disease.* New York: Cambridge University Press, 1998.

Gross, Charles G. *Brain Vision Memory: Tales in the History of Neuroscience.* Cambridge, Mass.: MIT Press, 1998.

Porter, Roy. *The Greatest Benefit to Mankind: A Medical History of Humanity.* New York: W.W. Norton, 1997.

Quétel, Claude. *The History of Syphilis.* Translated by Judith Braddock and Brian Pike. Baltimore: Johns Hopkins University Press, 1992.

Rosenberg, Charles E., and Janet Golden, eds. *Framing Disease: Studies in Cultural History.* New Brunswick, N.J.: Rutgers University Press, 1992.

Shorter, Edward. *A History of Psychiatry: From the Era of the Asylum to the Age of Prozac.* New York: John Wiley & Sons, 1997.

Temkin, Oswei. *The Double Face of Janus and Other Essays in the History of Medicine.* Baltimore: Johns Hopkins University Press, 1977.

Shift from "Senility" to "Alzheimer's Disease"

Cecil, Russell L., and Robert F. Loeb. *A Textbook of Medicine.* Philadelphia: W.B. Saunders, 1955.

Dillman, Rob. *Alzheimer's Disease: The Concept of Disease and the Construction of Medical Knowledge.* Amsterdam: Thesis Publishers, 1990.

Fox, Patrick. "From Senility to Alzheimer's Disease: The Rise of the Alzheimer's Disease Movement." *Milbank Quarterly* 67, Issue 1 (1989).

HISTNEUR-L, The History of Neuroscience Internet Forum: http:www.melsch.ucla.edu/sam/bri/archives/histneur.htm

Neumann, Meta A., and Robert Cohn. "Incidence of Alzheimer's Disease in a Large Mental Hospital." *Archives of Neurology and Psychiatry* 69 (May 1953).

White, Lon. "Alzheimer's Disease: The Evolution of a Diagnosis." *Public Health Reports,* November-December 1997.

Alzheimer's Caregiving

Henderson, Cary Smith. *Partial View: An Alzheimer's Journal.* Dallas: Southern Methodist University Press, 1998.

Kuhn, Daniel. *Alzheimer's Early Stages: First Steps in Caring and Treatment.* Salt Lake City: Publishers Press, 1999.

Mace, Nancy L., and Peter V. Rabins. *The 36-Hour Day.* New York: Warner, 1992.

Michaud, Paulette. *Early Stages: Changing Our Views of Alzheimer's.* New York: Alzheimer's Association, 1998.

Murphy, Beverly Bigtree. *He Used to Be Somebody.* Boulder, Colo.: Gibbs Associates, 1995.

Snyder, Lisa. *Speaking Our Minds: Personal Reflections from Individuals with Alzheimer's.* New York: W.H. Freeman, 1999.

Stephenson, Crocker. "The Vanishing Man." *Milwaukee Journal Sentinel,* 27 December 1998.

King Lear

Bullough, Geoffrey, ed. *Narrative and Dramatic Sources of Shakespeare.* Vol. 8. New York: Columbia University Press, 1973.

Bullough, Geoffrey. *"King Lear* and the Annesley Case: A Reconsideration." *Festchrift Rudolf Stamm.* Munich: Francke Verlag Bern, 1969.

Shakespeare, William. *King Lear.* Edited by Alfred Harbage. New York: Penguin Books, 1970.

———. *King Lear.* Edited by Kenneth Muir. London: Methuen & Co., 1978.

Morris Friedell

The essays "Introduction to Myself and My Plight," "Incipient Dementia: A Victim's Perspective," "Love in the Twilight Zone," and "The Road to Alzheimer's" are published, among many others, on Morris's Internet home page: http://members.aol.com/MorrisFF.

Human Suffering

Becker, Ernest. *The Denial of Death.* New York: Free Press, 1973.

Frankl, Viktor E. *Man's Search for Meaning.* New York: Washington Square Press, 1985.

Post, Stephen G. *The Moral Challenge of Alzheimer's Disease.* Baltimore: Johns Hopkins University Press, 1995.

Sontag, Susan. *Illness as Metaphor & AIDS and Its Metaphors.* New York: Anchor Books, 1990.

Alzheimer's Disease and Science

Baddeley, Alan D., Barbara A. Wilson, and Fraser N. Watts, eds. *Handbook of Memory Disorders.* New York: John Wiley & Sons, 1998.

Braak, Heiko, and Eva Braak. "Temporal Sequence of Alzheimer's Disease-Related Pathology." Vol. 14. *Cerebral Cortex.* Edited by Peters and Morrison. New York: Kluwer Academic/Plenum Publishers, 1999.

Clark, Cheryl. "Irony and Illness Hit Alzheimer's Researcher." *San Diego Union-Tribune,* 6 April 1995.

Dalton, Rex. "Researchers Caught in Dispute Over Transgenic Mice Patents." *Nature,* 23 March 2000.

Duff, Karen. "Alzheimer Transgenic Mouse Models Come of Age." *Trends in Neurosciences* 20, no. 7 (July 20, 1997).

———. "Curing Amyloidosis: Will It Work in Humans?" *Trends in Neurosciences* 22, no. 11 (November 1999).

Folstein, M. F., *et al.* "Mini-Mental State: A Practical Method for Grading the State of Patients for the Clinician." *Journal of Psychiatric Research* 12, pp. 196–198 (1975).

Franssen, Emile H., and Barry Reisberg. "Neurologic Markers of the Progression of Alzheimer's Disease." *International Psychogeriatrics* 9, suppl. 1 (1997).

Franssen, Emile H., *et al.* "Utility of Developmental Reflexes in the Differential Diagnosis and Prognosis of Incontinence in Alzheimer's Disease." *Journal of Geriatric Psychiatry and Neurology* 10 (January 1997).

Hyman, B. T. "The Neuropathological Diagnosis of Alzheimer's Disease: Clinical-Pathological Studies." *Neurobiology of Aging* 18, no. S4 (1997).

Iqbal, Khalid, *et al. Alzheimer's Disease and Related Disorders: Etiology, Pathogenesis and Therapeutics.* New York: John Wiley & Sons, 1999.

Itzhaki, Ruth F. "Viruses and Alzheimer's Disease." *Science Spectra* no. 14 (1998).

Katzman, Robert, and Katherine Bick. *Alzheimer's Disease: The Changing View.* New York: Academic Press, 2000.

Khachaturian, Zaven S. "Plundered Memories." *The Sciences,* July/August 1997.

Langreth, Robert. "To Fight Alzheimer's, Drug Firms Place Bets on an Unproven Theory." *Wall Street Journal,* 8 July 1999.

Marshall, Eliot. "Allen Roses: From 'Street Fighter' to Corporate Insider." *Science,* 15 May 1998.

Marx, Jean. "New 'Alzheimer's Mouse' Produced." *Science,* 11 October 1996.

Masters, Colin L., and Konrad Beyreuther. "Science, Medicine, and the Future: Alzheimer's Disease." *British Medical Journal,* 7 February 1998.

National Institute on Aging. *Alzheimer's Disease: Unraveling the Mystery.* October 1995. Available at www.alzheimers.org/unravel.html

Nelson, Peter. Interview with Karen Duff, 24 May 1999. Available at www.alzforum.org/members/forums/interview/karen_duff.html

Pollen, Daniel A. *Hannah's Heirs: The Quest for the Genetic Origins of Alzheimer's Disease.* New York: Oxford University Press, 1996.

Reisberg, Barry. *Alzheimer's Disease: The Standard Reference.* New York: Free Press, 1983.

———, *et al.* "Towards a Science of Alzheimer's Disease Management: A Model Based Upon Current Knowledge of Retrogenesis." *International Psychogeriatrics* 11, no. 1 (1999).

———. "Retrogenesis: Clinical, Physiologic, and Pathologic Mechanisms in Brain Aging, Alzheimer's and Other Dementing Processes." *European Archive of Psychiatry in Clinical Neurosciences* 249, suppl. 3 (1999).

Rovner, Sandy. "Aluminum Foiled." *Washington Post,* 9 March 1984.

Singer, Dorothy G., and Tracey A. Revenson. *How a Child Thinks: A Piaget Primer*. New York: Plume, 1978.

Longevity

Alexander, Brian. "Don't Die, Stay Pretty." *Wired*, January 2000.

Anderson, Robert N. "United States Abridged Life Tables, 1996." National Vital Statistics Reports, 24 December 1998.

Brookmeyer, Ron, *et al.* "Projections of Alzheimer's Disease in the United States and the Public Health Impact of Delaying Disease Onset." *American Journal of Public Health*, September 1998.

Eckholm, Erik. "An Aging Nation Grapples with Care for Old and Ill." *New York Times*, 27 March 1990. *(Note:* This is the first of four articles in the series: "Care of the Elderly; Private Burdens, Public Choices.")

Kirkland, Richard I. "Why We Will Live Longer . . . and What It Will Mean." *Fortune*, 21 February 1994.

Kristof, Nicholas D. "Aging World, New Wrinkles." *New York Times*, 22 September 1996.

Moody, Harry R. "Four Scenarios for an Aging Society." *The Hastings Center Report* 24, no. 5 (September 1994).

Olshansky, S. Jay, Bruce A. Carnes, and Christine K. Cassel. "The Aging of the Human Species." *Scientific American*, April 1993.

Olshansky, S. Jay, Bruce A. Carnes, and Douglas Grahn. "Confronting the Boundaries of Human Longevity." *American Scientist*, 11 January 1998.

Population Institute. "1998 World Population Overview and Outlook 1999." December 30, 1998. Available at http://www.populationinstitute.org/overview98.html

Rice, Dorothy P., *et al.* "The Economic Burden of Alzheimer's Disease Care." *Health Affairs*, Summer 1993.

U.S. Census Bureau. *Sixty-Five Plus in the United States.* May 1995.

———. "Estimated Number of People with Alzheimer's Now and Projections for 2025 (Broken Down by State)." Available at www.census.gov/population/www/projections/pp147.html

West, Maureen. "Turning Back Time." *Denver Rocky Mountain News,* 20 July 1999.

Jonathan Swift

Ehrenpreis, Irvin. *The Personality of Jonathan Swift.* Cambridge: Harvard University Press, 1958.

Glendinning, Victoria. *Jonathan Swift.* New York: Henry Holt, 1998.

Swift, Jonathan. *Gulliver's Travels.* 1726. Reprint, Boston: Houghton Mifflin, 1960.

———. *Prose Writings of Swift.* Chosen and Arranged by Walter Lewin. London: Walter Scott, Ltd., 1896.

Wilde, W. R. *The Closing Years of Dean Swift's Life.* Dublin: Hodges and Smith, 1849.

Willem de Kooning

Abbe, Mary. "Portrait of the Artist as an Old Man." *(Minneapolis) Star Tribune,* 4 February 1996.

de Kooning, Willem. *The Late Paintings: The 1980s.* San Francisco: San Francisco Museum of Modern Art/Minneapolis: Walker Art Center, 1995.

Espinel, Carlos Hugo. "De Kooning's Late Colours and Forms: Dementia, Creativity, and the Healing Power of Art." *Lancet,* 20 April 1996.

Larson, Kay. "Alzheimer's Expressionism." *Village Voice,* 31 May 1994.

Pepper, Curtis Bill. "The Indomitable De Kooning." *New York Times,* 20 November 1983.

Scaruffi, Piero. "Thinking About Thought." *Science's Last Frontiers: Consciousness, Life and Meaning.* Available at www.thymos.com/tat/consc2.html

Mnemonics

Yates, Frances A. *The Art of Memory.* Chicago: University of Chicago Press, 1966.

Frederick Law Olmsted

Roper, Laura Wood. *FLO: A Biography of Frederick Law Olmsted.* Baltimore: Johns Hopkins University Press, 1983.

Rybczynski, Witold. *A Clearing in the Distance: Frederick Law Olmsted and America in the Nineteenth Century.* New York: Scribner, 1999.

Stevenson, Elizabeth. *Park Maker: A Life of Frederick Law Olmsted.* New York: Macmillan, 1977.

Soliloquies

Page 9: Michaud, Paulette. *Early Stages: Changing Our Views of Alzheimer's.* New York: Alzheimer's Association, 1998.

Page 27: Michaud, Paulette. *Early Stages: Changing Our Views of Alzheimer's.* New York: Alzheimer's Association, 1998.

Page 43: Henderson, Cary Smith. *Partial View: An Alzheimer's Journal.* Dallas: Southern Methodist University Press, 1998.

Page 61: Snyder, Lisa. *Speaking Our Minds: Personal Reflections from Individuals with Alzheimer's.* New York: W.H. Freeman, 1999.

Page 71: Rose, Larry. *Show Me the Way to Go Home.* Forest Knolls, California: Elder Books, 1995.

Page 85: Toward, Jeffrey. Interviews with early-stage patients (unpublished). Houston: University of Texas Center on Aging, 1997.

Page 111: Snyder, Lisa. *Speaking Our Minds: Personal Reflections from Individuals with Alzheimer's.* New York: W.H. Freeman, 1999.

Page 131: Originally posted on Alzheimer List, 1998, at http://www.adrc.wustl.edu/alzheimer

Page 147: Originally posted on Alzheimer List, 1998.

Page 161: Originally posted on Alzheimer List, 1998.

Page 177: Originally posted on Alzheimer List, 1999.

Page 191: Originally posted on Alzheimer List, 1999.

Page 215: Originally posted on Alzheimer List, 1998.

Page 227: Petrovski, Sue. *Return Journey.* Book in progress.

Page 241: Morris Friedell, "The Loneliness of a Person with Early Alzheimer's Disease," published online at http://members.aol.com/MorrisFF/

INDEX

Abstract Expressionism, 195–206
abstract thinking, 36, 37, 125
acetylcholine, 62–63
Addison, Thomas, 80
Addison's disease, 80
adrenal glands, 80
adrenalin, 46
agnosia, 119
AIDS, 38, 80
alcoholism, 38, 195–96, 197, 229
Alcott, Bronson, 83
Alcott, Louisa May, 217–19
alpha rhythm, 38
aluminum, 138–40
Aluminum Association, 139
Alzheimer, Alois, 12–15, 22–26, 64,
       68–69, 74–84, 102, 133, 143,
       162–63, 182, 245
Alzheimer Disease Research Center, 91
Alzheimer List (website), 91–97, 121,
       223
Alzheimer Research Forum, 63–64
Alzheimer's Association, 32, 209
Alzheimer's disease:
   aesthetic experience in, 192–206
   awareness stage of, 94–97, 103–4,
       192–94

causes of, 68–70, 73, 118–20,
       137–40, 151, 155–56
cellular ultrastructure of, 133–34,
       143–46
childlike behavior in, 121–30
coping mechanisms for, 32–33, 114
costs of, 5, 65, 66, 88–89
cure for, 39, 62, 67, 97, 146, 178,
       209–14, 228, 235, 243–46, 251
death from, 4, 22, 37, 40, 62, 223–26
as degenerative condition, 19–22, 40,
       97, 112–30, 141
diagnosis and testing of, 19–22, 31,
       35–39, 94–97, 115, 116,
       127–28, 192
as disease, 74–84, 129–30, 133,
       137–38, 140, 142, 152–53, 250
early stages of, 31–33, 36, 37–42, 47,
       63, 94–97, 114, 154, 231
environmental factors in, 155–56
identification of, 12–15, 22–26,
       74–84
immunity to, 68, 137
incidence of, 5, 30–31, 65–67,
       73–74, 132–34, 163–65
insidious onset of, 17–22, 32–35, 67,
       103, 200, 221, 250

late stages of, 21–22, 37, 69, 119,
128, 130, 201, 216–26
in men vs. women, 67
middle stages of, 36–37, 39–40, 63,
103–4, 112–18, 119, 130
name of, 78–84, 183
neurological basis of, 21–26, 70–78,
118–20, 209–24; *see also*
neurons
postawareness stage of, 103–4, 113,
120, 198–99
prevention of, 228–29
as process, 64–65, 79–80, 221–24
public awareness of, 136–43
as public health problem, 5, 30–32,
65–67, 132–38, 163
reality of, 27, 93–94, 114–16, 147
rehabilitation in, 94–95, 247–52
research on, *see* research, Alzheimer's
resources for, 261–64
retrogenesis in, 117–30, 221–24
symptoms of, 13, 19–21, 63, 115,
142
treatment for, 39, 137, 209–14,
243–46
vaccine for, 209–14, 243–46
Alzheimer's Weekly, 63
American Association of Retired Persons
(AARP), 132
amino acids, 50
amnesia, 46–49, 201, 218–19
amygdala, 45–46, 118, 125
amyloid cascade hypothesis, 152, 155
amyloid precursor protein (APP), 144,
184, 246
amylum, 144
Angell, Roger, 34
anger, 12, 13, 118, 121–22, 129–30
animal rights, 184–85
Annesley, Bryan, 89–90, 169–70
Annesley, Cordell, 90, 169
anosognosia, 120
AN 1792, 209–14
Antabuse, 195–96
anterograde amnesia, 46–49, 218–19
antibodies, 209–14, 243–46
anti-inflammatory drugs, 229
antioxidants, 228
anxiety, 129–30
aphasia, 13, 41, 97, 112–13, 117, 118,
169, 221
ApoE gene, 153, 189, 245
Archives of Neurology and Psychiatry, 84

Area One, 46
Area Two, 46
Aricept, 62–63, 246, 250
Aristophanes, 112
As You Like It (Shakespeare), 83
Atlantic Monthly, 1
auditory hallucinations, 13–14, 119
Auguste D., 12–15, 21, 22–26, 74–75,
76, 77–78, 163
Augustine, Saint, 45, 231–32
Auschwitz concentration camp, 96
autoimmune response, 213–14
autonomy, 33
autopsies, 22–26, 35, 139
autotoxins, 76, 102
axons, 124, 145

Babinski, Joseph François Felix, 222
Babinski sign, 222
baby boomers, 5, 65–67, 172
Bacon, Roger, 15
Barney, 40, 115
Bataan Hall, 4, 67
beta-amyloid, 143–46, 152–53, 155–57,
184, 209–14, 243–46
biopsies, 35
Biser, Sam, 140
blindness, temporary, 38
blood-brain barrier, 139, 211–12, 244
Bok, Edward, 217–21
Bonetti, David, 203
Bonhoeffer, Karl, 76
Borchelt, David, 186
Borges, Jorge Luis, 192
bovine spongiform encephalopathy
("mad cow disease"), 148–50
Boyle, John, 168, 171–72
"Brahma" (Emerson), 2
brain:
autopsies of, 22–26, 72–74, 124–25
deterioration of, 20–22, 30, 37–38,
204
as electrochemical engine, 11–12
evolution of, 23, 53, 56–57
functional areas of, 21–22, 45–49
injuries to, 38, 201, 228
modular theory of, 45–49
neurons of, *see* neurons
nonhuman, 178–89
pathology of, 72–84, 102, 118–20
size of, 11, 21, 37–38, 204
tumors of, 34–35
ventricular theory of, 45

weight of, 23
"white matter" of, 124
see also specific brain areas
brainstem, 24, 49, 222–24
brain waves, 38, 184
Brickman, Irving, 28, 29, 31–32, 39, 113, 114
Broca's area, 46
Brooks, Phillips, 217, 218
Buber, Martin, 95
Buddhism, 96
Buschke Selective Reminding Test, 37
Butler, Robert, 135

Cabot, James Elliot, 107–8
Cairns-Smith, A. G., 52
calcium, 34–35, 64
camera lucida, 26
Campbell, Joseph, 238
Canada, 5
cancer, 62, 65–66, 95–96, 134, 135, 164, 176, 236
caregivers, 86–97
    Internet support for, 91–97, 121, 142, 223
    professional, 29, 66, 88, 92–93, 129
    reverse parenting by, 66, 88, 121–22, 126–30
"caregiver's dementia," 88, 94
Carlyle, Thomas, 108, 166, 219–20
Catania, Jennifer W., 247
cells:
    debris around, 21–22, 24–26
    place, 230–31
    ultrastructure of, 133–34, 143–46
    see also neurons
cerebellum, 24
cerebral arteriosclerosis, 73
cerebral cortex, 21, 24, 25, 69, 75, 77–78, 118, 124, 198, 200, 222, 223
cerebral localization, 45–49
cerebral palsy, 41
Charcot, Jean-Martin, 80
Charlotte's Web (White), 33
Cherokee Indians, 68
child development, 121–30
chromosome 19, 153
chromosome 21, 154
chromosomes, 150, 153
Churchill, Winston, 150
Cicero, 15
Clinton, Bill, 4–5, 40–41, 148

Clock Test, 37
cognitive impairment, 36–37, 117–30, 201, 202, 234, 249–52
Cohn, Robert, 74, 84
cold sores, 69
compassion, 96
competence, 33
comprehension, reduced, 13, 39, 41–42
concentration:
    development of, 125, 198
    loss of, 3, 118, 204
concentration camps, 16, 96, 182
Conel, J. L., 124
Confessions (St. Augustine), 231–32
confusion, 12, 19, 33, 34, 115, 196, 216
congestive heart failure, 223
consciousness, 51, 192–94, 202–6
constructional praxis, 36
coronary heart disease, 155
Cree Indians, 68
Creutzfeldt-Jakob disease, 148–50
Crick, Francis, 50, 183
Curry, Ann, 116

Dachau concentration camp, 16
Darwin, Charles, 166, 180–81
day care, 114
daydreams, 55
"Dear Abby," 136
death rate, 4, 62, 175–76
degeneration theory, 181–83
de Kooning, Elaine, 196
de Kooning, Willem, 195–206, 248, 252
delirium, 13–14
démence, 15
dementia, 15
dementia praecox, 14
dendrites, 145
denial, 27, 114–16, 147
depression, 38, 88, 95–96
diabetes, 38
diet, 34, 228–29
dignity, human, 94–97, 192–93, 248
Dillman, Rob, 82
diseases, hidden, 163–65, 175
disorientation, 12–13, 19, 36
Distl, R., 247
DNA, 50, 149, 150, 153, 183, 188, 238
dogs, 179
Doody, Rachel, 246
dopamine, 64
dotage, 15, 165

Down's syndrome, 97
driving, 33, 67, 115
drug abuse, 38
drug companies, 153, 158–59, 185–89,
  209–14, 246
Duff, Karen, 151, 186

Ecclesiasticus, Book of, 82–84
education, 229, 250–51
Elan Pharmaceuticals, 158–59, 186–87,
  209–14
elderly:
  hidden diseases of, 163–65, 175
  mental deterioration of, 15, 163
  political influence of, 132, 134,
    135–36, 137
  population of, 5, 30–31, 65–67, 132,
    134, 163–65
electroencephalogram (EEG), 38, 94,
  123
electrolytes, 34–35
Elizabeth I, Queen of England, 89
Emerson, Edward, 83, 105–6, 107, 108,
  216
Emerson, Ellen, 3, 102, 105–6, 107,
  218, 230
Emerson, Ralph Waldo, 1–3, 16–17, 55,
  83–84, 101–10, 172, 199, 206,
  216–21, 226, 232–33, 238, 249,
  252, 254, 255
emotions:
  expression of, 12, 14, 95–97, 118,
    121–22, 129–30, 170–71,
    202–3, 224
  memory and, 125
  negative, 12, 13, 118, 121–22,
    129–30
Engelhardt, H. Tristram, Jr., 79
engrams, 52, 55
enzymes, 236, 246
"Eos and Tithonus" myth, 166–68
epilepsy, 22, 46, 47
Erasmus, Desiderius, 121, 206
Espinel, Carlos Hugo, 205, 206
Esquirol, Jean Étienne, 15
"Essay on the Shaking Palsy"
  (Parkinson), 80
estates, 89–91
estrogen replacement therapy, 229
Everett, C. C., 101
evolution, 23, 53, 56–57, 173–75,
  180–83
Excavation (de Kooning), 202

executive function skills, 204
exercise, 34, 229
eye movements, 38
eyewitnesses, 56

faces, 59, 230, 238
families, 32, 33, 39, 66, 86–97, 116–17,
  120, 223, 224
fatty acids, 229
fatuity, 15
fear, 45–46, 118
feng shui, 251
fetal position, 14
Final Solution, 182
finances, 88–91
Flaherty, Carla, 91–92
flatworms, 49
flies, transgenic, 236
Florentine Codex, 165–66
fluorescent protein tagging, 64
folic acid, 229
Food and Drug Administration, U.S.,
  141–42
Forbes, John, 108–9
forebrain, 63
formalin, 23, 24
Frankl, Viktor, 16, 95, 96, 224, 234,
  248, 249
free association, 53–54
free-radical molecules, 228
Freud, Sigmund, 76–77
Freund House, 28–33, 39–42, 112–16
Friedell, Morris, 94–97, 192–94, 203,
  241, 247–52
Friedreich's ataxia, 14
friends, 40, 87, 114, 116–17, 120
frontal lobes, 119–20, 125, 250
frustration, 113, 115, 195, 199

Galen, 45
Galileo Galilei, 245–46
Garrels, Gary, 198, 199–200, 205
Gaupp, Robert, 76
genetics:
  in Alzheimer's research, 53, 63, 64,
    69–70, 124, 150–55, 178–89,
    243–46
  "dustbin" of, 175
  knock-out technology in, 183–89,
    235–39, 243, 246
  transgenics in, 151, 178–89, 209–14,
    236, 243, 246
  see also DNA

genome, 150
germline engineering, 235–39
Geron, 236
gingko, 142
Giuliani, Rudolph, 40
Glaxo Wellcome, 152, 187–89
Glenner, George, 137, 143–46, 149
glial cells, 25
glucose, 21, 35, 38, 123, 211
goal-setting, 204
Gompertz, Benjamin, 172–76
Grant, Ulysses S., 217
Green, Kevin, 56
Gross, Otto, 77
gross motor functions, 221–22
Gulliver's Travels (Swift), 167–68, 237

habits, 200–2, 203
hallucinations, 13–14, 34, 89, 119
Handbook of Psychiatry (Kraepelin),
    75–84
Hardy, John, 152, 210
Hasegawa, Tohru, 247
Haseltine, William, 236–37
Hawaii, 68
Hayes, Rutherford B., 217
Hayworth, Rita, 136
health insurance, 66, 88
hearing, 125
heart disease, 62, 65–66, 73, 135, 155,
    176
Henry IV, King of France, 121
herbal remedies, 140–43, 234
heredity, 180
herpes simplex virus 1 (HSV1), 69–70,
    245
high-order processing, 118–19
Hinckley, John, Jr., 72, 242
hippocampus, 37–38, 46–49, 69, 118,
    119, 125, 200, 218, 219, 223, 229,
    230–31, 246
Hitler, Adolf, 182
Hoche, Alfred, 75, 76, 182
Holmes, Oliver Wendell, 217
hormones, 46
Howells, William Dean, 1
Hsiao, Karen, 151, 184, 185–87
Huntington, George, 80
Huntington's disease, 14, 80
Hutton, John, 20–21
hyperphosphorylated tau, 145, 156
hypertension, 155

ibuprofen, 229
immortality, 109, 166–68, 236–39
"Immortality" (Emerson), 109
immune system, 69, 149, 209–14,
    243–46
immunization, 67, 69–70, 209–14,
    243–46
immuno-lesioning, 64
influenza, 80
information, 232–34, 238–39
insomnia, 92
intelligence, 53, 119–20, 201
Internet, 91–97, 121, 142, 223, 261
"Introduction to Myself and My Plight"
    (Friedell), 192–94
introspection, 120
Iqbal, Khalid, 155–56
Itzhaki, Ruth, 69–70, 156, 245

Japan, 5, 68
Johns, Jasper, 200
Johnson, Samuel, 169–70
Joosse, Barbara M., 129
Joseph, Judy, 29, 31–32, 39, 40, 114
Journal of Neuropsychiatry, 49
judgment, impairment of, 36, 57,
    114–15, 121
Juvenal, 44–45

Katzman, Robert, 132–33
Khachaturian, Zaven, 5, 65–66, 135–36,
    137, 143, 144, 145–46, 155
King Lear (Shakespeare), 89–90
knock-out technology, 183–89, 235–39,
    243, 246
Korsakoff's syndrome, 14
Kraepelin, Emil, 23, 75–84, 102, 162,
    182
Krimsky, Stanley,

language:
    development of, 46, 119, 120, 125
    impairment of, 13, 14, 36, 41, 97,
        112–13, 117, 118, 169, 221,
        230
Lao-tzu, 248
Larson, Kay, 198, 202, 203–4
Lasker, Mary, 134–35
Last Chance Health Report, The, 140
Law of Mortality, 172–76
Lee, Virginia, 155
legal issues, 88–89, 92–93
Leitz, Ernst, 24

Lewinsky, Monica, 4–5, 40–41, 148
Lieberburg, Ivan, 158–59, 243–44
life span, 31, 162–76
limbic system, 118
literature, children's, 129–30
Loftus, Elizabeth, 56
logic, 120, 128
Long, Russell, 18
longevity, 174–76
Longfellow, Henry Wadsworth, 106,
    109–10, 216, 217
long-term potentiation (LTP), 52
Lorenz, Konrad, 182, 183
loss, meaning of, 224–26, 234–35
Lowell, James Russell, 3
Lucullus, Lucius Licinius, 86–87
Lucullus, Marcus, 86–87
lunatics, 90, 93
Luria, A. R., 58–60, 236, 238–39, 248
"Lycidas" (Milton), 17

McConnell, James, 49
McLean Asylum, 255
mad cow disease (bovine spongiform
    encephalopathy), 148–50
magnetic resonance imaging (MRI),
    37–38, 94
Mahoney, Florence, 134–35
Mama, Do You Love Me? (Joosse), 129
Man's Search for Meaning (Frankl), 16,
    96, 224
marriage, 229
Maurer, Konrad, 182
Max's New Suit (Wells), 129
Mayo Clinic, 186, 246
means-ends ability, 127
Medicare, 88, 132
medication, 30, 34, 91, 141–42, 229
medicine:
    clinical, 22–24
    diagnostic, 14
    specialization in, 248–49
Memorabilia (Xenophon), 82
memory, 44–60
    acute deterioration of, 15, 46–49,
        201, 218–19
    ant-farm analogy for, 52
    character and, 53–55, 59
    constellation theory of, 51–56, 225
    emotional, 125
    episodic, 47–48
    external, 16–17, 106–7, 232–34
    false, 55–56

forgetting and, 44, 48–49, 56–60, 88,
    94–95, 113, 114–15, 116, 120,
    192–95, 198–99, 204–5,
    237–39
formation of, 47–48, 51–54, 102,
    118, 196–97, 218–19, 229, 252
immediate, 218–19
importance of, 16–17, 101–2,
    237–39
individual, 49–50
involuntary, 55
lapses of, 17–18, 19, 27, 234
long-term, 47, 49, 52–54, 125,
    192–94, 196–97, 218–19
meaning and, 57, 59–60
"mind," 200, 201
muscle (procedural), 200–2
neurological basis of, 21–22, 46–49,
    51–52, 55, 135, 145, 230–31,
    233
"palaces" of, 231–32
process of, 44–60, 229–34
progressive deterioration of, 3, 12–13,
    14, 39, 135–36, 138, 168–72,
    203, 218–19, 226, 254–56
retrieval of, 52–60, 119, 229–34
semantic, 47, 48, 119
short-term (working), 3, 13, 21–22,
    29, 36, 47, 48, 218–19, 254
testing of, 35–36, 38, 95
total recall in, 57–60, 236, 238–39
traces of (engrams), 52, 55
transfer of, 49–51, 56
use of, 229–34
visual, 230–31
word/number, 230
"Memory" (Emerson), 101–2, 107
"Memory Transfer Through Cannibalism
    in Planaria" (McConnell), 49
Mendel, Gregor, 180–81
Ménière's disease, 168
menopause, 229
mental illness, 75–84, 182
Meske, V., 247
metabolism, 155, 189, 198
Metaman: The Merging of Humans and
    Machines into a Global
    Superorganism (Stock), 235
mice, transgenic, 151, 178–89, 209–14,
    236, 243, 246
microglia, 213
microscopes, 22, 24–26, 64, 143–46,
    178

microtubule transports, 118
mild cognitive impairment (MCI), 234
Milton, John, 17
Mini Mental State Examination
    (MMSE), 35–36, 95
mitochondria, 64
mnemonics, 230–32
"Molecular Mechanisms in Alzheimer's
    Disease" (conference), 4–5, 62–70,
    148–59
molecules, memory, 49–51, 56
Montessori method, 250–51
mood changes, 14, 121–22
Moody, Harry, 164
Morel, Augustin, 181
morosis, 15
Morrison-Bogorad, Marcelle, 209, 246
mortality, 4, 62, 109, 166–69, 172–76,
    224–26, 236–39
mortality curve, 172–76
motor skills, 37, 38, 53, 200–202
mourning, 224–26
Muir, John, 110
multi-infarct dementia, 33–34
music, 40, 115, 130
mutations, presenilin, 151
myelin insulation, 124–25, 222

names, 106–7, 135, 195, 232
Nation, 41
National Alzheimer's Month, 136–37
National Institute on Aging (NIA), 134,
    135–36
National Institutes of Health (NIH),
    134
"Natural History of the Intellect"
    (Emerson), 107–8
natural selection, 23, 173, 175, 180–81
Nature (Emerson), 3, 232–33
Nature (journal), 50, 153
Nature Neuroscience, 64
Nazism, 182
Nedivi, E., 64
Nemesius, 45
Neumann, Meta, 72–74, 84, 133, 245
neurons:
    cellular debris among, 21–22, 24–26;
        see also plaques; tangles
    loss of, 52, 64, 118–20, 124–25, 137,
        143–46, 156, 221–24, 255
    membranes of, 145
    for memory, 21–22, 46–49, 51–52,
        55, 135, 145, 230–31, 233

myelinization of, 124–25, 222
    networks of, 11, 51–52, 143–46,
        200–201, 218–19, 233, 255
    synapses of, 21, 51–52, 62–63, 118,
        145
neuroses, 76
neurotransmitters, 21, 62–63
New Brunswick (N.J.) *Daily Times,* 102
New Yorker, 54, 57
New York Times, 20, 34, 198
Nietzsche, Friedrich, 16, 44, 238
Nissl, Franz, 24, 102
Nissl method, 24, 102
Nixon, Richard M., 135
nosology, psychiatric, 75–84
nurses, 92–93
nursing homes, 29, 88, 129

object permanence, 127
object registration, 36
oblivio, 15
occipital lobes, 46, 124–25
Olmsted, Frederick Law, 253–56
Olmsted, John, 254–55
Olshansky, S. Jay, 163, 174, 175, 176
Ordinal Scales of Psychological
    Development (OSPD), 127–28
Orrery, John Boyle, Earl of, 168,
    171–72
Our Town (Wilder), 241
oxygen flow, 38, 221, 223–24

painting, 195–206
paranoia, 13
parenthood, reverse, 66, 88, 121–22,
    126–30
paresis, 14
parietal lobes, 46, 49, 119, 124
Parkinson, James, 80
Parkinson's disease, 14, 40, 68, 80
patents, 157–58, 185–87
patients' rights, 94–95
pattern recognition, 37, 60, 117
"Peculiar Disease of the Cerebral Cortex,
    A" (Alzheimer), 75
Pepper, Curtis Bill, 198
peptides, 50
perception, 46, 124–25, 230–31
persistent vegetative state, 222–24
Perusini, Gaetano, 25–26
Piaget, Jean, 127, 128
pituitary gland, 46
plague, 80

planning, 37, 119–20, 125
plantar response, 222
plaques:
  beta-amyloid in, 143–46, 152–53,
    155–57, 184, 209–14, 243–46
  discovery of, 21–22, 24–26, 32, 35
  elimination of, 209–14, 243–46
  research on, 68–69, 70, 73–78, 102,
    118, 132–34, 137, 143–46,
    152–53, 179, 184
  spread of, 21–22, 24–26, 73–78,
    143–46, 152–57, 184, 201, 204,
    209–14, 218–24, 243–46
  tangles vs., 21–22, 24–26, 152–53,
    155–57
plasticity, 53
Plato, 15, 45, 233, 238
Plutarch, 86–87
polio, 67, 210
"politics of anguish," 134, 137
polymer pellets, 63
Porteus Mazes, 37
positron emission tomography (PET),
  38, 94, 193, 248
posthumanism, 235–39
Pound, Ezra, 72
prefrontal cortex, 46, 49, 246
"Preoperational" stage, 128
primary sensory area, 124
prions, 148–50, 245
prisoners-of-war, 95–96
problem-solving, 250
products, Alzheimer-related, 29–30
"prolongation of morbidity," 164
Prospect Park, 253–56
Prospect Park Residence, 256
proteins, 64, 144, 146, 148–50, 156,
  184, 245, 246
Prusinger, Stanley, 4, 148–50, 156, 245
psychiatry, 75–84
psychoanalysis, 76–77
psychomotor skills, 37
psychosis, 38
Pullman, George, 109
puzzles, 37, 117
Pyramid Texts, 44

qEEG, 94

Ra, 44
rats, 49–50
Reagan, Maureen, 116, 117, 242–43
Reagan, Nancy, 20, 21, 87, 117, 231

Reagan, Ronald, 17–22, 72, 87, 116–17,
  136–37, 143, 231, 242
reflexes, 14, 123, 222
rehabilitation, 94–95, 247–52
Reisberg, Barry, 122–24, 127
rejuvenation theory, 202–6
reproduction, sexual, 173–75
research, Alzheimer's:
  animal, 151, 178–89, 209–14, 243
  breakthroughs in, 63–64, 209–14
  conferences on, 4–5, 62–70, 148–59,
    242–52
  conventional wisdom in, 150,
    156–57, 244–46
  developmental, 117–30, 221–24
  drug, 62–63, 153, 158–59, 178,
    185–89, 209–14, 246, 250
  funding for, 68, 134–36, 157–60,
    187–89, 212, 242–43
  genetic, 53, 63, 64, 69–70, 124,
    150–55, 178–89, 243–46
  marketization of, 185–89
  molecular, 4–5, 63, 64, 143–46,
    148–50
  rivalry in, 148–50, 152–55
Research on Aging Act, 135
residual cognitive capacities, 128
retirement, 95
retrogenesis, 117–30, 221–24
Roethke, Theodore, 193
Rose, Michael, 236
Rose, Steven, 185
Roses, Allen, 152–55, 156, 187–89, 245
Royal Psychiatric Clinic, 22–23
Ruedin, Ernst, 182
Ruskin, John, 219
Russell, Phillips, 103

Sabin, Albert, 67, 210
safety issues, 33, 67, 121
Sahagún, Bernardino de, 166
St. Elizabeth's Hospital (Washington,
  D.C.), 72–74
Salk, Jonas, 67
Schacter, Daniel, 51
Scheck, Barry, 56
Scheffler, Israel, 202
Schellenberg, Gerard, 151
Schenk, Dale, 210–14, 243–46
schistosomiasis, 80
schizophrenia, 14
Schulze, Richard, 140–43
Science, 49

Scipio, L., 17, 230
Scorsese, Martin, 54–55, 57
scotophobin, 50
Scoville, William Beecher, 46
seizures, 22, 38, 46, 47
self-identity, 46, 55, 119, 128, 169–70,
    192–93, 196, 198–99, 202–3, 204
"Self-Reliance" (Emerson), 3
Seneca, 17, 230
senile dementia:
    Alzheimer's vs., 81–82, 84
    in animals, 179
    causes of, 73–74
    definition of, 15
    as disease, 74, 89–90, 101–2, 133,
        165–66
    progression of, 29–31, 33–34, 103,
        168–72
senility:
    aging and, 82–84
    Alzheimer's as form of, 5, 15, 17,
        29–35, 73–74, 75
    as disease, 30, 32, 81, 83–84, 137–38
    historical descriptions of, 15, 44,
        82–84, 89–90, 121, 165–68,
        206
senium praecox, 81
sensory input, 47, 119–20, 124
sequoias, 109
Seurat, Georges, 202
sexuality, 77, 173–75
Shakespeare, William, xi, 83, 89–90,
    206, 231
Shultz, George, 116–17
signatures, mortality, 175–76
sign language, 41
Simonides of Ceos, 230, 231
Singer, Mark, 54–55, 57
single nucleotide polymorphisms
    (SNPs), 187–88
single photon emission computed
    tomography (SPECT), 38
Sioli, Emil, 163
Sisodia, Sangram, 209, 210
sleep, 55, 29, 179, 229
smallpox, 80
smoking, 68
SNP mapping, 187–88
Snyder, Lisa, 252
social contact, 229
Society for Racial Hygiene, 182
Solon, 165
Song, H. J., 63

South Florida, University of, 243
spatial relations, 127
spinal cord, 24
Springsteen, Bruce, 253
Städtische Irrenanstalt, 12
"State of World Health" (1997 report),
    164
Stephanie (group facilitator), 114
Stern, Yaakov, 246
Stock, Gregory, 235–36
Storr, Robert, 205
stovetop fire extinguishers, 30
stress, 69, 88, 129–30
strokes, 14, 33–35, 62, 201, 250
Struldbruggs, 167–68, 171, 172
suffering, 171–72, 184–85, 238–39
Sulla, 86
Sunday Afternoon on the Island of La
    Grande Jatte (Seurat), 202
"sundowning," 92
support groups, 28–33, 39–42, 66,
    112–16
Swift, Jonathan, 167–72, 226, 237
symbolic thinking, 125, 128
Symbolic Worlds (Scheffler), 202
synapses, neural, 21, 51–52, 62–63,
    118, 145
syphilis, 14, 38
systemic senile amyloidosis, 146, 149
Szántó, András, 204–5

tangles:
    discovery of, 21–22, 24–26, 32, 35
    elimination of, 246, 247
    "ghost," 145
    plaques vs., 21–22, 24–26, 152–53,
        155–57
    research on, 68–69, 73–78, 102,
        118–20, 132–34, 137, 143–46,
        179
    spread of, 21–22, 24–26, 73–78,
        144–45, 155, 156, 201, 204,
        206, 218–19, 221–24
    tau in, 144–45, 155, 156
tantrums, 121–22
Taos, N. Mex., Alzheimer's conference
    (1999), 4–5, 62–70, 148–59
tau, 144–45, 155, 156
telomerase, 236
temporal lobes, 37, 46, 119, 125
"Terminus" (Emerson), 104–5, 107, 172
Terry, Robert, 132–34
Thackeray, William Makepeace, 169–70

Thatcher, Margaret, 20
Thayer, James Bradley, 109, 110
Thies, Bill, 209
Thomas, Lewis, 149
Thoreau, Henry David, 3, 55, 166, 248, 251
Thousand and One Nights, A, 165
thyroid condition, 34–35
time, manufactured, 176
tissue-staining, 24, 102
Today, 116
Tolstoy, Leo, 166
touch, sense of, 119, 124
tracking devices, 30
Trail Making Test, 37
Transcendentalism, 108
transgenics, 151, 178–89, 209–14, 236, 243, 246
"transubstantiated future," 236–37
tremors, 38
tuberculosis, 80
Tully, Tim, 236
tumors, brain, 34–35
Twain, Mark, 1–3, 101

Ungar, George, 50, 51

vaccine, Alzheimer's, 209–14, 243–46
Van Buren, Abigail, 136
Vanderbilt, George, 254
Vaux, Calvert, 253–54
"Verses on the Death of Dr. Swift" (Swift), 169
Virchow, Rudolf, 163
Virgil, 30
viruses, 149
vision, 46, 50, 124–25, 127–28, 222, 230–31
Vital Spirit, 45
vitamins, 34–35, 229

Walters, Barbara, 5

Wang, C. Y., 64
War and Peace (Tolstoy), 166
Warhol, Andy, 202
Washington, D.C., conference (2000), 242–52
Washington Post, 140
Watson, James, 183
Weber, Matthias M., 78
Wells, Rosemary, 129
Wenders, Wim, 238
Wernicke's area, 46
western blot analysis, 64
White, E. B., 33–34
Whiteaway, Martha, 169, 170, 171
Whitman, Walt, 106
"Wide World" journals (Emerson), 106
Wiesel, Elie, 95, 96
Wiesel, Torsten, 138–40
Wilder, Thornton, 241
willfulness, 46, 204
Wilson, Francis, 170–71
Wings of Desire, 238
Wired, 236
Wisconsin Card Sorting Test, 37
Women (de Kooning), 202
words, 36, 41, 230
Wordsworth, William, 17
World Health Organization, 164
"Wreck of the Hesperus, The" (Longfellow), 109–10
writing, 233

Xenophon, 82

Yates, Frances, 231
yellow fever, 80
Young, Brigham, 109
Young, Edward, 168
Younkin, Steven, 186

Zeiss, Carl, 24
Zeman, Stephanie, 223

Self

Self-im-age (self-im-ij) n. one's mental concept of oneself or one's position in relation to others; how one sees oneself.

ALTERNATE DEFINITION
what you think about your looks when you wake up in the morning with a huge zit on the end of your nose

Who's right about you? Are you the way your friends see you? Your parents or teachers? Or is everybody wrong? If you're still growing up and maturing, does anybody know the true you?

"You have taken off your old self with its practices and have put on the new self, which is being renewed in knowledge in the image of its Creator."
COLOSSIANS 3:9-10

The true you is the new you that you're becoming!

How can you build a positive self-image? Remember God made you the way you are. And God doesn't make junk. Don't spend time concentrating on what you think are your bad points. Work on your good ones. Build on your strengths, and stop focusing on your weaknesses. Most important—make good decisions. Stick to what you know is right, and you'll have a great reason to feel good about yourself.

Still worried about your looks? Remember they're temporary. They'll change. "So we fix our eyes not on what is seen, but on what is unseen. For what is seen is temporary, but what is unseen is eternal."
2 CORINTHIANS 4:18

Church 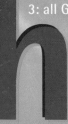 (church) n.

1: a congregation; 2: a specific Christian denomination (the Presbyterian Church); 3: all God's people everywhere; God's family.

Church

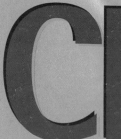

Presbyterian. Baptist. Pentecostal. Methodist. Lutheran. Church of Christ. Catholic. Assembly of God. Why are there so many different churches?

While we're at it, why so many athletic shoes? Adidas. Converse. Nike. Is one of them wrong? Or is it just a matter of preference?

What unites different churches? The conviction that Jesus is God's Son and our Savior. Churches differ on whether you should baptize babies or just adults and whether or not speaking in tongues is important—lots of things. But all true Christian churches look to Jesus for salvation and trust the Bible as God's Word.

ALTERNATE DEFINITION
what you have to get dressed up for so you can be bored for an hour at a morning service

Want to stop being bored in church? First, listen to the sermon until you hear one thing God wants you to do this week or one thing you didn't know before. Second, pay attention to the words of the songs and prayers until you hear one thing you want to say to God. Third, try to say or do one thing to encourage some other person.

"Let us consider how we may spur one another on toward love and good deeds. Let us not give up meeting together, as some are in the habit of doing, but let us encourage one another."
HEBREWS 10:24-25

Did you know that until about 300 A.D. there weren't any church buildings? Christians met in small groups in homes. Sometimes larger groups met outdoors for special praise services. But what made church special then can make it special now: meeting with Jesus.

Paul and Timothy, servants of Christ Jesus,

To all the saints in Christ Jesus at Philippi, together with the overseers[a] and deacons:

[2]Grace and peace to you from God our Father and the Lord Jesus Christ.

Thanksgiving and Prayer   [3]I thank my God every time I remember you. [4]In all my prayers for all of you, I always pray with joy [5]because of your partnership in the gospel from the first day until now, [6]being confident of this, that he who began a good work in you will carry it on to completion until the day of Christ Jesus.

[7]It is right for me to feel this way about all of you, since I have you in my heart; for whether I am in chains or defending and confirming the gospel, all of you share in God's grace with me. [8]God can testify how I long for all of you with the affection of Christ Jesus.

[9]And this is my prayer: that your love may abound more and more in knowledge and depth of insight, [10]so that you may be able to discern what is best and may be pure and blameless until the day of Christ, [11]filled with the fruit of righteousness that comes through Jesus Christ—to the glory and praise of God.

> He who began a good work in you will carry it on to completion until the day of Christ Jesus (Philippians 1:6).

Paul's Chains Advance the Gospel   [12]Now I want you to know, brothers, that what has happened to me has really served to advance the gospel. [13]As a result, it has become clear throughout the whole palace guard[b] and to everyone else that I am in chains for Christ. [14]Because of my chains, most of the brothers in the Lord have been encouraged to speak the word of God more courageously and fearlessly.

[15]It is true that some preach Christ out of envy and rivalry, but others out of goodwill. [16]The latter do so in love, knowing that I am put here for the defense of the gospel. [17]The former preach Christ out of selfish ambition, not sincerely, supposing that they can stir up trouble for me while I am in chains.[c] [18]But what does it matter? The important thing is that in every way, whether from false motives or true, Christ is preached. And because of this I rejoice.

Yes, and I will continue to rejoice, [19]for I know that through your prayers and the help given by the Spirit of Jesus Christ, what has happened to me will turn out for my deliverance.[d] [20]I eagerly expect and hope that I will in no way be ashamed, but will have sufficient courage so that now as always Christ will be exalted in my body, whether by life or by death. [21]For to me, to live is Christ and to die is gain. [22]If I am to go on living in the body, this will mean fruitful labor for me. Yet what shall I choose? I do not know! [23]I am torn between the two: I desire to depart and be with Christ, which is better by far; [24]but it is more necessary for you that I remain in the body. [25]Convinced of this, I know that I will remain, and I will continue with all of you for your progress and joy in the faith, [26]so that through my being with you again your joy in Christ Jesus will overflow on account of me.

[27]Whatever happens, conduct yourselves in a manner worthy of the gospel of Christ. Then, whether I come and see you or only hear about you in my absence, I will know that you stand firm in one spirit, contending as one man for the faith of the gospel [28]without being frightened in any way by those who oppose you. This is a sign to them that they will be destroyed, but that you will be saved—and that by God. [29]For it has been granted to you on be-

---

[a]1 Traditionally *bishops*   [b]13 Or *whole palace*   [c]16,17 Some late manuscripts have verses 16 and 17 in reverse order.   [d]19 Or *salvation*

half of Christ not only to believe on him, but also to suffer for him, ³⁰since you are going through the same struggle you saw I had, and now hear that I still have.

Imitating Christ's Humility   If you have any encouragement from being united with Christ, if any comfort from his love, if any fellowship with the Spirit, if any tenderness and compassion, ²then make my joy complete by being like-minded, having the same love, being one in spirit and purpose. ³Do nothing out of selfish ambition or vain conceit, but in humility consider others better than yourselves. ⁴Each of you should look not only to your own interests, but also to the interests of others.

⁵Your attitude should be the same as that of Christ Jesus:

⁶Who, being in very nature*ᵃ* God,
   did not consider equality with God something to be grasped,
⁷but made himself nothing,
   taking the very nature*ᵇ* of a servant,
   being made in human likeness.
⁸And being found in appearance as a man,
   he humbled himself
   and became obedient to death—
      even death on a cross!
⁹Therefore God exalted him to the highest place
   and gave him the name that is above every name,
¹⁰that at the name of Jesus every knee should bow,
   in heaven and on earth and under the earth,
¹¹and every tongue confess that Jesus Christ is Lord,
   to the glory of God the Father.

Shining as Stars   ¹²Therefore, my dear friends, as you have always obeyed— not only in my presence, but now much more in my absence—continue to work out your salvation with fear and trembling, ¹³for it is God who works in you to will and to act according to his good purpose.

¹⁴Do everything without complaining or arguing, ¹⁵so that you may become blameless and pure, children of God without fault in a crooked and depraved generation, in which you shine like stars in the universe ¹⁶as you hold out*ᶜ* the word of life—in order that I may boast on the day of Christ that I did not run or labor for nothing. ¹⁷But even if I am being poured out like a drink offering on the sacrifice and service coming from your faith, I am glad and rejoice with all of you. ¹⁸So you too should be glad and rejoice with me.

Timothy and Epaphroditus   ¹⁹I hope in the Lord Jesus to send Timothy to you soon, that I also may be cheered when I receive news about you. ²⁰I have no one else like him, who takes a genuine interest in your welfare. ²¹For everyone looks out for his own interests, not those of Jesus Christ.

Direct Line

PHILIPPIANS 2:12–18

Know any complainers? Those who gripe about folding clothes or doing dishes? Who nag to go shopping when Mom's busy or who want to make a federal case every time someone uses the phone one minute more than the limit? It's about just such things that this passage says, "Do everything without complaining or arguing" (Philippians 2:14). God is ready to work in your life. But a complaining, ornery attitude blocks what he is eager to do. So, if you're one of those negative types, always complaining and arguing, now is a good time to change. A negative attitude makes life miserable for those around you. And it makes you miserable too.

ᵃ6 Or in the form of ᵇ7 Or the form ᶜ16 Or hold on to

Siblings

Sib-ling (sib-ling) n. one of two or more persons having one or both parents in common: a brother or sister.

ALTERNATE DEFINITION
a monster, younger or older than you are, who lives in your house but couldn't possibly be related to you or any other human being

They borrow your sweater without asking and spill peanut butter and jelly on it. Then they hide it so you won't find out, and it rots. They listen in on your phone calls. They pound on the door when you're in the bathroom. Mom and Dad always believe them and not you, so you get in trouble for things they do. Ugh! Who can stand brothers and sisters!

Of course, you're stuck with your brothers and sisters. Your parents have to let them in the door when they come home.

What do teens say about their brothers and sisters? Mostly they ask: How can I get along better with them? Which reveals, of course, the fact that they aren't getting along.

They also ask: Why can't brothers and sisters be nice? Why do my brothers beat me up? Why can't they learn to behave? Why is my sister so annoying? Why do we fight? Why are they the ones who get spoiled?

And, why did my parents have them?

There is one way to get back at them though. It's really nasty, but have you got any choice? Here's the secret:

"Do not take revenge, my friends...on the contrary: 'if your enemy is hungry, feed him; if he is thirsty, give him something to drink. In doing this, you will heap burning coals on his head.' Do not be overcome by evil, but overcome evil with good."
ROMANS 12:19-21

Isn't that sneaky? They do something rotten to you, and you just smile and offer to help with their homework. Or you ask what TV channel they want to watch. It would drive them wild. Who knows? After a while, they might even give up and begin to act human.

Parents

Par-ents (pare-unts) n.
one that produces or brings forth offspring.

Curfews. Clean rooms. Homework. Allowances. Dishes. Little brothers. Little sisters. Yard work. Are these the ammunition that parents use to make life miserable for their teenagers? Or are they simply the (often frustrating) parts of life that everyone, no matter what age, must learn to deal with? You answer.

Most parents really do love their kids. Sure, they'll sometimes admit that you drive them crazy, but that doesn't mean they don't care. Do all that you can to make your relationship with your parents a good one. Be as open and respectful and loving as you can be. And be prepared for them to be open and respectful and loving in return.

Is your house a battleground? Does it seem like there is constant fighting? Check it out: How many battles do you cause? How many could you prevent?

"Honor your father and mother...that it may go well with you and that you may enjoy long life on the earth."
EPHESIANS 6:2-3

So you don't always get along with your parents as great as you'd like? They just don't understand at all what it's like to be a teenager today? Well, it's been a few years since they were teenagers and the world has changed tremendously. So why not be their "teacher"? Talk to them. Fill them in on all the honest-to-goodness truth about your world.

Friends

Friends (frenz) n.
those who know, like and trust
one another; those who support
and sympathize.

How can you tell if
you have true friends?
Why do your friends
sometimes leave you
out? Why are some
friends two-faced?
Why do they lie? Is it
good or bad to be
friends with non-
Christians? Why are
some friends caring
and others aren't?

The Greek philosopher Aristotle said we
choose friends who are useful to us, friends
whose company we enjoy, friends
whose qualities we admire and
who admire us in return. How
do you choose your friends?

*Jesus chose you to be
his friend. "Accept one
another, then, just as
Christ accepted you,
in order to bring
praise to God."*
ROMANS 15:7

*Maybe it's more important
to be a friend than to have
one. How can you be a
friend? Proverbs gives these
guidelines:*

—Love unconditionally
PROVERBS 17:17

—Be available for advice
PROVERBS 27:9

—Speak the truth
PROVERBS 27:5-6

—Be loyal
PROVERBS 16:28

Check it off. What's the goal of having
friends, anyway?

a. to have someone to talk with at school.
b. to keep from being lonely.
c. to let their popularity rub off on you.
d. to learn how to be a friend.
e. to have someone to talk about behind
   his or her back.
f. to let them know how much Christ
   cares for them.
g. to learn and grow together
   as Christians.

Dating

Dat-ing (day-ting) n.
meeting someone socially at a particular
time, especially a member of the opposite sex.

Why is it so scary to ask someone for a date? How old should you be to go out on a date? If a guy spends a lot of money on you, do you have to let him kiss you? Do you get embarrassed when your parents want to meet the person you're dating?

Lots of adults will give you advice. Even when you don't ask for it. Here's some. Which do you think is good advice?
—Look for friendship, not love.
—Go out with groups. Don't isolate yourselves.
—Avoid getting too close too soon.
—Don't stay together just for security.
—Don't feel you have to pay for dates with physical intimacy.

"Each of you should learn to control his own body in a way that is holy and honorable, not in passionate lust like the heathen, who do not know God...No one should wrong his brother or take advantage of him."
1 THESSALONIANS 4:4-6

What can you do on a date? Ride a bike. Visit a beach. Take a walk. Share a pizza. Watch TV. Bake cookies. Listen to music. Do homework together. Play tennis. Hang out at the mall. Talk. Hold hands.

Actually, 50 percent of the girls and 40 percent of the guys graduate from high school without ever having had a date! Surprised? If you're a "late bloomer," it's good to know you're not alone.

In India Christian marriages are often still arranged by the families. The bride and groom may never even see each other until the wedding. Yet divorce between such couples is rare. Do you think their way is better than ours? Why, or why not?

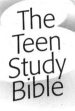

The
Teen
Study
Bible

**New
International
Version**

PROJECT MANAGEMENT AND EDITORIAL
JEAN E. SYSWERDA, EDITORIAL & PUBLISHING SERVICES, ALLENDALE, MI

INTERIOR DESIGN
SHARON WRIGHT, BELMONT, MI

CARTOONS
CARL MEINKE, GRAND RAPIDS, MI

COVER DESIGN
CINDY TOBEY, GRAND RAPIDS, MI

TIP-IN COLOR PAGES
PAZ DESIGN GROUP, SALEM, OR

TYPESETTING
COMCOM AN RR DONNELLEY & SONS COMPANY, ALLENTOWN, PA

PROOFREADING
PEACHTREE EDITORIAL AND PROOFREADING SERVICE, PEACHTREE CITY, GA

²²But you know that Timothy has proved himself, because as a son with his father he has served with me in the work of the gospel. ²³I hope, therefore, to send him as soon as I see how things go with me. ²⁴And I am confident in the Lord that I myself will come soon.

²⁵But I think it is necessary to send back to you Epaphroditus, my brother, fellow worker and fellow soldier, who is also your messenger, whom you sent to take care of my needs. ²⁶For he longs for all of you and is distressed because you heard he was ill. ²⁷Indeed he was ill, and almost died. But God had mercy on him, and not on him only but also on me, to spare me sorrow upon sorrow. ²⁸Therefore I am all the more eager to send him, so that when you see him again you may be glad and I may have less anxiety. ²⁹Welcome him in the Lord with great joy, and honor men like him, ³⁰because he almost died for the work of Christ, risking his life to make up for the help you could not give me.

3

No Confidence in the Flesh   Finally, my brothers, rejoice in the Lord! It is no trouble for me to write the same things to you again, and it is a safeguard for you.

²Watch out for those dogs, those men who do evil, those mutilators of the flesh. ³For it is we who are the circumcision, we who worship by the Spirit of God, who glory in Christ Jesus, and who put no confidence in the flesh— ⁴though I myself have reasons for such confidence.

If anyone else thinks he has reasons to put confidence in the flesh, I have more: ⁵circumcised on the eighth day, of the people of Israel, of the tribe of Benjamin, a Hebrew of Hebrews; in regard to the law, a Pharisee; ⁶as for zeal, persecuting the church; as for legalistic righteousness, faultless.

⁷But whatever was to my profit I now consider loss for the sake of Christ. ⁸What is more, I consider everything a loss compared to the surpassing greatness of knowing Christ Jesus my Lord, for whose sake I have lost all things. I consider them rubbish, that I may gain Christ ⁹and be found in him, not having a righteousness of my own that comes from the law, but that which is through faith in Christ—the righteousness that comes from God and is by faith. ¹⁰I want to know Christ and the power of his resurrection and the fellowship of sharing in his sufferings, becoming like him in his death, ¹¹and so, somehow, to attain to the resurrection from the dead.

Pressing on Toward the Goal   ¹²Not that I have already obtained all this, or have already been made perfect, but I press on to take hold of that for which Christ Jesus took hold of me. ¹³Brothers, I do not consider myself yet to have taken hold of it. But one thing I do: Forgetting what is behind and straining toward what is ahead, ¹⁴I press on toward the goal to win the prize for which God has called me heavenward in Christ Jesus.

¹⁵All of us who are mature should take such a view of things. And if on some point you think differently, that too God will make clear to you. ¹⁶Only let us live up to what we have already attained.

¹⁷Join with others in following my ex-

PHILIPPIANS 3:17–21

When you're a little kid, the place you live determines who your friends are. When all you have for wheels is a tricycle, you just about have to play with kids who live on your block. When you become a teen, things change. Then you meet kids from all over, and you get to choose your friends. Of course, along with that privilege comes responsibility. You get to choose your friends, but you need to choose wisely. Paul's advice is to take note of the way others live. Note the way they talk about others. And pick as your friends teens who live "according to the pattern" God outlines in the Bible.

Direct Line

ample, brothers, and take note of those who live according to the pattern we gave you. [18]For, as I have often told you before and now say again even with tears, many live as enemies of the cross of Christ. [19]Their destiny is destruction, their god is their stomach, and their glory is in their shame. Their mind is on earthly things. [20]But our citizenship is in heaven. And we eagerly await a Savior from there, the Lord Jesus Christ, [21]who, by the power that enables him to bring everything under his control, will transform our lowly bodies so that they will be like his glorious body.

4 Therefore, my brothers, you whom I love and long for, my joy and crown, that is how you should stand firm in the Lord, dear friends!

Exhortations [2]I plead with Euodia and I plead with Syntyche to agree with each other in the Lord. [3]Yes, and I ask you, loyal yokefellow,[a] help these women who have contended at my side in the cause of the gospel, along with Clement and the rest of my fellow workers, whose names are in the book of life.

[4]Rejoice in the Lord always. I will say it again: Rejoice! [5]Let your gentleness be evident to all. The Lord is near. [6]Do not be anxious about anything, but in everything, by prayer and petition, with thanksgiving, present your requests to God. [7]And the peace of God, which transcends all understanding, will guard your hearts and your minds in Christ Jesus.

[8]Finally, brothers, whatever is true, whatever is noble, whatever is right, whatever is pure, whatever is lovely, whatever is admirable—if anything is excellent or praiseworthy—think about such things. [9]Whatever you have learned or received or heard from me, or seen in me—put it into practice. And the God of peace will be with you.

Thanks for Their Gifts [10]I rejoice greatly in the Lord that at last you have renewed your concern for me. Indeed, you have been concerned, but you had no opportunity to show it. [11]I am not saying this because I am in need, for I have learned to be content whatever the circumstances. [12]I know what it is to be in need, and I know what it is to have plenty. I have learned the secret of being content in any and every situation, whether well fed or hungry, whether living in plenty or in want. [13]I can do everything through him who gives me strength.

[14]Yet it was good of you to share in my troubles. [15]Moreover, as you Philippians know, in the early days of your acquaintance with the gospel, when I set out from Macedonia, not one church shared with me in the matter of giving and receiving, except you only; [16]for even when I was in Thessalonica, you sent me aid again and again when I was in need. [17]Not that I am looking for a gift, but I am looking for what may be credited to your account. [18]I have received full payment and even more; I am amply supplied, now that I have received from Epaphroditus the gifts you sent. They are a fragrant offering, an acceptable sacrifice, pleasing

---

Direct Line

PHILIPPIANS 4:10-13

You get a bike, and you want a moped. Get a moped, and you want an old car. Get an old car, and you want a new car. You need the latest in athletic shoes too, right? Sometimes Mom and Dad try to make you feel guilty by saying things like, "I only had two dresses," or "I had to walk 23 miles in snow over my head." But that misses the point. When Paul talks about contentment, he's reminding you that the never-satisfied person is miserable. Why settle for misery? Enjoy that bike now. When the old car comes, enjoy it too. Enjoy life's good gifts. It really isn't fun being a "gotta-have-more" type. No fun at all.

[a]3 Or *loyal Syzygus*

Dear Sam,

Movies, music videos and modern music didn't exist in Bible times, so how can the Bible say anything about them?

Ray in Rapid City

---

100 Advice Lane, Anywhere, USA

Dear Sam, Inc.

Dear Ray,

You're right. There's not a verse that says, "Thou shall not watch any naughty music videos." But if you study God's Word, your answer is just as clear as if it did. Paul tells you what to focus your mind on (Philippians 4:8): "Whatever is true, whatever is noble, whatever is right, whatever is pure, whatever is lovely, whatever is admirable—if anything is excellent or praiseworthy—think about such things." If the movies, music and videos you enjoy fall into these categories, great. Enjoy!

But be very careful. Don't just pass it off and say, "Oh, the stuff I listen to isn't so bad." Examine what you see and hear very carefully. Do the words (or their meanings) in the music and movies fit with the description in Philippians 4:8? You decide. But remember, you will be responsible directly to God for your choices, and your life will reflect what you're thinking about (Matthew 12:36-37).

Sam

to God. [19]And my God will meet all your needs according to his glorious riches in Christ Jesus.

[20]To our God and Father be glory for ever and ever. Amen.

Final Greetings [21]Greet all the saints in Christ Jesus. The brothers who are with me send greetings. [22]All the saints send you greetings, especially those who belong to Caesar's household.

[23]The grace of the Lord Jesus Christ be with your spirit. Amen.[a]

[a]*23 Some manuscripts do not have* Amen.

Introduction

to the

book of # Colossians

HOROSCOPES. MEDIUMS. PALM READERS.
Ouija boards. Psychics. People who say they talk
with a "friendly spirit." Past lives people claim to
remember. All these ideas about what's real can be
confusing.

The Colossians were confused too. Some of them
believed they had to go through spirits to reach God.
Some said Jesus was a spirit but not a very important
one. Paul wrote Colossians to explain who Jesus is
and how you can stay close to God. Anyone who
understands what Colossians teaches won't be confused any longer!

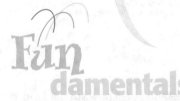

Fundamentals

*How important is Christ (Colossians
1:15-20)?*

*Are you a better Christian just
because you don't do the things
other kids do (Colossians 2:20-23)?*

*Do you ever get mad when someone
doesn't keep a promise to you
(Colossians 3:12-14)?*

FAST FACTS

*Colosse was an important
city in what is now Turkey.*

*Paul did not start the church
in Colosse.*

*Some people in Colosse said
the physical body is evil.*

*If Jesus had a real, physical body,
how can the body be evil?*

*The body is neither bad nor good.
It's what you do with your body that
makes the difference.*

Paul, an apostle of Christ Jesus by the will of God, and Timothy our brother,

²To the holy and faithful*a* brothers in Christ at Colosse:

Grace and peace to you from God our Father.*b*

Thanksgiving and Prayer ³We always thank God, the Father of our Lord Jesus Christ, when we pray for you, ⁴because we have heard of your faith in Christ Jesus and of the love you have for all the saints— ⁵the faith and love that spring from the hope that is stored up for you in heaven and that you have already heard about in the word of truth, the gospel ⁶that has come to you. All over the world this gospel is bearing fruit and growing, just as it has been doing among you since the day you heard it and understood God's grace in all its truth. ⁷You learned it from Epaphras, our dear fellow servant, who is a faithful minister of Christ on our*c* behalf, ⁸and who also told us of your love in the Spirit.

⁹For this reason, since the day we heard about you, we have not stopped praying for you and asking God to fill you with the knowledge of his will through all spiritual wisdom and understanding. ¹⁰And we pray this in order that you may live a life worthy of the Lord and may please him in every way: bearing fruit in every good work, growing in the knowledge of God, ¹¹being strengthened with all power according to his glorious might so that you may have great endurance and patience, and joyfully ¹²giving thanks to the Father, who has qualified you*d* to share in the inheritance of the saints in the kingdom of light. ¹³For he has rescued us from the dominion of darkness and brought us into the kingdom of the Son he loves, ¹⁴in whom we have redemption,*e* the forgiveness of sins.

The Supremacy of Christ ¹⁵He is the image of the invisible God, the firstborn over all creation. ¹⁶For by him all things were created: things in heaven and on earth, visible and invisible, whether thrones or powers or rulers or authorities; all things were created by him and for him. ¹⁷He is before all things, and in him all things hold together. ¹⁸And he is the head of the body, the church; he is the beginning and the firstborn from among the dead, so that in everything he might have the supremacy. ¹⁹For God was pleased to have

---

a2 Or *believing*   *b2* Some manuscripts *Father and the Lord Jesus Christ*   *c7* Some manuscripts *your*
d12 Some manuscripts *us*   *e14* A few late manuscripts *redemption through his blood*

The Bible Says

Jesus Is Supreme

Many passages in the New Testament tell how special Jesus is:

* Jesus is "far above all rule and authority" (Ephesians 1:20–22).
* Jesus is "in very nature God" (Philippians 2:6).
* Jesus created all things (Colossians 1:16).
* Jesus is supreme (Colossians 1:18).
* All God's fullness dwells in Jesus (Colossians 1:19).
* Jesus is "the radiance of God's glory and the exact representation of his being" (Hebrews 1:3).
* Jesus sustains "all things by his powerful word." Without Jesus the universe would dissolve (Hebrews 1:3).

Christians are familiar with what Jesus did while he was here on earth. But it's good to think about who Jesus is.

all his fullness dwell in him, ²⁰and through him to reconcile to himself all things, whether things on earth or things in heaven, by making peace through his blood, shed on the cross.

²¹Once you were alienated from God and were enemies in your minds because of*ᵃ* your evil behavior. ²²But now he has reconciled you by Christ's physical body through death to present you holy in his sight, without blemish and free from accusation— ²³if you continue in your faith, established and firm, not moved from the hope held out in the gospel. This is the gospel that you heard and that has been proclaimed to every creature under heaven, and of which I, Paul, have become a servant.

Paul's Labor for the Church ²⁴Now I rejoice in what was suffered for you, and I fill up in my flesh what is still lacking in regard to Christ's afflictions, for the sake of his body, which is the church. ²⁵I have become its servant by the commission God gave me to present to you the word of God in its fullness— ²⁶the mystery that has been kept hidden for ages and generations, but is now disclosed to the saints. ²⁷To them God has chosen to make known among the Gentiles the glorious riches of this mystery, which is Christ in you, the hope of glory.

²⁸We proclaim him, admonishing and teaching everyone with all wisdom, so that we may present everyone perfect in Christ. ²⁹To this end I labor, struggling with all his energy, which so powerfully works in me.

2 I want you to know how much I am struggling for you and for those at Laodicea, and for all who have not met me personally. ²My purpose is that they may be encouraged in heart and united in love, so that they may have the full riches of complete understanding, in order that they may know the mystery of God, namely, Christ, ³in whom are hidden all the treasures of wisdom and knowledge. ⁴I tell you this so that no one may deceive you by fine-sounding arguments. ⁵For though I am absent from you in body, I am present with you in spirit and delight to see how orderly you are and how firm your faith in Christ is.

Freedom From Human Regulations Through Life With Christ ⁶So then, just as you received Christ Jesus as Lord, continue to live in him, ⁷rooted and built up in him, strengthened in the faith as you were taught, and overflowing with thankfulness.

⁸See to it that no one takes you captive through hollow and deceptive philosophy, which depends on human tradition and the basic principles of this world rather than on Christ.

⁹For in Christ all the fullness of the Deity lives in bodily form, ¹⁰and you have been given fullness in Christ, who is the head over every power and authority. ¹¹In him you were also circumcised, in the putting off of the sinful nature,*ᵇ* not with a circumcision done by the hands of men but with the circumcision done by Christ, ¹²having been buried with him in baptism and raised with him through your faith in the power of God, who raised him from the dead.

¹³When you were dead in your sins and in the uncircumcision of your sinful nature,*ᶜ* God made you*ᵈ* alive with Christ. He forgave us all our sins, ¹⁴having canceled the written code, with its regulations, that was against us and that stood opposed to us; he took it away, nailing it to the cross. ¹⁵And having disarmed the powers and authorities, he made a public spectacle of them, triumphing over them by the cross.*ᵉ*

¹⁶Therefore do not let anyone judge you by what you eat or drink, or with regard to a religious festival, a New Moon celebration or a Sabbath day.

ᵃ21 Or *minds, as shown by* *ᵇ11* Or *the flesh* *ᶜ13* Or *your flesh* *ᵈ13* Some manuscripts *us* *ᵉ15* Or *them in him*

[17]These are a shadow of the things that were to come; the reality, however, is found in Christ. [18]Do not let anyone who delights in false humility and the worship of angels disqualify you for the prize. Such a person goes into great detail about what he has seen, and his unspiritual mind puffs him up with idle notions. [19]He has lost connection with the Head, from whom the whole body, supported and held together by its ligaments and sinews, grows as God causes it to grow.

[20]Since you died with Christ to the basic principles of this world, why, as though you still belonged to it, do you submit to its rules: [21]"Do not handle! Do not taste! Do not touch!"? [22]These are all destined to perish with use, because they are based on human commands and teachings. [23]Such regulations indeed have an appearance of wisdom, with their self-imposed worship, their false humility and their harsh treatment of the body, but they lack any value in restraining sensual indulgence.

Rules for Holy Living   Since, then, you have been raised with Christ, set your hearts on things above, where Christ is seated at the right hand of God. [2]Set your minds on things above, not on earthly things. [3]For you died, and your life is now hidden with Christ in God. [4]When Christ, who is your[a] life, appears, then you also will appear with him in glory.

[5]Put to death, therefore, whatever belongs to your earthly nature: sexual immorality, impurity, lust, evil desires and greed, which is idolatry. [6]Because of these, the wrath of God is coming.[b] [7]You used to walk in these ways, in the life you once lived. [8]But now you must rid yourselves of all such things as these: anger, rage, malice, slander, and filthy language from your lips. [9]Do not lie to each other, since you have taken off your old self with its practices [10]and have put on the new self, which is being renewed in knowledge in the image of its Creator. [11]Here there is no Greek or Jew, circumcised or uncircumcised, barbarian, Scythian, slave or free, but Christ is all, and is in all.

[12]Therefore, as God's chosen people, holy and dearly loved, clothe yourselves with compassion, kindness, humility, gentleness and patience. [13]Bear with each other and forgive whatever grievances you may have against one another. Forgive as the Lord forgave you. [14]And over all these virtues put on love, which binds them all together in perfect unity.

[15]Let the peace of Christ rule in your hearts, since as members of one body you were called to peace. And be thankful. [16]Let the word of Christ dwell in you richly as you teach and admonish one another with all wisdom, and as you sing psalms, hymns and spiritual songs with gratitude in your hearts to God. [17]And whatever you do, whether in word or deed, do it all in the name of the Lord Jesus, giving thanks to God the Father through him.

Rules for Christian Households   [18]Wives, submit to your husbands, as is fitting in the Lord.

[19]Husbands, love your wives and do not be harsh with them.

[20]Children, obey your parents in everything, for this pleases the Lord.

Direct Line

COLOSSIANS 2:20–23

Have you ever gone on a crash diet? Your stomach twists. You're starving. If you're suffering that much, you *must* be losing weight. Then you get on the scales and find you've lost half an ounce! Some people take the same approach to spirituality. They figure if they cut out everything that's fun, they'll be more spiritual. Paul says such things "have an appearance of wisdom" but, like crash diets, "lack any value in restraining sensual indulgence"(Colossians 2:23). You feel spiritual without being spiritual. What's the true way to become a spiritual Christian? Check out Colossians 3:5–14.

---

[a]4 Some manuscripts *our* [b]6 Some early manuscripts *coming on those who are disobedient*

Dear Sam,

We want to have some fun! Isn't partying with designated drivers and practicing safe sex being responsible?

Patty in Pella

Dear Sam, Inc.

100 Advice Lane, Anywhere, USA

Dear Patty,

God is very fair. He doesn't expect you to guess at right and wrong. His Word tells you. And if you're honest, you usually know right from wrong deep inside because the Holy Spirit guides you if you let him.

Truly, there is no such thing as safe sex outside of marriage. If there were, God would have told you. He doesn't try to make you miserable. He tries to save you from misery. Having a designated driver is better than drunk driving, but car accidents aren't the only danger in drunkenness. Alcohol also kills inhibitions, sometimes with disastrous results.

Check out Colossians 3:5-10 and think how the Lord would answer your question. Then stand up for what is right. Perhaps your example will get others to do the same. Be a leader of what is right, not a follower of what is wrong.

Sam

²¹Fathers, do not embitter your children, or they will become discouraged. ²²Slaves, obey your earthly masters in everything; and do it, not only when their eye is on you and to win their favor, but with sincerity of heart and reverence for the Lord. ²³Whatever you do, work at it with all your heart, as working for the Lord, not for men, ²⁴since you know that you will receive an inheritance from the Lord as a reward. It is the Lord Christ you are serving. ²⁵Anyone who does wrong will be repaid for his wrong, and there is no favoritism.

4 Masters, provide your slaves with what is right and fair, because you know that you also have a Master in heaven.

Further Instructions ²Devote yourselves to prayer, being watchful and thankful. ³And pray for us, too, that God may open a door for our message, so that we may proclaim the mystery of Christ, for which I am in chains. ⁴Pray that I may proclaim it clearly, as I should. ⁵Be wise in the way you act toward outsiders; make the most of every opportunity. ⁶Let your conversation be always full of grace, seasoned with salt, so that you may know how to answer everyone.

Final Greetings ⁷Tychicus will tell you all the news about me. He is a dear brother, a faithful minister and fellow servant in the Lord. ⁸I am sending him to you for the express purpose that you may know about our*a* circumstances and that he may encourage your hearts. ⁹He is coming with Onesimus, our faithful and dear brother, who is one of you. They will tell you everything that is happening here.

¹⁰My fellow prisoner Aristarchus sends you his greetings, as does Mark, the cousin of Barnabas. (You have received instructions about him; if he comes to you, welcome him.) ¹¹Jesus, who is called Justus, also sends greetings. These are the only Jews among my fellow workers for the kingdom of God, and they have proved a comfort to me. ¹²Epaphras, who is one of you and a servant of Christ Jesus, sends greetings. He is always wrestling in prayer for you, that you may stand firm in all the will of God, mature and fully assured. ¹³I vouch for him that he is working hard for you and for those at Laodicea and Hierapolis. ¹⁴Our dear friend Luke, the doctor, and Demas send greetings. ¹⁵Give my greetings to the brothers at Laodicea, and to Nympha and the church in her house.

¹⁶After this letter has been read to you, see that it is also read in the church of the Laodiceans and that you in turn read the letter from Laodicea.

¹⁷Tell Archippus: "See to it that you complete the work you have received in the Lord."

¹⁸I, Paul, write this greeting in my own hand. Remember my chains. Grace be with you.

COLOSSIANS 3:18—4:1

Direct Line

So your parents are unfair. You do your work, and they still won't let you go out with your friends. Or you work hard at a grocery store, and the manager is crabby at you anyway. What do you do? Paul reminds you that if your boss or your parents are unfair, that doesn't mean you're released from your responsibility to them. How can you keep on being a good person when others are bad to you? Here's the secret: Remember that you are "working for the Lord," not for your unfair parent or boss. And because it is for the Lord, "you know that you will receive an inheritance" (Colossians 3:23–24). What you do right is appreciated. By God himself.

---

a8 Some manuscripts that he may know about your

1 Thessalonians

HARD TIMES.

Some of you will face hard times while you're young. A friend may get killed in a car accident. A mom or grandma may get cancer. Someone you know may commit suicide. How can you stand it when suffering or death comes?

Paul wrote to the Thessalonian Christians to encourage them. They'd been true to God in spite of sufferings. But they were worried about Christians who had died. Paul let them know that death isn't the end. When Jesus comes, you'll be reunited with the people you love.

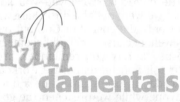

Fundamentals

How can you make real friends, not just have acquaintances (1 Thessalonians 2:6-12)?

Do your friends think sex is OK as long as you have "safe sex" (1 Thessalonians 4:3-8)?

Do you get depressed when you think about people you know who have died (1 Thessalonians 4:13-18)?

FAST FACTS

Thessalonica was the capital of the province of Macedonia. The Romans had a great naval base there.

Paul was in Thessalonica only a few weeks.

Paul left because anti-Paul riots threatened the lives of the new Christians (Acts 17:1-9).

The church grew despite opposition, and the gospel spread to all Macedonia.

1538

1 Paul, Silas*a* and Timothy,

To the church of the Thessalonians in God the Father and the Lord Jesus Christ:

Grace and peace to you.*b*

Thanksgiving for the Thessalonians' Faith ²We always thank God for all of you, mentioning you in our prayers. ³We continually remember before our God and Father your work produced by faith, your labor prompted by love, and your endurance inspired by hope in our Lord Jesus Christ.

⁴For we know, brothers loved by God, that he has chosen you, ⁵because our gospel came to you not simply with words, but also with power, with the Holy Spirit and with deep conviction. You know how we lived among you for your sake. ⁶You became imitators of us and of the Lord; in spite of severe suffering, you welcomed the message with the joy given by the Holy Spirit. ⁷And so you became a model to all the believers in Macedonia and Achaia. ⁸The Lord's message rang out from you not only in Macedonia and Achaia— your faith in God has become known everywhere. Therefore we do not need to say anything about it, ⁹for they themselves report what kind of reception you gave us. They tell how you turned to God from idols to serve the living and true God, ¹⁰and to wait for his Son from heaven, whom he raised from the dead—Jesus, who rescues us from the coming wrath.

2 *Paul's Ministry in Thessalonica* You know, brothers, that our visit to you was not a failure. ²We had previously suffered and been insulted in Philippi, as you know, but with the help of our God we dared to tell you his gospel in spite of strong opposition. ³For the appeal we make does not spring from error or impure motives, nor are we trying to trick you. ⁴On the contrary, we speak as men approved by God to be entrusted with the gospel. We are not trying to please men but God, who tests our hearts. ⁵You know we never used flattery, nor did we put on a mask to cover up greed—God is our witness. ⁶We were not looking for praise from men, not from you or anyone else.

As apostles of Christ we could have been a burden to you, ⁷but we were gentle among you, like a mother caring for her little children. ⁸We loved you so much that we were delighted to share with you not only the gospel of God but our lives as well, because you had become so dear to us. ⁹Surely you remember, brothers, our toil and hardship; we worked night and day in order not to be a burden to anyone while we preached the gospel of God to you.

¹⁰You are witnesses, and so is God, of how holy, righteous and blameless we were among you who believed. ¹¹For you know that we dealt with each of you as a father deals with his own children, ¹²encouraging, comforting and urging you to live lives worthy of God, who calls you into his kingdom and glory.

---

1 THESSALONIANS 2:5-12

Your friends are pretty important to you, aren't they? Oh yeah, Mom and Dad get upset at times because you're always on the phone. But, hey, they're your friends! Friends are so important that it's good to know how to make them and keep them. These verses tell how Paul made lasting friendships. He didn't flatter. He didn't say things just so others would like him better. He really cared about his friends. And he was willing to share personal things with them. You may not feel free to share with all the kids you know. But you can get close to a special few if you treat them as Paul treated his friends.

Direct Line

---

a1 Greek *Silvanus,* a variant of *Silas* *b1* Some early manuscripts *you from God our Father and the Lord Jesus Christ*

¹³And we also thank God continually because, when you received the word of God, which you heard from us, you accepted it not as the word of men, but as it actually is, the word of God, which is at work in you who believe. ¹⁴For you, brothers, became imitators of God's churches in Judea, which are in Christ Jesus: You suffered from your own countrymen the same things those churches suffered from the Jews, ¹⁵who killed the Lord Jesus and the prophets and also drove us out. They displease God and are hostile to all men ¹⁶in their effort to keep us from speaking to the Gentiles so that they may be saved. In this way they always heap up their sins to the limit. The wrath of God has come upon them at last.*a*

Paul's Longing to See the Thessalonians   ¹⁷But, brothers, when we were torn away from you for a short time (in person, not in thought), out of our intense longing we made every effort to see you. ¹⁸For we wanted to come to you—certainly I, Paul, did, again and again—but Satan stopped us. ¹⁹For what is our hope, our joy, or the crown in which we will glory in the presence of our Lord Jesus when he comes? Is it not you? ²⁰Indeed, you are our glory and joy.

So when we could stand it no longer, we thought it best to be left by ourselves in Athens. ²We sent Timothy, who is our brother and God's fellow worker*b* in spreading the gospel of Christ, to strengthen and encourage you in your faith, ³so that no one would be unsettled by these trials. You know quite well that we were destined for them. ⁴In fact, when we were with you, we kept telling you that we would be persecuted. And it turned out that way, as you well know. ⁵For this reason, when I could stand it no longer, I sent to find out about your faith. I was afraid that in some way the tempter might have tempted you and our efforts might have been useless.

Timothy's Encouraging Report   ⁶But Timothy has just now come to us from you and has brought good news about your faith and love. He has told us that you always have pleasant memories of us and that you long to see us, just as we also long to see you. ⁷Therefore, brothers, in all our distress and persecution we were encouraged about you because of your faith. ⁸For now we really live, since you are standing firm in the Lord. ⁹How can we thank God enough for you in return for all the joy we have in the presence of our God because of you? ¹⁰Night and day we pray most earnestly that we may see you again and supply what is lacking in your faith.

¹¹Now may our God and Father himself and our Lord Jesus clear the way for us to come to you. ¹²May the Lord make your love increase and overflow for each other and for everyone else, just as ours does for you. ¹³May he strengthen your hearts so that you will be blameless and holy in the presence of our God and Father when our Lord Jesus comes with all his holy ones.

Living to Please God   Finally, brothers, we instructed you how to live in order to please God, as in fact you are living. Now we ask you and urge you in the Lord Jesus to do this more and more. ²For you know what instructions we gave you by the authority of the Lord Jesus.

³It is God's will that you should be sanctified: that you should avoid sexual immorality; ⁴that each of you should learn to control his own body*c* in a way that is holy and honorable, ⁵not in passionate lust like the heathen, who do not know God; ⁶and that in this matter no one should wrong his brother or take advantage of him. The Lord will punish men for all such sins, as we have already told you and warned you. ⁷For God did not call us to be impure, but to live a holy life. ⁸Therefore, he who rejects this instruction does not reject man but God, who gives you his Holy Spirit.

---

a16 Or *them fully*   *b2* Some manuscripts *brother and fellow worker;* other manuscripts *brother and God's servant*   *c4* Or *learn to live with his own wife;* or *learn to acquire a wife*

Dear Sam,

All my friends think it's OK to have sex as long as you're smart and you use protection. What do you think?

Michelle in Mackinaw

100 Advice Lane, Anywhere, USA

Dear Sam, Inc.

Dear Michelle,

I have had many letters from teens just like you, struggling with either hormones or peer pressure or both. But Scripture gives only one answer to your question, and it's there over and over again because God understands the temptations and weaknesses of people. God wants you to be pure, using self-control over your physical desires (1 Thessalonians 4:3-8).

There is no mistaking God's directive. No one is safe having sex outside of marriage. No protection works 100 percent of the time. And even if you escape pregnancy and disease, there is no escaping being accountable for your actions on the day of judgment. Saving sex for your marriage partner is God's best gift for you to give your spouse. Sex in marriage is sacred. God doesn't want you to cheapen it. Staying pure before marriage may be one of the most difficult things you do, especially in this modern age; but you'll never regret it. I promise.

Sam

⁹Now about brotherly love we do not need to write to you, for you yourselves have been taught by God to love each other. ¹⁰And in fact, you do love all the brothers throughout Macedonia. Yet we urge you, brothers, to do so more and more.

¹¹Make it your ambition to lead a quiet life, to mind your own business and to work with your hands, just as we told you, ¹²so that your daily life may win the respect of outsiders and so that you will not be dependent on anybody.

The Coming of the Lord   ¹³Brothers, we do not want you to be ignorant about those who fall asleep, or to grieve like the rest of men, who have no hope. ¹⁴We believe that Jesus died and rose again and so we believe that God will bring with Jesus those who have fallen asleep in him. ¹⁵According to the Lord's own word, we tell you that we who are still alive, who are left till the coming of the Lord, will certainly not precede those who have fallen asleep. ¹⁶For the Lord himself will come down from heaven, with a loud command, with the voice of the archangel and with the trumpet call of God, and the dead in Christ will rise first. ¹⁷After that, we who are still alive and are left will be caught up together with them in the clouds to meet the Lord in the air. And so we will be with the Lord forever. ¹⁸Therefore encourage each other with these words.

Now, brothers, about times and dates we do not need to write to you, ²for you know very well that the day of the Lord will come like a thief in the night. ³While people are saying, "Peace and safety," destruction will come on them suddenly, as labor pains on a pregnant woman, and they will not escape.

⁴But you, brothers, are not in darkness so that this day should surprise you like a thief. ⁵You are all sons of the light and sons of the day. We do not belong to the night or to the darkness. ⁶So then, let us not be like others, who are asleep, but let us be alert and self-controlled. ⁷For those who sleep, sleep at night, and those who get drunk, get drunk at night. ⁸But since we belong to the day, let us be self-controlled, putting on faith and love as a breastplate, and the hope of salvation as a helmet. ⁹For God did not appoint us to suffer wrath but to receive salvation through our Lord Jesus Christ. ¹⁰He died for us so that, whether we are awake or asleep, we may live together with him. ¹¹Therefore encourage one another and build each other up, just as in fact you are doing.

It hurts when someone you love dies. You feel empty. You know things will never be the same again. Everybody grieves. But Paul says that Christians do not grieve "like the rest of men, who have no hope" (1 Thessalonians 4:13).

In the Bible hoping is not the same as wishing. It's not like hoping your parents will buy you a sports car. In the Bible hope is being sure about something for which you have to wait. You know that what you hope for will happen because God has promised it.

When Christians experience the death of someone they love, they also experience hope—hope that when Jesus returns he will bring that loved one with him. They will be caught up and reunited. They will "be with the Lord forever" (1 Thessalonians 4:17). Nothing will ever again separate them from those they love.

The Bible Says

You'll See Them Again

1542

Final Instructions ¹²Now we ask you, brothers, to respect those who work hard among you, who are over you in the Lord and who admonish you. ¹³Hold them in the highest regard in love because of their work. Live in peace with each other. ¹⁴And we urge you, brothers, warn those who are idle, encourage the timid, help the weak, be patient with everyone. ¹⁵Make sure that nobody pays back wrong for wrong, but always try to be kind to each other and to everyone else.

¹⁶Be joyful always; ¹⁷pray continually; ¹⁸give thanks in all circumstances, for this is God's will for you in Christ Jesus.

¹⁹Do not put out the Spirit's fire; ²⁰do not treat prophecies with contempt. ²¹Test everything. Hold on to the good. ²²Avoid every kind of evil.

²³May God himself, the God of peace, sanctify you through and through. May your whole spirit, soul and body be kept blameless at the coming of our Lord Jesus Christ. ²⁴The one who calls you is faithful and he will do it.

²⁵Brothers, pray for us. ²⁶Greet all the brothers with a holy kiss. ²⁷I charge you before the Lord to have this letter read to all the brothers.

²⁸The grace of our Lord Jesus Christ be with you.

2 Thessalonians

DRUGS. KILLINGS.

Things do look pretty bad. Fighting all over the world. Bombings. Drug wars and shootings in the streets. Maybe this is what the Bible talks about when it says things will get really bad just before Jesus comes back.

Paul wrote this letter to people who thought things couldn't get worse. He wrote that, yes, Satan is behind the terrible things that happen in our time. But the situation will get a lot worse when Satan really turns loose! So, how are you supposed to live in a world that's pretty bad already? You keep on loving God and hold tight to his Word.

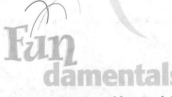

Fundamentals

Do you get persecuted for your faith and wonder if God even cares (2 Thessalonians 1:3-10)?

What are you supposed to do when you're ridiculed for your faith (2 Thessalonians 2:13-17)?

What do you do when a friend wants to copy your homework (2 Thessalonians 3:6)?

FAST FACTS

Paul wrote this letter to clear up misunderstandings about Jesus' second coming.

Man of lawlessness is a name for the antichrist.

Satan will work miracles to try to convince the world the antichrist is God.

Jesus will come to destroy the antichrist.

1 Paul, Silas[a] and Timothy,

To the church of the Thessalonians in God our Father and the Lord Jesus Christ:

[2]Grace and peace to you from God the Father and the Lord Jesus Christ.

Thanksgiving and Prayer [3]We ought always to thank God for you, brothers, and rightly so, because your faith is growing more and more, and the love every one of you has for each other is increasing. [4]Therefore, among God's churches we boast about your perseverance and faith in all the persecutions and trials you are enduring.

[5]All this is evidence that God's judgment is right, and as a result you will be counted worthy of the kingdom of God, for which you are suffering. [6]God is just: He will pay back trouble to those who trouble you [7]and give relief to you who are troubled, and to us as well. This will happen when the Lord Jesus is revealed from heaven in blazing fire with his powerful angels. [8]He will punish those who do not know God and do not obey the gospel of our Lord Jesus. [9]They will be punished with everlasting destruction and shut out from the presence of the Lord and from the majesty of his power [10]on the day he comes to be glorified in his holy people and to be marveled at among all those who have believed. This includes you, because you believed our testimony to you.

[11]With this in mind, we constantly pray for you, that our God may count you worthy of his calling, and that by his power he may fulfill every good purpose of yours and every act prompted by your faith. [12]We pray this so that the name of our Lord Jesus may be glorified in you, and you in him, according to the grace of our God and the Lord Jesus Christ.[b]

2 ***The Man of Lawlessness*** Concerning the coming of our Lord Jesus Christ and our being gathered to him, we ask you, brothers, [2]not to become easily unsettled or alarmed by some prophecy, report or letter supposed to have come from us, saying that the day of the Lord has already come. [3]Don't let anyone deceive you in any way, for that day will not come, until the rebellion occurs and the man of lawlessness[c] is revealed, the man doomed to destruction. [4]He will oppose and will exalt himself over everything that is called God or is worshiped, so that he sets himself up in God's temple, proclaiming himself to be God.

[a]1 Greek *Silvanus*, a variant of *Silas*   [b]12 Or *God and Lord, Jesus Christ*   [c]3 Some manuscripts *sin*

The Bible Says

God Plays Fair

So many things in life aren't fair. Untrue rumors ruin your reputation. A drunk driver smashes into a church bus filled with kids. A desperate drug addict robs a store and shoots an innocent person. A girl is date raped by a guy she trusted. Does it ever make you wonder: Where is God? Why doesn't he do something?

God does not cause terrible things like this. They're caused by people who choose to sin and in their sin hurt innocent people. God usually doesn't pay them back right away. But 2 Thessalonians 1:5–10 tells you that God surely will. It really isn't fair that people can sin against and hurt others. But they won't get away with it. Not in the end. When Jesus comes, "they will be punished . . . and shut out from the presence of the Lord" (2 Thessalonians 1:9).

⁵Don't you remember that when I was with you I used to tell you these things? ⁶And now you know what is holding him back, so that he may be revealed at the proper time. ⁷For the secret power of lawlessness is already at work; but the one who now holds it back will continue to do so till he is taken out of the way. ⁸And then the lawless one will be revealed, whom the Lord Jesus will overthrow with the breath of his mouth and destroy by the splendor of his coming. ⁹The coming of the lawless one will be in accordance with the work of Satan displayed in all kinds of counterfeit miracles, signs and wonders, ¹⁰and in every sort of evil that deceives those who are perishing. They perish because they refused to love the truth and so be saved. ¹¹For this reason God sends them a powerful delusion so that they will believe the lie ¹²and so that all will be condemned who have not believed the truth but have delighted in wickedness.

Stand Firm ¹³But we ought always to thank God for you, brothers loved by the Lord, because from the beginning God chose you*a* to be saved through the sanctifying work of the Spirit and through belief in the truth. ¹⁴He called you to this through our gospel, that you might share in the glory of our Lord Jesus Christ. ¹⁵So then, brothers, stand firm and hold to the teachings*b* we passed on to you, whether by word of mouth or by letter.

¹⁶May our Lord Jesus Christ himself and God our Father, who loved us and by his grace gave us eternal encouragement and good hope, ¹⁷encourage your hearts and strengthen you in every good deed and word.

3 ***Request for Prayer*** Finally, brothers, pray for us that the message of the Lord may spread rapidly and be honored, just as it was with you. ²And pray that we may be delivered from wicked and evil men, for not everyone has faith. ³But the Lord is faithful, and he will strengthen and protect you from the evil one. ⁴We have confidence in the Lord that you are doing and will continue to do the things we command. ⁵May the Lord direct your hearts into God's love and Christ's perseverance.

Warning Against Idleness ⁶In the name of the Lord Jesus Christ, we command you, brothers, to keep away from every brother who is idle and does not live according to the teaching*c* you received from us. ⁷For you yourselves know how you ought to follow our example. We were not idle when we were with you, ⁸nor did we eat anyone's food without paying for it. On the contrary, we worked night and day, laboring and toiling so that we would not be a burden to any of you. ⁹We did this, not because we do not have the right to such help, but in order to make ourselves a model for you to follow. ¹⁰For even when we were with you, we gave you this rule: "If a man will not work, he shall not eat."

> The Lord is faithful, and he will strengthen and protect you from the evil one (2 Thessalonians 3:3).

¹¹We hear that some among you are idle. They are not busy; they are busybodies. ¹²Such people we command and urge in the Lord Jesus Christ to settle down and earn the bread they eat. ¹³And as for you, brothers, never tire of doing what is right.

¹⁴If anyone does not obey our instruction in this letter, take special note of him. Do not associate with him, in order that he may feel ashamed. ¹⁵Yet do not regard him as an enemy, but warn him as a brother.

Final Greetings ¹⁶Now may the Lord of peace himself give you peace at all times and in every way. The Lord be with all of you.

¹⁷I, Paul, write this greeting in my own hand, which is the distinguishing mark in all my letters. This is how I write.

¹⁸The grace of our Lord Jesus Christ be with you all.

---

*a13 Some manuscripts *because God chose you as his firstfruits* *b15 Or *traditions* *c6 Or *tradition*

Dear Sam,

One of my friends keeps wanting to copy my homework. What should I do?

Randy in Redding

100 Advice Lane, Anywhere, USA

Dear Sam, Inc.

Dear Randy,

Unfortunately, this is a common problem in schools today. Many students don't even give a thought to whether copying homework is right or wrong.

Paul wrote that anyone who was not willing to work should not eat (2 Thessalonians 3:6-10). You can substitute the following words: "If a student will not do homework, he shall not get credit" (2 Thessalonians 3:10). Everyone has a job to do. Students have to keep up with their studies. Children have chores to do. Adults have to go to work every day. Each person is responsible to do his or her own work.

Tell your friend that if he doesn't understand the work, you'll try to explain it. But tell him you simply can't have him copy your work. Maybe you and your friend can get together at home or over the phone to go over the homework assignment. That way you'll be able to help your friend, your friend will be responsible for his own work, and you'll feel better about the whole situation.

Sam

TEENS.

Have you ever noticed how older people often look down on teens? Not all adults, of course. But many adults don't listen very closely to teenagers.

In this letter to a young follower, the apostle Paul tells him, "Don't let anyone look down on you because you are young" (1 Timothy 4:12). Better yet, Paul tells Timothy what to do to earn older people's respect! His words of wisdom may show you how to get more respect too!

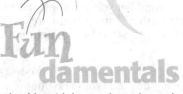

Fundamentals

Should a girl dress only to please the guys (1 Timothy 2:9-10)?

How do you get respect from people who are older (1 Timothy 4:11-16)?

Is money the root of all evil? If not, what is (1 Timothy 6:3-10)?

FAST FACTS

Paul wrote this letter near the end of his life.

Timothy had a Jewish mother and a Greek father.

Timothy traveled with Paul on two missionary journeys.

Even though Timothy was young and shy, Paul sent him on several important missions.

Timothy did not always succeed, but Paul didn't give up on him.

1 Paul, an apostle of Christ Jesus by the command of God our Savior and of Christ Jesus our hope,

²To Timothy my true son in the faith:

Grace, mercy and peace from God the Father and Christ Jesus our Lord.

Warning Against False Teachers of the Law   ³As I urged you when I went into Macedonia, stay there in Ephesus so that you may command certain men not to teach false doctrines any longer ⁴nor to devote themselves to myths and endless genealogies. These promote controversies rather than God's work— which is by faith. ⁵The goal of this command is love, which comes from a pure heart and a good conscience and a sincere faith. ⁶Some have wandered away from these and turned to meaningless talk. ⁷They want to be teachers of the law, but they do not know what they are talking about or what they so confidently affirm.

⁸We know that the law is good if one uses it properly. ⁹We also know that law*ᵃ* is made not for the righteous but for lawbreakers and rebels, the ungodly and sinful, the unholy and irreligious; for those who kill their fathers or mothers, for murderers, ¹⁰for adulterers and perverts, for slave traders and liars and perjurers—and for whatever else is contrary to the sound doctrine ¹¹that conforms to the glorious gospel of the blessed God, which he entrusted to me.

The Lord's Grace to Paul   ¹²I thank Christ Jesus our Lord, who has given me strength, that he considered me faithful, appointing me to his service. ¹³Even though I was once a blasphemer and a persecutor and a violent man, I was shown mercy because I acted in ignorance and unbelief. ¹⁴The grace of our Lord was poured out on me abundantly, along with the faith and love that are in Christ Jesus.

¹⁵Here is a trustworthy saying that deserves full acceptance: Christ Jesus came into the world to save sinners—of whom I am the worst. ¹⁶But for that very reason I was shown mercy so that in me, the worst of sinners, Christ Jesus might display his unlimited patience as an example for those who would believe on him and receive eternal life. ¹⁷Now to the King eternal, immortal, invisible, the only God, be honor and glory for ever and ever. Amen.

¹⁸Timothy, my son, I give you this instruction in keeping with the prophecies once made about you, so that by following them you may fight the good fight, ¹⁹holding on to faith and a good conscience. Some have rejected these and so have shipwrecked their faith. ²⁰Among them are Hymenaeus and Alexander, whom I have handed over to Satan to be taught not to blaspheme.

2 *Instructions on Worship*   I urge, then, first of all, that requests, prayers, intercession and thanksgiving be made for everyone— ²for kings and all those in authority, that we may live peaceful and quiet lives in all godliness and holiness. ³This is good, and pleases God our Savior, ⁴who wants all men to be saved and to come to a knowledge of the truth. ⁵For there is one God and one mediator between God and men, the man Christ Jesus, ⁶who gave himself as a ransom for all men—the testimony given in its proper time. ⁷And for this purpose I was appointed a herald and an apostle—I am telling the truth, I am not lying—and a teacher of the true faith to the Gentiles.

⁸I want men everywhere to lift up holy hands in prayer, without anger or disputing.

⁹I also want women to dress modestly, with decency and propriety, not

---

ᵃ9 Or that the law

Dear Sam,

Some of The Things I've done are so bad even ChrisT couldn'T forgive me. I sure don'T feel forgiven.

Joan in JamesTown

Dear Sam, Inc.

100 Advice Lane, Anywhere, USA

Dear Joan,

You may have done some terrible things, but you don't get the prize. Paul says he does. He claims he was the worst of sinners (1 Timothy 1:15). One of his favorite activities was persecuting Christians. But God spoke to Paul, and Paul had a change of heart. He realized what he was doing was wrong, and he stopped and asked for-giveness. Paul knew that if God could forgive him, God could forgive anyone (1 Timothy 1:13-14). And that means you too.

You say you know you aren't forgiven because you don't feel forgiven. If you believe that Christ died for your sins and you have asked for forgiveness, God has forgiven you regardless of your feelings. Perhaps it's time to forgive yourself. Let God help. Here are some verses to look up. Read and reread them until you can hear that "still small voice" telling you that you are loved and forgiven and that it's OK to feel that forgiveness: Psalm 103:11-13; 130:3-4; Isaiah 43:25; Jeremiah 33:8; Daniel 9:9.

Sam

with braided hair or gold or pearls or expensive clothes, [10]but with good deeds, appropriate for women who profess to worship God.

[11]A woman should learn in quietness and full submission. [12]I do not permit a woman to teach or to have authority over a man; she must be silent. [13]For Adam was formed first, then Eve. [14]And Adam was not the one deceived; it was the woman who was deceived and became a sinner. [15]But women[a] will be saved[b] through childbearing—if they continue in faith, love and holiness with propriety.

Overseers and Deacons Here is a trustworthy saying: If anyone sets his heart on being an overseer,[c] he desires a noble task. [2]Now the overseer must be above reproach, the husband of but one wife, temperate, self-controlled, respectable, hospitable, able to teach, [3]not given to drunkenness, not violent but gentle, not quarrelsome, not a lover of money. [4]He must manage his own family well and see that his children obey him with proper respect. [5](If anyone does not know how to manage his own family, how can he take care of God's church?) [6]He must not be a recent convert, or he may become conceited and fall under the same judgment as the devil. [7]He must also have a good reputation with outsiders, so that he will not fall into disgrace and into the devil's trap.

[8]Deacons, likewise, are to be men worthy of respect, sincere, not indulging in much wine, and not pursuing dishonest gain. [9]They must keep hold of the deep truths of the faith with a clear conscience. [10]They must first be tested; and then if there is nothing against them, let them serve as deacons.

[11]In the same way, their wives[d] are to be women worthy of respect, not malicious talkers but temperate and trustworthy in everything.

[12]A deacon must be the husband of but one wife and must manage his children and his household well. [13]Those who have served well gain an excellent standing and great assurance in their faith in Christ Jesus.

[14]Although I hope to come to you soon, I am writing you these instructions so that, [15]if I am delayed, you will know how people ought to conduct themselves in God's household, which is the church of the living God, the pillar and foundation of the truth. [16]Beyond all question, the mystery of godliness is great:

[a]15 Greek *she* [b]15 Or *restored* [c]1 Traditionally *bishop*, also in verse 2 [d]11 Or *way, deaconesses*

The Bible Says

Gifted Women

Do you ever wonder: "Is it OK to be female?" "What is my role in the church?" Some Bible passages (1 Corinthians 11; Ephesians 5; 1 Timothy 2) may make you think, "Paul had something against women." And then you learn more about the world in which Paul lived. Paul spoke a revolutionary message about women. When so many in his day said, "Women are inferior," Paul declared, "Men and women are one in Christ Jesus" (Galatians 3:28). Where so many said, "Women must not be educated," Paul declared, "A woman should learn in quietness and full submission" (1 Timothy 2:11).

Though interpretations of this passage differ, Christians can agree on two conclusions: Women are spiritually gifted members (not inferior members) of the body of Christ, the church. All of us, men and women, must stand quietly before God, submitting to his Word and to each other in love.

He[a] appeared in a body,[b]
    was vindicated by the Spirit,
   was seen by angels,
    was preached among the nations,
   was believed on in the world,
    was taken up in glory.

Instructions to Timothy The Spirit clearly says that in later times some will abandon the faith and follow deceiving spirits and things taught by demons. [2]Such teachings come through hypocritical liars, whose consciences have been seared as with a hot iron. [3]They forbid people to marry and order them to abstain from certain foods, which God created to be received with thanksgiving by those who believe and who know the truth. [4]For everything God created is good, and nothing is to be rejected if it is received with thanksgiving, [5]because it is consecrated by the word of God and prayer.

[6]If you point these things out to the brothers, you will be a good minister of Christ Jesus, brought up in the truths of the faith and of the good teaching that you have followed. [7]Have nothing to do with godless myths and old wives' tales; rather, train yourself to be godly. [8]For physical training is of some value, but godliness has value for all things, holding promise for both the present life and the life to come.

[9]This is a trustworthy saying that deserves full acceptance [10](and for this we labor and strive), that we have put our hope in the living God, who is the Savior of all men, and especially of those who believe.

[11]Command and teach these things. [12]Don't let anyone look down on you because you are young, but set an example for the believers in speech, in life, in love, in faith and in purity. [13]Until I come, devote yourself to the public reading of Scripture, to preaching and to teaching. [14]Do not neglect your gift, which was given you through a prophetic message when the body of elders laid their hands on you.

[15]Be diligent in these matters; give yourself wholly to them, so that everyone may see your progress. [16]Watch your life and doctrine closely. Persevere in them, because if you do, you will save both yourself and your hearers.

Advice About Widows, Elders and Slaves Do not rebuke an older man harshly, but exhort him as if he were your father. Treat younger men as brothers, [2]older women as mothers, and younger women as sisters, with absolute purity.

[3]Give proper recognition to those widows who are really in need. [4]But if a widow has children or grandchildren, these should learn first of all to put their religion into practice by caring for their own family and so repaying their parents and grandparents, for this is pleasing to God. [5]The widow who is really in need and left all alone puts her hope in God and continues night and day to pray and to ask God

[a]16 Some manuscripts *God* [b]16 Or *in the flesh*

---

1 TIMOTHY 4:11–16

Old Mr. Bronson is always yelling at you for cutting through his yard. You haven't, but he won't believe you. You sit with your friends in church, and some of the old folks watch every move, ready to criticize you if you say something to each other. Some of this comes with the territory. Many older people figure today's teens are a lot worse than they were. But you don't have to stand for it. Paul says so in 1 Timothy 4:12: "Set an example for the believers in speech, in life, in love, in faith and in purity." Live the Christian life consistently, and in time everyone will learn to respect you!

Direct Line

for help. ⁶But the widow who lives for pleasure is dead even while she lives. ⁷Give the people these instructions, too, so that no one may be open to blame. ⁸If anyone does not provide for his relatives, and especially for his immediate family, he has denied the faith and is worse than an unbeliever.

⁹No widow may be put on the list of widows unless she is over sixty, has been faithful to her husband,ᵃ ¹⁰and is well known for her good deeds, such as bringing up children, showing hospitality, washing the feet of the saints, helping those in trouble and devoting herself to all kinds of good deeds.

¹¹As for younger widows, do not put them on such a list. For when their sensual desires overcome their dedication to Christ, they want to marry. ¹²Thus they bring judgment on themselves, because they have broken their first pledge. ¹³Besides, they get into the habit of being idle and going about from house to house. And not only do they become idlers, but also gossips and busybodies, saying things they ought not to. ¹⁴So I counsel younger widows to marry, to have children, to manage their homes and to give the enemy no opportunity for slander. ¹⁵Some have in fact already turned away to follow Satan.

¹⁶If any woman who is a believer has widows in her family, she should help them and not let the church be burdened with them, so that the church can help those widows who are really in need.

¹⁷The elders who direct the affairs of the church well are worthy of double honor, especially those whose work is preaching and teaching. ¹⁸For the Scripture says, "Do not muzzle the ox while it is treading out the grain,"ᵇ and "The worker deserves his wages."ᶜ ¹⁹Do not entertain an accusation against an elder unless it is brought by two or three witnesses. ²⁰Those who sin are to be rebuked publicly, so that the others may take warning.

²¹I charge you, in the sight of God and Christ Jesus and the elect angels, to keep these instructions without partiality, and to do nothing out of favoritism.

²²Do not be hasty in the laying on of hands, and do not share in the sins of others. Keep yourself pure.

²³Stop drinking only water, and use a little wine because of your stomach and your frequent illnesses.

²⁴The sins of some men are obvious, reaching the place of judgment ahead of them; the sins of others trail behind them. ²⁵In the same way, good deeds are obvious, and even those that are not cannot be hidden.

6 All who are under the yoke of slavery should consider their masters worthy of full respect, so that God's name and our teaching may not be slandered. ²Those who have believing masters are not to show less respect for them because they are brothers. Instead, they are to serve them even better, because those who benefit from their service are believers, and dear to them. These are the things you are to teach and urge on them.

Direct Line

1 TIMOTHY 6:3–10

If money is the root of all evil, it must be that those without any money are better off than those with a lot. Right? Maybe. But the verse says "the *love* of money." Money itself isn't bad, but loving money can lead to making bad choices. A person who is poor and loves money may rob a store or sell drugs, yet refuse to buy medicine for a sick child. A person who is rich and loves money may be stingy and cheat others in business. It doesn't make any difference if you're rich or poor, young or old. Start loving money, and you'll make bad choices in life. Instead, use money, and use it wisely. But keep your love for God.

ᵃ9 Or *has had but one husband*   ᵇ18 Deut. 25:4
ᶜ18 Luke 10:7

Love of Money   ³If anyone teaches false doctrines and does not agree to the sound instruction of our Lord Jesus Christ and to godly teaching, ⁴he is conceited and understands nothing. He has an unhealthy interest in controversies and quarrels about words that result in envy, strife, malicious talk, evil suspicions ⁵and constant friction between men of corrupt mind, who have been robbed of the truth and who think that godliness is a means to financial gain.

⁶But godliness with contentment is great gain. ⁷For we brought nothing into the world, and we can take nothing out of it. ⁸But if we have food and clothing, we will be content with that. ⁹People who want to get rich fall into temptation and a trap and into many foolish and harmful desires that plunge men into ruin and destruction. ¹⁰For the love of money is a root of all kinds of evil. Some people, eager for money, have wandered from the faith and pierced themselves with many griefs.

Paul's Charge to Timothy   ¹¹But you, man of God, flee from all this, and pursue righteousness, godliness, faith, love, endurance and gentleness. ¹²Fight the good fight of the faith. Take hold of the eternal life to which you were called when you made your good confession in the presence of many witnesses. ¹³In the sight of God, who gives life to everything, and of Christ Jesus, who while testifying before Pontius Pilate made the good confession, I charge you ¹⁴to keep this command without spot or blame until the appearing of our Lord Jesus Christ, ¹⁵which God will bring about in his own time— God, the blessed and only Ruler, the King of kings and Lord of lords, ¹⁶who alone is immortal and who lives in unapproachable light, whom no one has seen or can see. To him be honor and might forever. Amen.

¹⁷Command those who are rich in this present world not to be arrogant nor to put their hope in wealth, which is so uncertain, but to put their hope in God, who richly provides us with everything for our enjoyment. ¹⁸Command them to do good, to be rich in good deeds, and to be generous and willing to share. ¹⁹In this way they will lay up treasure for themselves as a firm foundation for the coming age, so that they may take hold of the life that is truly life.

²⁰Timothy, guard what has been entrusted to your care. Turn away from godless chatter and the opposing ideas of what is falsely called knowledge, ²¹which some have professed and in so doing have wandered from the faith.
  Grace be with you.

2 Timothy

CHARACTER.

You'll probably read about it sooner or later in school. Young Ben Franklin made a list of things to work on to develop his character. If you made such a list, what would you put on it? What would you work on first?

Paul knew he was about to be executed when he wrote this second letter to Timothy. It was the last letter he ever wrote, so he jotted down things he thought were important to encourage and guide his young friend. Paul's last words can help you keep on the right path too.

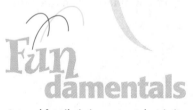

Fundamentals

A good family is important, but is it enough (2 Timothy 1:5-7)?

OK, so you fight with your brothers and sisters. That's normal, isn't it (2 Timothy 2:23-26)?

Do you really have to be so careful about the friends you pick (2 Timothy 3:1-5)?

FAST FACTS

Paul was executed in Rome about A.D. 67, shortly after sending this letter.

Timothy became a leader in the church after Paul died.

Timothy's father wasn't a Christian.

Timothy learned about the Lord from his mother and grandmother.

1 Paul, an apostle of Christ Jesus by the will of God, according to the promise of life that is in Christ Jesus,

²To Timothy, my dear son:

Grace, mercy and peace from God the Father and Christ Jesus our Lord.

Encouragement to Be Faithful   ³I thank God, whom I serve, as my forefathers did, with a clear conscience, as night and day I constantly remember you in my prayers. ⁴Recalling your tears, I long to see you, so that I may be filled with joy. ⁵I have been reminded of your sincere faith, which first lived in your grandmother Lois and in your mother Eunice and, I am persuaded, now lives in you also. ⁶For this reason I remind you to fan into flame the gift of God, which is in you through the laying on of my hands. ⁷For God did not give us a spirit of timidity, but a spirit of power, of love and of self-discipline.

⁸So do not be ashamed to testify about our Lord, or ashamed of me his prisoner. But join with me in suffering for the gospel, by the power of God, ⁹who has saved us and called us to a holy life—not because of anything we have done but because of his own purpose and grace. This grace was given us in Christ Jesus before the beginning of time, ¹⁰but it has now been revealed through the appearing of our Savior, Christ Jesus, who has destroyed death and has brought life and immortality to light through the gospel. ¹¹And of this gospel I was appointed a herald and an apostle and a teacher. ¹²That is why I am suffering as I am. Yet I am not ashamed, because I know whom I have believed, and am convinced that he is able to guard what I have entrusted to him for that day.

¹³What you heard from me, keep as the pattern of sound teaching, with faith and love in Christ Jesus. ¹⁴Guard the good deposit that was entrusted to you—guard it with the help of the Holy Spirit who lives in us.

¹⁵You know that everyone in the province of Asia has deserted me, including Phygelus and Hermogenes.

¹⁶May the Lord show mercy to the household of Onesiphorus, because he often refreshed me and was not ashamed of my chains. ¹⁷On the contrary, when he was in Rome, he searched hard for me until he found me. ¹⁸May the Lord grant that he will find mercy from the Lord on that day! You know very well in how many ways he helped me in Ephesus.

2 You then, my son, be strong in the grace that is in Christ Jesus. ²And the things you have heard me say in the presence of many witnesses entrust to reliable men who will also be qualified to teach others. ³Endure hardship with us like a good soldier of Christ Jesus. ⁴No one serving as a soldier gets involved in civilian affairs—he wants to please his commanding officer. ⁵Similarly, if anyone competes as an athlete, he does not receive the victor's crown unless he competes according to the rules. ⁶The hardworking farmer should be the first to receive a share of the crops. ⁷Reflect on what I am saying, for the Lord will give you insight into all this.

⁸Remember Jesus Christ, raised from the dead, descended from David. This is

---

2 TIMOTHY 1:5–7

If you have a mom and grandmother like Timothy's, you're fortunate. They each had a sincere faith, and they passed it on to Timothy, and it became his personal faith. There was no way their faith could do Timothy any good. That's one of the first lessons any person who comes from a Christian home needs to learn. You can't get to heaven on your parents' faith any more than you can get there on rollerblades. If you have Christian parents or grandparents, make their faith your own. Tell Jesus you accept him as your personal Savior. You'll be glad you did. And so will Mom and Dad.

Direct Line

my gospel, [9]for which I am suffering even to the point of being chained like a criminal. But God's word is not chained. [10]Therefore I endure everything for the sake of the elect, that they too may obtain the salvation that is in Christ Jesus, with eternal glory.

[11]Here is a trustworthy saying:

> If we died with him,
>   we will also live with him;
> [12]if we endure,
>   we will also reign with him.
> If we disown him,
>   he will also disown us;
> [13]if we are faithless,
>   he will remain faithful,
>   for he cannot disown himself.

A Workman Approved by God   [14]Keep reminding them of these things. Warn them before God against quarreling about words; it is of no value, and only ruins those who listen. [15]Do your best to present yourself to God as one approved, a workman who does not need to be ashamed and who correctly handles the word of truth. [16]Avoid godless chatter, because those who indulge in it will become more and more ungodly. [17]Their teaching will spread like gangrene. Among them are Hymenaeus and Philetus, [18]who have wandered away from the truth. They say that the resurrection has already taken place, and they destroy the faith of some. [19]Nevertheless, God's solid foundation stands firm, sealed with this inscription: "The Lord knows those who are his,"[a] and, "Everyone who confesses the name of the Lord must turn away from wickedness."

> The Lord knows those who are his
> (2 Timothy 2:19).

[20]In a large house there are articles not only of gold and silver, but also of wood and clay; some are for noble purposes and some for ignoble. [21]If a man cleanses himself from the latter, he will be an instrument for noble purposes, made holy, useful to the Master and prepared to do any good work.

[22]Flee the evil desires of youth, and pursue righteousness, faith, love and peace, along with those who call on the Lord out of a pure heart. [23]Don't have anything to do with foolish and stupid arguments, because you know they produce quarrels. [24]And the Lord's servant must not quarrel; instead, he must be kind to everyone, able to teach, not resentful. [25]Those who oppose him he must gently instruct, in the hope that God will grant them repentance leading them to a knowledge of the truth, [26]and that they will come to their senses and escape from the trap of the devil, who has taken them captive to do his will.

Godlessness in the Last Days   But mark this: There will be terrible times in the last days. [2]People will be lovers of themselves, lovers of money, boastful, proud, abusive, disobedient to their parents, ungrateful, unholy, [3]without love, unforgiving, slanderous, without self-control, brutal, not lovers of the good, [4]treacherous, rash, conceited, lovers of pleasure rather than lovers of God— [5]having a form of godliness but denying its power. Have nothing to do with them.

[6]They are the kind who worm their way into homes and gain control over weak-willed women, who are loaded down with sins and are swayed by all kinds of evil desires, [7]always learning but never able to acknowledge the truth. [8]Just as Jannes and Jambres opposed Moses, so also these men oppose

---

[a]*19* Num. 16:5 (see Septuagint)

the truth—men of depraved minds, who, as far as the faith is concerned, are rejected. [9]But they will not get very far because, as in the case of those men, their folly will be clear to everyone.

Paul's Charge to Timothy [10]You, however, know all about my teaching, my way of life, my purpose, faith, patience, love, endurance, [11]persecutions, sufferings—what kinds of things happened to me in Antioch, Iconium and Lystra, the persecutions I endured. Yet the Lord rescued me from all of them. [12]In fact, everyone who wants to live a godly life in Christ Jesus will be persecuted, [13]while evil men and impostors will go from bad to worse, deceiving and being deceived. [14]But as for you, continue in what you have learned and have become convinced of, because you know those from whom you learned it, [15]and how from infancy you have known the holy Scriptures, which are able to make you wise for salvation through faith in Christ Jesus. [16]All Scripture is God-breathed and is useful for teaching, rebuking, correcting and training in righteousness, [17]so that the man of God may be thoroughly equipped for every good work.

In the presence of God and of Christ Jesus, who will judge the living and the dead, and in view of his appearing and his kingdom, I give you this charge: [2]Preach the Word; be prepared in season and out of season; correct, rebuke and encourage—with great patience and careful instruction. [3]For the time will come when men will not put up with sound doctrine. Instead, to suit their own desires, they will gather around them a great number of teachers to say what their itching ears want to hear. [4]They will turn their ears away from the truth and turn aside to myths. [5]But you, keep your head in all situations, endure hardship, do the work of an evangelist, discharge all the duties of your ministry.

[6]For I am already being poured out like a drink offering, and the time has come for my departure. [7]I have fought the good fight, I have finished the race, I have kept the faith. [8]Now there is in store for me the crown of righteousness, which the Lord, the righteous Judge, will award to me on that day—and not only to me, but also to all who have longed for his appearing.

Personal Remarks [9]Do your best to come to me quickly, [10]for Demas, because he loved this world, has deserted me and has gone to Thessalonica. Crescens has gone to Galatia, and Titus to Dalmatia. [11]Only Luke is with me.

Everything in the Bible is not necessarily interesting or inspiring. But it is "inspired": God was at work making sure that what the writer put down was God's message.

Even if everything in the Bible may not seem interesting, it's there for a purpose. And when you read the Bible, you should look for these things (2 Timothy 3:16):

* Teaching. What truths can you discover that will help you understand God and other people?
* Rebuking. What have you been doing wrong that you need to change?
* Correcting. What can you do to become more Christ-like?
* Training. What can you discover that will equip you for good deeds?

The Bible Says

All Scripture Is Inspired

Get Mark and bring him with you, because he is helpful to me in my ministry. [12]I sent Tychicus to Ephesus. [13]When you come, bring the cloak that I left with Carpus at Troas, and my scrolls, especially the parchments.

[14]Alexander the metalworker did me a great deal of harm. The Lord will repay him for what he has done. [15]You too should be on your guard against him, because he strongly opposed our message.

[16]At my first defense, no one came to my support, but everyone deserted me. May it not be held against them. [17]But the Lord stood at my side and gave me strength, so that through me the message might be fully proclaimed and all the Gentiles might hear it. And I was delivered from the lion's mouth. [18]The Lord will rescue me from every evil attack and will bring me safely to his heavenly kingdom. To him be glory for ever and ever. Amen.

Final Greetings [19]Greet Priscilla[a] and Aquila and the household of Onesiphorus. [20]Erastus stayed in Corinth, and I left Trophimus sick in Miletus. [21]Do your best to get here before winter. Eubulus greets you, and so do Pudens, Linus, Claudia and all the brothers.

[22]The Lord be with your spirit. Grace be with you.

---

[a]19 Greek *Prisca*, a variant of *Priscilla*

to the

book of **Titus**

LEADERSHIP.

Are you an officer in your youth group? Do you ever get frustrated or feel like most of the other kids are lazy? And when you try to help, do they get angry at you? Well, this book of the New Testament may be just for you.

Paul wrote this short letter to Titus, a young leader he sent to Crete because of problems in that church. Paul reminds young Titus of the best way to influence others. Paul also reminds Titus that people who know Jesus should concentrate on doing good.

FAST FACTS

Crete is an island 160 miles long and 35 miles wide. It is in the Mediterranean Sea southwest of Greece.

Cretans had a reputation for being immoral and stubborn.

Titus was a Gentile Christian.

Titus is mentioned 14 times in the New Testament.

Titus was sent on many missions by Paul.

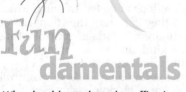

Fundamentals

Who should get elected to office in any church group (Titus 1:5-9)?

How can you influence other kids to be better followers of Jesus (Titus 2)?

Did you think good works had nothing to do with being a Christian (Titus 3)?

Paul, a servant of God and an apostle of Jesus Christ for the faith of God's elect and the knowledge of the truth that leads to godliness— ²a faith and knowledge resting on the hope of eternal life, which God, who does not lie, promised before the beginning of time, ³and at his appointed season he brought his word to light through the preaching entrusted to me by the command of God our Savior,

⁴To Titus, my true son in our common faith:

Grace and peace from God the Father and Christ Jesus our Savior.

Titus' Task on Crete   ⁵The reason I left you in Crete was that you might straighten out what was left unfinished and appoint*ᵃ* elders in every town, as I directed you. ⁶An elder must be blameless, the husband of but one wife, a man whose children believe and are not open to the charge of being wild and disobedient. ⁷Since an overseer*ᵇ* is entrusted with God's work, he must be blameless—not overbearing, not quick-tempered, not given to drunkenness, not violent, not pursuing dishonest gain. ⁸Rather he must be hospitable, one who loves what is good, who is self-controlled, upright, holy and disciplined. ⁹He must hold firmly to the trustworthy message as it has been taught, so that he can encourage others by sound doctrine and refute those who oppose it.

¹⁰For there are many rebellious people, mere talkers and deceivers, especially those of the circumcision group. ¹¹They must be silenced, because they are ruining whole households by teaching things they ought not to teach—and that for the sake of dishonest gain. ¹²Even one of their own prophets has said, "Cretans are always liars, evil brutes, lazy gluttons." ¹³This testimony is true. Therefore, rebuke them sharply, so that they will be sound in the faith ¹⁴and will pay no attention to Jewish myths or to the commands of those who reject the truth. ¹⁵To the pure, all things are pure, but to those who are corrupted and do not believe, nothing is pure. In fact, both their minds and consciences are corrupted. ¹⁶They claim to know God, but by their actions they deny him. They are detestable, disobedient and unfit for doing anything good.

What Must Be Taught to Various Groups   You must teach what is in accord with sound doctrine. ²Teach the older men to be temperate, worthy of respect, self-controlled, and sound in faith, in love and in endurance.

³Likewise, teach the older women to be reverent in the way they live, not to be slanderers or addicted to much wine, but to teach what is good. ⁴Then they can train the younger women to love their husbands and children, ⁵to be self-controlled and pure, to be busy at home, to be kind, and to be subject to their husbands, so that no one will malign the word of God.

⁶Similarly, encourage the young men to be self-controlled. ⁷In everything set them an example by doing what is good. In your teaching show integrity, seriousness ⁸and soundness of speech that cannot be condemned, so that those who oppose you may be ashamed because they have nothing bad to say about us.

⁹Teach slaves to be subject to their masters in everything, to try to please them, not to talk back to them, ¹⁰and not to steal from them, but to show that they can be fully trusted, so that in every way they will make the teaching about God our Savior attractive.

¹¹For the grace of God that brings salvation has appeared to all men. ¹²It teaches us to say "No" to ungodliness and worldly passions, and to live self-controlled, upright and godly lives in this present age, ¹³while we

> We wait for the blessed hope— the glorious appearing of our great God and Savior, Jesus Christ (Titus 2:13).

*ᵃ5 Or *ordain*   *ᵇ7 Traditionally *bishop*

wait for the blessed hope—the glorious appearing of our great God and Savior, Jesus Christ, [14]who gave himself for us to redeem us from all wickedness and to purify for himself a people that are his very own, eager to do what is good.

[15]These, then, are the things you should teach. Encourage and rebuke with all authority. Do not let anyone despise you.

Doing What Is Good Remind the people to be subject to rulers and authorities, to be obedient, to be ready to do whatever is good, [2]to slander no one, to be peaceable and considerate, and to show true humility toward all men.

[3]At one time we too were foolish, disobedient, deceived and enslaved by all kinds of passions and pleasures. We lived in malice and envy, being hated and hating one another. [4]But when the kindness and love of God our Savior appeared, [5]he saved us, not because of righteous things we had done, but because of his mercy. He saved us through the washing of rebirth and renewal by the Holy Spirit, [6]whom he poured out on us generously through Jesus Christ our Savior, [7]so that, having been justified by his grace, we might become heirs having the hope of eternal life. [8]This is a trustworthy saying. And I want you to stress these things, so that those who have trusted in God may be careful to devote themselves to doing what is good. These things are excellent and profitable for everyone.

[9]But avoid foolish controversies and genealogies and arguments and quarrels about the law, because these are unprofitable and useless. [10]Warn a divisive person once, and then warn him a second time. After that, have nothing to do with him. [11]You may be sure that such a man is warped and sinful; he is self-condemned.

Final Remarks [12]As soon as I send Artemas or Tychicus to you, do your best to come to me at Nicopolis, because I have decided to winter there. [13]Do everything you can to help Zenas the lawyer and Apollos on their way and see that they have everything they need. [14]Our people must learn to devote themselves to doing what is good, in order that they may provide for daily necessities and not live unproductive lives.

[15]Everyone with me sends you greetings. Greet those who love us in the faith.

Grace be with you all.

The Bible says you're not saved by doing good deeds (Ephesians 2:8–9). But it also says that people who are saved should "devote themselves to doing what is good" (Titus 3:14). The Greek word used here for *good* means "right and beneficial." Good deeds are actions you take to benefit others.

You don't have to look too far to find good deeds to do. You can help out at home. Help a friend with studies. Volunteer as an aide at a hospital or retirement home. Give the clothes you outgrow to a thrift store. Help a neighbor with yard work or shopping. The opportunities are all around you. And they really are opportunities. Be devoted to doing good, and the greatest blessing of all will be yours!

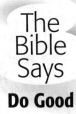

The
Bible
Says

Do Good

FAVORS.

Have you ever asked someone for a favor? Maybe you felt someone owed you a favor? You'll be more likely to get what you want if you ask the right way.

Paul wanted a special favor from a Christian friend named Philemon. A slave of Philemon's named Onesimus had stolen Philemon's property and run away. Later Onesimus met Paul in prison and became a Christian. In this letter Paul asks Philemon to welcome back his returning slave as a Christian brother.

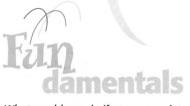

Fundamentals

What would you do if someone who hurt you wanted to be friends again (Philemon 17)?

What's the best way to ask for a favor you know a person doesn't want to grant (Philemon 8-9)?

FAST FACTS

Onesimus means "useful."

In many first-century cities, half of the population were slaves.

Some doctors and teachers in the Roman empire were slaves.

So many slaves were being freed in the first century that the empire taxed owners five percent of a freed slave's value.

Many slaves at this time had better food and housing than those who were free.

¹Paul, a prisoner of Christ Jesus, and Timothy our brother,

To Philemon our dear friend and fellow worker, ²to Apphia our sister, to Archippus our fellow soldier and to the church that meets in your home:

³Grace to you and peace from God our Father and the Lord Jesus Christ.

Thanksgiving and Prayer   ⁴I always thank my God as I remember you in my prayers, ⁵because I hear about your faith in the Lord Jesus and your love for all the saints. ⁶I pray that you may be active in sharing your faith, so that you will have a full understanding of every good thing we have in Christ. ⁷Your love has given me great joy and encouragement, because you, brother, have refreshed the hearts of the saints.

Paul's Plea for Onesimus   ⁸Therefore, although in Christ I could be bold and order you to do what you ought to do, ⁹yet I appeal to you on the basis of love. I then, as Paul—an old man and now also a prisoner of Christ Jesus— ¹⁰I appeal to you for my son Onesimus,ᵃ who became my son while I was in chains. ¹¹Formerly he was useless to you, but now he has become useful both to you and to me.

¹²I am sending him—who is my very heart—back to you. ¹³I would have liked to keep him with me so that he could take your place in helping me while I am in chains for the gospel. ¹⁴But I did not want to do anything without your consent, so that any favor you do will be spontaneous and not forced. ¹⁵Perhaps the reason he was separated from you for a little while was that you might have him back for good— ¹⁶no longer as a slave, but better than a slave, as a dear brother. He is very dear to me but even dearer to you, both as a man and as a brother in the Lord.

¹⁷So if you consider me a partner, welcome him as you would welcome me. ¹⁸If he has done you any wrong or owes you anything, charge it to me. ¹⁹I, Paul, am writing this with my own hand. I will pay it back—not to mention that you owe me your very self. ²⁰I do wish, brother, that I may have some benefit from you in the Lord; refresh my heart in Christ. ²¹Confident of your obedience, I write to you, knowing that you will do even more than I ask.

²²And one thing more: Prepare a guest room for me, because I hope to be restored to you in answer to your prayers.

²³Epaphras, my fellow prisoner in Christ Jesus, sends you greetings. ²⁴And so do Mark, Aristarchus, Demas and Luke, my fellow workers.

²⁵The grace of the Lord Jesus Christ be with your spirit.

ᵃ10 Onesimus means useful.

Dear Sam,

Two of my good friends, both Christians, got into a big argument. They haven't spoken to each other for over a month. Should I just stay out of it?

Melinda in Mansfield

Dear Sam, Inc.

100 Advice Lane, Anywhere, USA

Dear Melinda,

Since both of your friends are Christians, there is a Biblical example that you may want to examine. Paul wrote a short letter to his friend Philemon. Philemon's slave Onesimus had run away and had probably also stolen from his master to pay his expenses along the way. (We assume this because in Philemon 18 Paul offered to pay for anything that Onesimus owed Philemon.) After running away Onesimus met Paul and became a Christian.

In his letter Paul said he could command Philemon to do what was right in the eyes of God (forgive Onesimus). But instead Paul reminded Philemon that he was a loving Christian and asked him to do what was right. He also sent Onesimus back to Philemon to ask for forgiveness.

If you know who started this whole thing, encourage him or her to take the first step in apologizing. If this friend agrees, encourage the other friend to be gracious and accept the apology. Through this process, pray that your friends will get back together and let Christ's Spirit work in their hearts.

Sam

CHURCHES.

There are lots of different Christian churches. Maybe you're a Baptist Christian. Or a Methodist Christian. Or a Catholic Christian. You think your own church is special, and it probably is. But more important than the brand is that word *Christian*.

First-century Jews who accepted Jesus as their Savior saw themselves as Jewish Christians. As God's chosen people they felt special. Some began to think that "Jewish" was special enough without the "Christian"! The book of Hebrews is a reminder that what's so special about "Christian" is Jesus Christ himself.

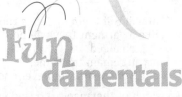

Fun
damentals

Are you ever ashamed to even think about God after you've sinned (Hebrews 4:14–5:10)?

What's "new" about the New Testament (Hebrews 8:7-13)?

If you have enough faith, does that mean everything in your life will go just great (Hebrews 11)?

FAST FACTS

This letter was written to Jewish Christians.

No one knows who wrote Hebrews.

A Christian writer who wrote in A.D. 96 mentioned this book.

Hebrews was probably written before the Jerusalem temple was destroyed in A.D. 70.

The Son Superior to Angels In the past God spoke to our forefathers through the prophets at many times and in various ways, ²but in these last days he has spoken to us by his Son, whom he appointed heir of all things, and through whom he made the universe. ³The Son is the radiance of God's glory and the exact representation of his being, sustaining all things by his powerful word. After he had provided purification for sins, he sat down at the right hand of the Majesty in heaven. ⁴So he became as much superior to the angels as the name he has inherited is superior to theirs.

⁵For to which of the angels did God ever say,

> "You are my Son;
>   today I have become your Father*ᵃ*"ᵇ?

Or again,

> "I will be his Father,
>   and he will be my Son"ᶜ?

⁶And again, when God brings his firstborn into the world, he says,

> "Let all God's angels worship him."ᵈ

⁷In speaking of the angels he says,

> "He makes his angels winds,
>   his servants flames of fire."ᵉ

⁸But about the Son he says,

> "Your throne, O God, will last for ever and ever,
>   and righteousness will be the scepter of your kingdom.
> ⁹You have loved righteousness and hated wickedness;
>   therefore God, your God, has set you above your
>   companions
>   by anointing you with the oil of joy."ᶠ

¹⁰He also says,

> "In the beginning, O Lord, you laid the foundations of the earth,
>   and the heavens are the work of your hands.
> ¹¹ They will perish, but you remain;
>   they will all wear out like a
>   garment.
> ¹² You will roll them up like a robe;
>   like a garment they will be
>   changed.
> But you remain the same,
>   and your years will never end."ᵍ

¹³To which of the angels did God ever say,

> "Sit at my right hand
> until I make your enemies
>   a footstool for your feet"ʰ?

¹⁴Are not all angels ministering spirits sent to serve those who will inherit salvation?

HEBREWS 1:14

Who are these "angels" and where are they? They are "ministering spirits" whom God sends to serve you as one of "those who will inherit salvation." And they're right there beside and around you. That's comforting to know when you're facing some bully. Or wavering over a hard choice. You feel all alone, but remember— you're not! God doesn't say a lot about angels, but he does let you know that these powerful spiritual beings are with you. Whatever the situation, you're really not alone.

Direct Line

ᵃ5 Or *have begotten you* ᵇ5 Psalm 2:7 ᶜ5 2 Samuel 7:14; 1 Chron. 17:13 ᵈ6 Deut. 32:43 (see Dead Sea Scrolls and Septuagint) ᵉ7 Psalm 104:4 ᶠ9 Psalm 45:6,7 ᵍ12 Psalm 102:25-27 ʰ13 Psalm 110:1

2 *Warning to Pay Attention* We must pay more careful attention, therefore, to what we have heard, so that we do not drift away. ²For if the message spoken by angels was binding, and every violation and disobedience received its just punishment, ³how shall we escape if we ignore such a great salvation? This salvation, which was first announced by the Lord, was confirmed to us by those who heard him. ⁴God also testified to it by signs, wonders and various miracles, and gifts of the Holy Spirit distributed according to his will.

Jesus Made Like His Brothers ⁵It is not to angels that he has subjected the world to come, about which we are speaking. ⁶But there is a place where someone has testified:

> "What is man that you are mindful of him,
>   the son of man that you care for him?
> ⁷You made him a little*ᵃ* lower than the angels;
>   you crowned him with glory and honor
> ⁸   and put everything under his feet."*ᵇ*

In putting everything under him, God left nothing that is not subject to him. Yet at present we do not see everything subject to him. ⁹But we see Jesus, who was made a little lower than the angels, now crowned with glory and honor because he suffered death, so that by the grace of God he might taste death for everyone.

¹⁰In bringing many sons to glory, it was fitting that God, for whom and through whom everything exists, should make the author of their salvation perfect through suffering. ¹¹Both the one who makes men holy and those who are made holy are of the same family. So Jesus is not ashamed to call them brothers. ¹²He says,

> "I will declare your name to my brothers;
>   in the presence of the congregation I will sing your praises."*ᶜ*

¹³And again,

> "I will put my trust in him."*ᵈ*

And again he says,

> "Here am I, and the children God has given me."*ᵉ*

¹⁴Since the children have flesh and blood, he too shared in their humanity so that by his death he might destroy him who holds the power of death—that is, the devil— ¹⁵and free those who all their lives were held in slavery by their fear of death. ¹⁶For surely it is not angels he helps, but Abraham's descendants. ¹⁷For this reason he had to be made like his brothers in every way, in order that he might become a merciful and faithful high priest in service to God, and that he might make atonement for*ᶠ* the sins of the people. ¹⁸Because he himself suffered when he was tempted, he is able to help those who are being tempted.

3 *Jesus Greater Than Moses* Therefore, holy brothers, who share in the heavenly calling, fix your thoughts on Jesus, the apostle and high priest whom we confess. ²He was faithful to the one who appointed him, just as Moses was faithful in all God's house. ³Jesus has been found worthy of greater honor than Moses, just as the builder of a house has greater honor than the house itself. ⁴For every house is built by someone, but God is the builder of everything. ⁵Moses was faithful as a servant in all God's house, tes-

ᵃ7 Or him for a little while; also in verse 9   ᵇ8 Psalm 8:4-6   ᶜ12 Psalm 22:22   ᵈ13 Isaiah 8:17   ᵉ13 Isaiah 8:18   ᶠ17 Or and that he might turn aside God's wrath, taking away

tifying to what would be said in the future. ⁶But Christ is faithful as a son over God's house. And we are his house, if we hold on to our courage and the hope of which we boast.

Warning Against Unbelief   ⁷So, as the Holy Spirit says:

> "Today, if you hear his voice,
> ⁸ do not harden your hearts
> as you did in the rebellion,
>   during the time of testing in the desert,
> ⁹where your fathers tested and tried me
>   and for forty years saw what I did.
> ¹⁰That is why I was angry with that generation,
>   and I said, 'Their hearts are always going astray,
>   and they have not known my ways.'
> ¹¹So I declared on oath in my anger,
>   'They shall never enter my rest.' "ᵃ

¹²See to it, brothers, that none of you has a sinful, unbelieving heart that turns away from the living God. ¹³But encourage one another daily, as long as it is called Today, so that none of you may be hardened by sin's deceitfulness. ¹⁴We have come to share in Christ if we hold firmly till the end the confidence we had at first. ¹⁵As has just been said:

> "Today, if you hear his voice,
>   do not harden your hearts
> as you did in the rebellion."ᵇ

¹⁶Who were they who heard and rebelled? Were they not all those Moses led out of Egypt? ¹⁷And with whom was he angry for forty years? Was it not with those who sinned, whose bodies fell in the desert? ¹⁸And to whom did God swear that they would never enter his rest if not to those who disobeyedᶜ? ¹⁹So we see that they were not able to enter, because of their unbelief.

A Sabbath-Rest for the People of God   Therefore, since the promise of entering his rest still stands, let us be careful that none of you be found to have fallen short of it. ²For we also have had the gospel preached to us, just as they did; but the message they heard was of no value to them, because those who heard did not combine it with faith.ᵈ ³Now we who have believed enter that rest, just as God has said,

> "So I declared on oath in my anger,
>   'They shall never enter my rest.' "ᵉ

And yet his work has been finished since the creation of the world. ⁴For somewhere he has spoken about the seventh day in these words: "And on the seventh day God rested from all his work."ᶠ ⁵And again in the passage above he says, "They shall never enter my rest."

⁶It still remains that some will enter that rest, and those who formerly had the gospel preached to them did not go in, because of their disobedience. ⁷Therefore God again set a certain day, calling it Today, when a long time later he spoke through David, as was said before:

> "Today, if you hear his voice,
>   do not harden your hearts."ᵇ

⁸For if Joshua had given them rest, God would not have spoken later about another day. ⁹There remains, then, a Sabbath-rest for the people of God;

ᵃ*11* Psalm 95:7-11   ᵇ*15,7* Psalm 95:7,8   ᶜ*18* Or *disbelieved*   ᵈ*2* Many manuscripts *because they did not share in the faith of those who obeyed*   ᵉ*3* Psalm 95:11; also in verse 5   ᶠ*4* Gen. 2:2

¹⁰for anyone who enters God's rest also rests from his own work, just as God did from his. ¹¹Let us, therefore, make every effort to enter that rest, so that no one will fall by following their example of disobedience.

¹²For the word of God is living and active. Sharper than any double-edged sword, it penetrates even to dividing soul and spirit, joints and marrow; it judges the thoughts and attitudes of the heart. ¹³Nothing in all creation is hidden from God's sight. Everything is uncovered and laid bare before the eyes of him to whom we must give account.

Jesus the Great High Priest ¹⁴Therefore, since we have a great high priest who has gone through the heavens,*ᵃ* Jesus the Son of God, let us hold firmly to the faith we profess. ¹⁵For we do not have a high priest who is unable to sympathize with our weaknesses, but we have one who has been tempted in every way, just as we are—yet was without sin. ¹⁶Let us then approach the throne of grace with confidence, so that we may receive mercy and find grace to help us in our time of need.

Every high priest is selected from among men and is appointed to represent them in matters related to God, to offer gifts and sacrifices for sins. ²He is able to deal gently with those who are ignorant and are going astray, since he himself is subject to weakness. ³This is why he has to offer sacrifices for his own sins, as well as for the sins of the people.

⁴No one takes this honor upon himself; he must be called by God, just as Aaron was. ⁵So Christ also did not take upon himself the glory of becoming a high priest. But God said to him,

> "You are my Son;
>   today I have become your Father.*ᵇ"ᶜ*

⁶And he says in another place,

> "You are a priest forever,
>   in the order of Melchizedek."*ᵈ*

⁷During the days of Jesus' life on earth, he offered up prayers and petitions with loud cries and tears to the one who could save him from death, and he was heard because of his reverent submission. ⁸Although he was a son, he learned obedience from what he suffered ⁹and, once made perfect, he became the source of eternal salvation for all who obey him ¹⁰and was designated by God to be high priest in the order of Melchizedek.

Warning Against Falling Away ¹¹We have much to say about this, but it is hard to explain because you are slow to learn. ¹²In fact, though by this time you ought to be teachers, you need someone to teach you the elementary truths of God's word all over again. You need milk, not solid food! ¹³Anyone who lives on milk, being still an infant, is not acquainted with the teaching about righteousness.

ᵃ14 Or *gone into heaven*   ᵇ5 Or *have begotten you*
ᶜ5 Psalm 2:7   ᵈ6 Psalm 110:4

HEBREWS 4:15

Life is pretty tough at times, isn't it? There's pressure on every side to conform to what the world around you wants rather than to what God wants. There's pressure to wear the right thing, act the right way, go to the right places. Life is not easy. This verse says Jesus "has been tempted in every way, just as we are." Yeah. Sure. He didn't live in the 90s. How could he know what it's like? Because Jesus was a true human being as well as God. He felt every pressure you feel. He knew disappointment and heartbreak. That's why you can bring everything to him. He does know what you're going through. And he cares.

Direct Line

[14]But solid food is for the mature, who by constant use have trained themselves to distinguish good from evil.

Therefore let us leave the elementary teachings about Christ and go on to maturity, not laying again the foundation of repentance from acts that lead to death,[a] and of faith in God, [2]instruction about baptisms, the laying on of hands, the resurrection of the dead, and eternal judgment. [3]And God permitting, we will do so.

[4]It is impossible for those who have once been enlightened, who have tasted the heavenly gift, who have shared in the Holy Spirit, [5]who have tasted the goodness of the word of God and the powers of the coming age, [6]if they fall away, to be brought back to repentance, because[b] to their loss they are crucifying the Son of God all over again and subjecting him to public disgrace.

[7]Land that drinks in the rain often falling on it and that produces a crop useful to those for whom it is farmed receives the blessing of God. [8]But land that produces thorns and thistles is worthless and is in danger of being cursed. In the end it will be burned.

[9]Even though we speak like this, dear friends, we are confident of better things in your case—things that accompany salvation. [10]God is not unjust; he will not forget your work and the love you have shown him as you have helped his people and continue to help them. [11]We want each of you to show this same diligence to the very end, in order to make your hope sure. [12]We do not want you to become lazy, but to imitate those who through faith and patience inherit what has been promised.

The Certainty of God's Promise   [13]When God made his promise to Abraham, since there was no one greater for him to swear by, he swore by himself, [14]saying, "I will surely bless you and give you many descendants."[c] [15]And so after waiting patiently, Abraham received what was promised.

[16]Men swear by someone greater than themselves, and the oath confirms what is said and puts an end to all argument. [17]Because God wanted to make the unchanging nature of his purpose very clear to the heirs of what was promised, he confirmed it with an oath. [18]God did this so that, by two unchangeable things in which it is impossible for God to lie, we who have fled to take hold of the hope offered to us may be greatly encouraged. [19]We have this hope as an anchor for the soul, firm and secure. It enters the inner sanctuary behind the curtain, [20]where Jesus, who went before us, has entered on our behalf. He has become a high priest forever, in the order of Melchizedek.

Melchizedek the Priest   This Melchizedek was king of Salem and priest of God Most High. He met Abraham returning from the defeat of the kings and blessed him, [2]and Abraham gave him a tenth of everything. First, his name means "king of righteousness"; then also,

HEBREWS 5:14

Most teens want to grow up fast. If you're 12, you want to be 15. If you're 15, you want to be 18. Well, if you really want to grow up faster, this verse tells you how! It says that a person becomes mature by using the Bible's teachings to see the difference between good and evil. Here's how it works. Instead of taking your friend's word on whether something is right or wrong, good or bad, you follow God's direction. In other words, you learn to take responsibility for your decisions. And you make your decisions using God's Word as your guide. Show that kind of maturity, and you can call yourself truly grown up.

Direct Line

[a]1 Or from useless rituals   [b]6 Or repentance while   [c]14 Gen. 22:17

"king of Salem" means "king of peace." ³Without father or mother, without genealogy, without beginning of days or end of life, like the Son of God he remains a priest forever.

⁴Just think how great he was: Even the patriarch Abraham gave him a tenth of the plunder! ⁵Now the law requires the descendants of Levi who become priests to collect a tenth from the people—that is, their brothers—even though their brothers are descended from Abraham. ⁶This man, however, did not trace his descent from Levi, yet he collected a tenth from Abraham and blessed him who had the promises. ⁷And without doubt the lesser person is blessed by the greater. ⁸In the one case, the tenth is collected by men who die; but in the other case, by him who is declared to be living. ⁹One might even say that Levi, who collects the tenth, paid the tenth through Abraham, ¹⁰because when Melchizedek met Abraham, Levi was still in the body of his ancestor.

Jesus Like Melchizedek ¹¹If perfection could have been attained through the Levitical priesthood (for on the basis of it the law was given to the people), why was there still need for another priest to come—one in the order of Melchizedek, not in the order of Aaron? ¹²For when there is a change of the priesthood, there must also be a change of the law. ¹³He of whom these things are said belonged to a different tribe, and no one from that tribe has ever served at the altar. ¹⁴For it is clear that our Lord descended from Judah, and in regard to that tribe Moses said nothing about priests. ¹⁵And what we have said is even more clear if another priest like Melchizedek appears, ¹⁶one who has become a priest not on the basis of a regulation as to his ancestry but on the basis of the power of an indestructible life. ¹⁷For it is declared:

> "You are a priest forever,
>   in the order of Melchizedek."[a]

¹⁸The former regulation is set aside because it was weak and useless ¹⁹(for the law made nothing perfect), and a better hope is introduced, by which we draw near to God.

²⁰And it was not without an oath! Others became priests without any oath, ²¹but he became a priest with an oath when God said to him:

> "The Lord has sworn
>   and will not change his mind:
> 'You are a priest forever.' "[a]

²²Because of this oath, Jesus has become the guarantee of a better covenant.

²³Now there have been many of those priests, since death prevented them from continuing in office; ²⁴but because Jesus lives forever, he has a permanent priesthood. ²⁵Therefore he is able to save completely[b] those who come to God through him, because he always lives to intercede for them.

²⁶Such a high priest meets our need—one who is holy, blameless, pure, set apart from sinners, exalted above the heavens. ²⁷Unlike the other high priests, he does not need to offer sacrifices day after day, first for his own sins, and then for the sins of the people. He sacrificed for their sins once for all when he offered himself. ²⁸For the law appoints as high priests men who are weak; but the oath, which came after the law, appointed the Son, who has been made perfect forever.

The High Priest of a New Covenant The point of what we are saying is this: We do have such a high priest, who sat down at the right hand of the throne of the Majesty in heaven, ²and who serves in the sanctuary, the true tabernacle set up by the Lord, not by man.

a17,21 Psalm 110:4 b25 Or forever

³Every high priest is appointed to offer both gifts and sacrifices, and so it was necessary for this one also to have something to offer. ⁴If he were on earth, he would not be a priest, for there are already men who offer the gifts prescribed by the law. ⁵They serve at a sanctuary that is a copy and shadow of what is in heaven. This is why Moses was warned when he was about to build the tabernacle: "See to it that you make everything according to the pattern shown you on the mountain."ᵃ ⁶But the ministry Jesus has received is as superior to theirs as the covenant of which he is mediator is superior to the old one, and it is founded on better promises.

⁷For if there had been nothing wrong with that first covenant, no place would have been sought for another. ⁸But God found fault with the people and saidᵇ:

> "The time is coming, declares the Lord,
>   when I will make a new covenant
> with the house of Israel
>   and with the house of Judah.
> ⁹It will not be like the covenant
>   I made with their forefathers
> when I took them by the hand
>   to lead them out of Egypt,
> because they did not remain faithful to my covenant,
>   and I turned away from them,
>   declares the Lord.
> ¹⁰This is the covenant I will make with the house of Israel
>   after that time, declares the Lord.
> I will put my laws in their minds
>   and write them on their hearts.
> I will be their God,
>   and they will be my people.
> ¹¹No longer will a man teach his neighbor,
>   or a man his brother, saying, 'Know the Lord,'
> because they will all know me,
>   from the least of them to the greatest.

ᵃ5 Exodus 25:40   ᵇ8 Some manuscripts may be translated *fault and said to the people.*

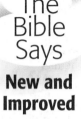

The Bible Says

New and Improved

The prophet Jeremiah announced that one day God would replace the law with a "new covenant" (Jeremiah 31:31–34). The law told people what good was, but the law couldn't make anyone good! A change from within was needed, not some command saying, "Do this!"

When Jesus died on the cross, the promised "new covenant" became a reality. God began to work in believers in a new way:

* God writes his laws on your heart (Hebrews 8:10). Believers are changed from the inside to become more and more like Jesus.
* God becomes yours and you become his (Hebrews 8:10–11). The Holy Spirit comes to live in you, bonding you to God forever.
* God forgives you completely (Hebrews 8:12). Your sins are forgotten, and you can look ahead to a new, better life.

¹²For I will forgive their wickedness
    and will remember their sins no more."ᵃ

¹³By calling this covenant "new," he has made the first one obsolete; and what is obsolete and aging will soon disappear.

9 *Worship in the Earthly Tabernacle* Now the first covenant had regulations for worship and also an earthly sanctuary. ²A tabernacle was set up. In its first room were the lampstand, the table and the consecrated bread; this was called the Holy Place. ³Behind the second curtain was a room called the Most Holy Place, ⁴which had the golden altar of incense and the gold-covered ark of the covenant. This ark contained the gold jar of manna, Aaron's staff that had budded, and the stone tablets of the covenant. ⁵Above the ark were the cherubim of the Glory, overshadowing the atonement cover.ᵇ But we cannot discuss these things in detail now.

⁶When everything had been arranged like this, the priests entered regularly into the outer room to carry on their ministry. ⁷But only the high priest entered the inner room, and that only once a year, and never without blood, which he offered for himself and for the sins the people had committed in ignorance. ⁸The Holy Spirit was showing by this that the way into the Most Holy Place had not yet been disclosed as long as the first tabernacle was still standing. ⁹This is an illustration for the present time, indicating that the gifts and sacrifices being offered were not able to clear the conscience of the worshiper. ¹⁰They are only a matter of food and drink and various ceremonial washings—external regulations applying until the time of the new order.

The Blood of Christ ¹¹When Christ came as high priest of the good things that are already here,ᶜ he went through the greater and more perfect tabernacle that is not man-made, that is to say, not a part of this creation. ¹²He did not enter by means of the blood of goats and calves; but he entered the Most Holy Place once for all by his own blood, having obtained eternal redemption. ¹³The blood of goats and bulls and the ashes of a heifer sprinkled on those who are ceremonially unclean sanctify them so that they are outwardly clean. ¹⁴How much more, then, will the blood of Christ, who through the eternal Spirit offered himself unblemished to God, cleanse our consciences from acts that lead to death,ᵈ so that we may serve the living God!

¹⁵For this reason Christ is the mediator of a new covenant, that those who are called may receive the promised eternal inheritance—now that he has died as a ransom to set them free from the sins committed under the first covenant.

¹⁶In the case of a will,ᵉ it is necessary to prove the death of the one who made it, ¹⁷because a will is in force only when somebody has died; it never takes effect while the one who made it is living. ¹⁸This is why even the first covenant was not put into effect without blood. ¹⁹When Moses had proclaimed every commandment of the law to all the people, he took the

ᵃ12 Jer. 31:31-34 ᵇ5 Traditionally *the mercy seat*
ᶜ11 Some early manuscripts *are to come* ᵈ14 Or *from useless rituals* ᵉ16 Same Greek word as *covenant*; also in verse 17

HEBREWS 9:14

Some choices can have tragic results. You drink and drive, and a friend is injured. You have sex with your boyfriend, and you get pregnant or you get a disease. And your conscience constantly reminds you of your guilt and says how useless you are. Well, it's true bad choices often have tragic results. But you don't have to live with a guilty conscience. Hebrews 9:14 says that the blood of Christ cleanses. You see, you can't go back and undo your past mistakes. But you can be forgiven for them. Your guilt is gone, and God is with you to make your future bright.

Direct Line

blood of calves, together with water, scarlet wool and branches of hyssop, and sprinkled the scroll and all the people. ²⁰He said, "This is the blood of the covenant, which God has commanded you to keep."ᵃ ²¹In the same way, he sprinkled with the blood both the tabernacle and everything used in its ceremonies. ²²In fact, the law requires that nearly everything be cleansed with blood, and without the shedding of blood there is no forgiveness.

²³It was necessary, then, for the copies of the heavenly things to be purified with these sacrifices, but the heavenly things themselves with better sacrifices than these. ²⁴For Christ did not enter a man-made sanctuary that was only a copy of the true one; he entered heaven itself, now to appear for us in God's presence. ²⁵Nor did he enter heaven to offer himself again and again, the way the high priest enters the Most Holy Place every year with blood that is not his own. ²⁶Then Christ would have had to suffer many times since the creation of the world. But now he has appeared once for all at the end of the ages to do away with sin by the sacrifice of himself. ²⁷Just as man is destined to die once, and after that to face judgment, ²⁸so Christ was sacrificed once to take away the sins of many people; and he will appear a second time, not to bear sin, but to bring salvation to those who are waiting for him.

Christ's Sacrifice Once for All The law is only a shadow of the good things that are coming—not the realities themselves. For this reason it can never, by the same sacrifices repeated endlessly year after year, make perfect those who draw near to worship. ²If it could, would they not have stopped being offered? For the worshipers would have been cleansed once for all, and would no longer have felt guilty for their sins. ³But those sacrifices are an annual reminder of sins, ⁴because it is impossible for the blood of bulls and goats to take away sins.

⁵Therefore, when Christ came into the world, he said:

> "Sacrifice and offering you did not desire,
>   but a body you prepared for me;
> ⁶with burnt offerings and sin offerings
>   you were not pleased.
> ⁷Then I said, 'Here I am—it is written about me in the
>   scroll—
> I have come to do your will, O God.' "ᵇ

⁸First he said, "Sacrifices and offerings, burnt offerings and sin offerings you did not desire, nor were you pleased with them" (although the law required them to be made). ⁹Then he said, "Here I am, I have come to do your will." He sets aside the first to establish the second. ¹⁰And by that will, we have been made holy through the sacrifice of the body of Jesus Christ once for all.

¹¹Day after day every priest stands and performs his religious duties; again and again he offers the same sacrifices, which can never take away sins. ¹²But when this priest had offered for all time one sacrifice for sins, he sat down at the right hand of God. ¹³Since that time he waits for his enemies to be made his footstool, ¹⁴because by one sacrifice he has made perfect forever those who are being made holy.

¹⁵The Holy Spirit also testifies to us about this. First he says:

> ¹⁶"This is the covenant I will make with them
>   after that time, says the Lord.
> I will put my laws in their hearts,
>   and I will write them on their minds."ᶜ

ᵃ20 Exodus 24:8   ᵇ7 Psalm 40:6-8 (see Septuagint)   ᶜ16 Jer. 31:33

¹⁷Then he adds:

> "Their sins and lawless acts
> I will remember no more."ᵃ

¹⁸And where these have been forgiven, there is no longer any sacrifice for sin.

A Call to Persevere ¹⁹Therefore, brothers, since we have confidence to enter the Most Holy Place by the blood of Jesus, ²⁰by a new and living way opened for us through the curtain, that is, his body, ²¹and since we have a great priest over the house of God, ²²let us draw near to God with a sincere heart in full assurance of faith, having our hearts sprinkled to cleanse us from a guilty conscience and having our bodies washed with pure water. ²³Let us hold unswervingly to the hope we profess, for he who promised is faithful. ²⁴And let us consider how we may spur one another on toward love and good deeds. ²⁵Let us not give up meeting together, as some are in the habit of doing, but let us encourage one another—and all the more as you see the Day approaching.

²⁶If we deliberately keep on sinning after we have received the knowledge of the truth, no sacrifice for sins is left, ²⁷but only a fearful expectation of judgment and of raging fire that will consume the enemies of God. ²⁸Anyone who rejected the law of Moses died without mercy on the testimony of two or three witnesses. ²⁹How much more severely do you think a man deserves to be punished who has trampled the Son of God under foot, who has treated as an unholy thing the blood of the covenant that sanctified him, and who has insulted the Spirit of grace? ³⁰For we know him who said, "It is mine to avenge; I will repay,"ᵇ and again, "The Lord will judge his people."ᶜ ³¹It is a dreadful thing to fall into the hands of the living God.

³²Remember those earlier days after you had received the light, when you stood your ground in a great contest in the face of suffering. ³³Sometimes you were publicly exposed to insult and persecution; at other times you stood side by side with those who were so treated. ³⁴You sympathized with those in prison and joyfully accepted the confiscation of your property, because you knew that you yourselves had better and lasting possessions.

³⁵So do not throw away your confidence; it will be richly rewarded. ³⁶You need to persevere so that when you have done the will of God, you will receive what he has promised. ³⁷For in just a very little while,

> "He who is coming will come
> and will not delay.
> ³⁸ But my righteous oneᵈ will
> live by faith.
> And if he shrinks back,
> I will not be pleased with
> him."ᵉ

³⁹But we are not of those who shrink back and are destroyed, but of those who believe and are saved.

ᵃ*17* Jer. 31:34 ᵇ*30* Deut. 32:35 ᶜ*30* Deut. 32:36; Psalm 135:14 ᵈ*38* One early manuscript *But the righteous* ᵉ*38* Hab. 2:3,4

HEBREWS 10:24–25

Living a Christian life isn't easy. It can be really hard. That's when you need the support of Christian friends. But how do you get that support? First of all, make sure you get together regularly. Maybe at church. Maybe at an after-school club. Or maybe on your own with two or three Christian friends. What can you do when you get together? Talk about what's happening in your lives. Encourage each other. And "spur one another on toward love and good deeds" (Hebrews 10:24). It's a lot easier to stand firm in your Christian commitment if you know other teens are standing beside you.

Direct Line

11 *By Faith* Now faith is being sure of what we hope for and certain of what we do not see. ²This is what the ancients were commended for.

³By faith we understand that the universe was formed at God's command, so that what is seen was not made out of what was visible.

⁴By faith Abel offered God a better sacrifice than Cain did. By faith he was commended as a righteous man, when God spoke well of his offerings. And by faith he still speaks, even though he is dead.

⁵By faith Enoch was taken from this life, so that he did not experience death; he could not be found, because God had taken him away. For before he was taken, he was commended as one who pleased God. ⁶And without faith it is impossible to please God, because anyone who comes to him must believe that he exists and that he rewards those who earnestly seek him.

⁷By faith Noah, when warned about things not yet seen, in holy fear built an ark to save his family. By his faith he condemned the world and became heir of the righteousness that comes by faith.

⁸By faith Abraham, when called to go to a place he would later receive as his inheritance, obeyed and went, even though he did not know where he was going. ⁹By faith he made his home in the promised land like a stranger in a foreign country; he lived in tents, as did Isaac and Jacob, who were heirs with him of the same promise. ¹⁰For he was looking forward to the city with foundations, whose architect and builder is God.

¹¹By faith Abraham, even though he was past age—and Sarah herself was barren—was enabled to become a father because he*a* considered him faithful who had made the promise. ¹²And so from this one man, and he as good as dead, came descendants as numerous as the stars in the sky and as countless as the sand on the seashore.

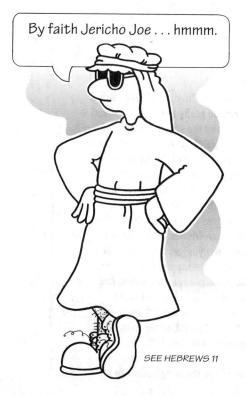

By faith Jericho Joe . . . hmmm.

SEE HEBREWS 11

¹³All these people were still living by faith when they died. They did not receive the things promised; they only saw them and welcomed them from a distance. And they admitted that they were aliens and strangers on earth. ¹⁴People who say such things show that they are looking for a country of their own. ¹⁵If they had been thinking of the country they had left, they would have had opportunity to return. ¹⁶Instead, they were longing for a better country—a heavenly one. Therefore God is not ashamed to be called their God, for he has prepared a city for them.

¹⁷By faith Abraham, when God tested him, offered Isaac as a sacrifice. He who had received the promises was about to sacrifice his one and only son, ¹⁸even though God had said to him, "It is through Isaac that your offspring*b* will be reckoned."*c* ¹⁹Abraham reasoned that God could raise the dead, and figuratively speaking, he did receive Isaac back from death.

²⁰By faith Isaac blessed Jacob and Esau in regard to their future.

²¹By faith Jacob, when he was dying, blessed each of Joseph's sons, and worshiped as he leaned on the top of his staff.

²²By faith Joseph, when his end was near,

a11 Or By faith even Sarah, who was past age, was enabled to bear children because she b18 Greek seed c18 Gen. 21:12

spoke about the exodus of the Israelites from Egypt and gave instructions about his bones.

²³By faith Moses' parents hid him for three months after he was born, because they saw he was no ordinary child, and they were not afraid of the king's edict.

²⁴By faith Moses, when he had grown up, refused to be known as the son of Pharaoh's daughter. ²⁵He chose to be mistreated along with the people of God rather than to enjoy the pleasures of sin for a short time. ²⁶He regarded disgrace for the sake of Christ as of greater value than the treasures of Egypt, because he was looking ahead to his reward. ²⁷By faith he left Egypt, not fearing the king's anger; he persevered because he saw him who is invisible. ²⁸By faith he kept the Passover and the sprinkling of blood, so that the destroyer of the firstborn would not touch the firstborn of Israel.

²⁹By faith the people passed through the Red Sea*a* as on dry land; but when the Egyptians tried to do so, they were drowned.

³⁰By faith the walls of Jericho fell, after the people had marched around them for seven days.

³¹By faith the prostitute Rahab, because she welcomed the spies, was not killed with those who were disobedient.*b*

³²And what more shall I say? I do not have time to tell about Gideon, Barak, Samson, Jephthah, David, Samuel and the prophets, ³³who through faith conquered kingdoms, administered justice, and gained what was promised; who shut the mouths of lions, ³⁴quenched the fury of the flames, and escaped the edge of the sword; whose weakness was turned to strength; and who became powerful in battle and routed foreign armies. ³⁵Women received back their dead, raised to life again. Others were tortured and refused to be released, so that they might gain a better resurrection. ³⁶Some faced jeers and flogging, while still others were chained and put in prison. ³⁷They were stoned*c*; they were sawed in two; they were put to death by the sword. They went about in sheepskins and goatskins, destitute, persecuted and mistreated— ³⁸the world was not worthy of them. They wandered in deserts and mountains, and in caves and holes in the ground.

³⁹These were all commended for their faith, yet none of them received what had been promised. ⁴⁰God had planned something better for us so that only together with us would they be made perfect.

12 *God Disciplines His Sons* Therefore, since we are surrounded by such a great cloud of witnesses, let us throw off everything that hinders and the sin that so easily entangles, and let us run with perseverance the race marked out for us. ²Let us fix our eyes on Jesus, the author and perfecter of our faith, who for the joy set before him endured the cross, scorning its shame, and sat down at the right hand of the throne of God. ³Consider him who endured such opposition from sinful men, so that you will not grow weary and lose heart.

⁴In your struggle against sin, you have not yet resisted to the point of shedding your blood. ⁵And you have forgotten that word of encouragement that addresses you as sons:

> "My son, do not make light of the Lord's discipline,
>   and do not lose heart when he rebukes you,
> ⁶because the Lord disciplines those he loves,
>   and he punishes everyone he accepts as a son."*d*

⁷Endure hardship as discipline; God is treating you as sons. For what son is not disciplined by his father? ⁸If you are not disciplined (and everyone under-

a29 That is, Sea of Reeds b31 Or unbelieving c37 Some early manuscripts stoned; they were put to the test; d6 Prov. 3:11,12

goes discipline), then you are illegitimate children and not true sons. [9]Moreover, we have all had human fathers who disciplined us and we respected them for it. How much more should we submit to the Father of our spirits and live! [10]Our fathers disciplined us for a little while as they thought best; but God disciplines us for our good, that we may share in his holiness. [11]No discipline seems pleasant at the time, but painful. Later on, however, it produces a harvest of righteousness and peace for those who have been trained by it.

[12]Therefore, strengthen your feeble arms and weak knees. [13]"Make level paths for your feet,"[a] so that the lame may not be disabled, but rather healed.

Warning Against Refusing God   [14]Make every effort to live in peace with all men and to be holy; without holiness no one will see the Lord. [15]See to it that no one misses the grace of God and that no bitter root grows up to cause trouble and defile many. [16]See that no one is sexually immoral, or is godless like Esau, who for a single meal sold his inheritance rights as the oldest son. [17]Afterward, as you know, when he wanted to inherit this blessing, he was rejected. He could bring about no change of mind, though he sought the blessing with tears.

[18]You have not come to a mountain that can be touched and that is burning with fire; to darkness, gloom and storm; [19]to a trumpet blast or to such a voice speaking words that those who heard it begged that no further word be spoken to them, [20]because they could not bear what was commanded: "If even an animal touches the mountain, it must be stoned."[b] [21]The sight was so terrifying that Moses said, "I am trembling with fear."[c]

[22]But you have come to Mount Zion, to the heavenly Jerusalem, the city of the living God. You have come to thousands upon thousands of angels in joyful assembly, [23]to the church of the firstborn, whose names are written in heaven. You have come to God, the judge of all men, to the spirits of righteous men made perfect, [24]to Jesus the mediator of a new covenant, and to the sprinkled blood that speaks a better word than the blood of Abel.

[25]See to it that you do not refuse him who speaks. If they did not escape when they refused him who warned them on earth, how much less will we, if we turn away from him who warns us from heaven? [26]At that time his voice shook the earth, but now he has promised, "Once more I will shake not only the earth but also the heavens."[d] [27]The words "once more" indicate the removing of what can be shaken—that is, created things—so that what cannot be shaken may remain.

[28]Therefore, since we are receiving a kingdom that cannot be shaken, let us be thankful, and so worship God acceptably with reverence and awe, [29]for our "God is a consuming fire."[e]

13 *Concluding Exhortations*   Keep on loving each other as brothers. [2]Do not forget to entertain strangers, for by so doing some people have enter-

---

Direct Line

HEBREWS 12:1–13

You break your leg a week before the big ski trip. Your mom gets sick just before you graduate. Hebrews 12 says to look at some of the painful things that happen to you as "God's discipline." No, not "God's punishment." Discipline means training, helping you grow up, preparing you to be strong. Some people fight any kind of discipline. Like squalling babies, they want what they want, and they want it now. What a terrible way to live! God thinks far too much of you to let you remain a baby, so he sometimes lets hard things happen to you. When they do, see them as God's discipline— and as a sign of his love for you (Hebrews 12:6).

---

[a]*13* Prov. 4:26   [b]*20* Exodus 19:12,13   [c]*21* Deut. 9:19
[d]*26* Haggai 2:6   [e]*29* Deut. 4:24

Dear Sam,

I'm only 15 years old, but I'm pregnant. My parents say abortion is wrong, and I agree. But I'm scared. What do I do?

Kira in Kennewick

100 Advice Lane, Anywhere, USA

Dear Sam, Inc.

Dear Kira,

It makes me sad to get letters like yours. So many girls are finding themselves in this very situation. And they're scared too. You have already made some good choices in dealing with your problem. You have told your parents. You no longer have to handle this alone. They can give you a lot of support. You've chosen not to have an abortion because it is wrong. There are counseling centers that can give you advice on what choices you do have.

I would advise you to pray for wisdom in making this difficult decision. Whether you give your baby up for adoption or try to raise it yourself, it will be difficult. But God is with you, holding your hand, holding you up. He has promised never to forsake you (Hebrews 13:5). You can count on him. God will use even this painful experience for good in your life (Romans 8:28).

God knows your weaknesses and understands them. You were forgiven the first time you asked.

Sam

tained angels without knowing it. ³Remember those in prison as if you were their fellow prisoners, and those who are mistreated as if you yourselves were suffering.

⁴Marriage should be honored by all, and the marriage bed kept pure, for God will judge the adulterer and all the sexually immoral. ⁵Keep your lives free from the love of money and be content with what you have, because God has said,

> "Never will I leave you;
> never will I forsake you."ᵃ

⁶So we say with confidence,

> "The Lord is my helper; I will not be afraid.
> What can man do to me?"ᵇ

⁷Remember your leaders, who spoke the word of God to you. Consider the outcome of their way of life and imitate their faith. ⁸Jesus Christ is the same yesterday and today and forever.

⁹Do not be carried away by all kinds of strange teachings. It is good for our hearts to be strengthened by grace, not by ceremonial foods, which are of no value to those who eat them. ¹⁰We have an altar from which those who minister at the tabernacle have no right to eat.

> *Jesus Christ is the same yesterday and today and forever (Hebrews 13:8).*

¹¹The high priest carries the blood of animals into the Most Holy Place as a sin offering, but the bodies are burned outside the camp. ¹²And so Jesus also suffered outside the city gate to make the people holy through his own blood. ¹³Let us, then, go to him outside the camp, bearing the disgrace he bore. ¹⁴For here we do not have an enduring city, but we are looking for the city that is to come.

¹⁵Through Jesus, therefore, let us continually offer to God a sacrifice of praise—the fruit of lips that confess his name.

¹⁶And do not forget to do good and to share with others, for with such sacrifices God is pleased.

¹⁷Obey your leaders and submit to their authority. They keep watch over you as men who must give an account. Obey them so that their work will be a joy, not a burden, for that would be of no advantage to you.

¹⁸Pray for us. We are sure that we have a clear conscience and desire to live honorably in every way. ¹⁹I particularly urge you to pray so that I may be restored to you soon.

²⁰May the God of peace, who through the blood of the eternal covenant brought back from the dead our Lord Jesus, that great Shepherd of the sheep, ²¹equip you with everything good for doing his will, and may he work in us what is pleasing to him, through Jesus Christ, to whom be glory for ever and ever. Amen.

²²Brothers, I urge you to bear with my word of exhortation, for I have written you only a short letter.

²³I want you to know that our brother Timothy has been released. If he arrives soon, I will come with him to see you.

²⁴Greet all your leaders and all God's people. Those from Italy send you their greetings.

²⁵Grace be with you all.

ᵃ5 Deut. 31:6   ᵇ6 Psalm 118:6,7

CHRISTIAN.

Just saying so doesn't make you Christian. It's not just saying you believe the Bible. Or that you believe in Jesus. Being a real Christian will make a difference in the way you live. Not that you'll suddenly be perfect. Not at all.

James wrote this book to remind Christians to practice their faith. His letter is very practical. James talks about things like temptation, anger, showing favoritism, watching your mouth, fighting, boasting and patience. God doesn't expect you to be perfectly good. But he doesn't expect you to be perfectly awful either.

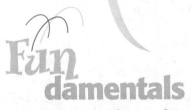

Fundamentals

How can you stop getting angry? You don't want to get mad, but . . . (James 1:19-25).

Loving my neighbor is all right. But who's my neighbor (James 2:1-13)?

Do you go crazy when you don't have control over the things that happen to you (James 5:7-11)?

FAST FACTS

The James who wrote this book was Jesus' brother, the son of Mary and Joseph.

James was a leader of the church in Jerusalem.

James was probably martyred in A.D. 62. This book was probably written about A.D. 45-48.

James was probably the first book of the New Testament to be written.

James, a servant of God and of the Lord Jesus Christ,

To the twelve tribes scattered among the nations:

Greetings.

Trials and Temptations ²Consider it pure joy, my brothers, whenever you face trials of many kinds, ³because you know that the testing of your faith develops perseverance. ⁴Perseverance must finish its work so that you may be mature and complete, not lacking anything. ⁵If any of you lacks wisdom, he should ask God, who gives generously to all without finding fault, and it will be given to him. ⁶But when he asks, he must believe and not doubt, because he who doubts is like a wave of the sea, blown and tossed by the wind. ⁷That man should not think he will receive anything from the Lord; ⁸he is a double-minded man, unstable in all he does.

⁹The brother in humble circumstances ought to take pride in his high position. ¹⁰But the one who is rich should take pride in his low position, because he will pass away like a wild flower. ¹¹For the sun rises with scorching heat and withers the plant; its blossom falls and its beauty is destroyed. In the same way, the rich man will fade away even while he goes about his business.

¹²Blessed is the man who perseveres under trial, because when he has stood the test, he will receive the crown of life that God has promised to those who love him.

¹³When tempted, no one should say, "God is tempting me." For God cannot be tempted by evil, nor does he tempt anyone; ¹⁴but each one is tempted when, by his own evil desire, he is dragged away and enticed. ¹⁵Then, after desire has conceived, it gives birth to sin; and sin, when it is full-grown, gives birth to death.

¹⁶Don't be deceived, my dear brothers. ¹⁷Every good and perfect gift is from above, coming down from the Father of the heavenly lights, who does not change like shifting shadows. ¹⁸He chose to give us birth through the word of truth, that we might be a kind of firstfruits of all he created.

Listening and Doing ¹⁹My dear brothers, take note of this: Everyone should be quick to listen, slow to speak and slow to become angry, ²⁰for man's anger does not bring about the righteous life that God desires. ²¹Therefore, get rid of all moral filth and the evil that is so prevalent and humbly accept the word planted in you, which can save you.

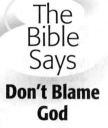

The Bible Says

Don't Blame God

Did your mom ever bake cookies and tell you not to eat any? You smell those cookies, and you want one. You're even a little angry with your mom. Like she baked those cookies just to tempt you!

Some people feel the same way about God. They want something they know is wrong, and they wonder why God is tempting them. But God doesn't tempt anyone! Their own "evil desire" makes them want what is wrong (James 1:13–15). Like those cookies. If that were a spinach casserole, would you want any?

When you're tempted, it's because something inside you likes to do the wrong thing you know you shouldn't do. The problem is in you, not in the thing you want to do. God has made you new in Jesus. You may still like what you know is wrong—but you will like pleasing God better.

²²Do not merely listen to the word, and so deceive yourselves. Do what it says. ²³Anyone who listens to the word but does not do what it says is like a man who looks at his face in a mirror ²⁴and, after looking at himself, goes away and immediately forgets what he looks like. ²⁵But the man who looks intently into the perfect law that gives freedom, and continues to do this, not forgetting what he has heard, but doing it—he will be blessed in what he does.

²⁶If anyone considers himself religious and yet does not keep a tight rein on his tongue, he deceives himself and his religion is worthless. ²⁷Religion that God our Father accepts as pure and faultless is this: to look after orphans and widows in their distress and to keep oneself from being polluted by the world.

Favoritism Forbidden My brothers, as believers in our glorious Lord Jesus Christ, don't show favoritism. ²Suppose a man comes into your meeting wearing a gold ring and fine clothes, and a poor man in shabby clothes also comes in. ³If you show special attention to the man wearing fine clothes and say, "Here's a good seat for you," but say to the poor man, "You stand there" or "Sit on the floor by my feet," ⁴have you not discriminated among yourselves and become judges with evil thoughts?

⁵Listen, my dear brothers: Has not God chosen those who are poor in the eyes of the world to be rich in faith and to inherit the kingdom he promised those who love him? ⁶But you have insulted the poor. Is it not the rich who are exploiting you? Are they not the ones who are dragging you into court? ⁷Are they not the ones who are slandering the noble name of him to whom you belong?

⁸If you really keep the royal law found in Scripture, "Love your neighbor as yourself,"ᵃ you are doing right. ⁹But if you show favoritism, you sin and are convicted by the law as lawbreakers. ¹⁰For whoever keeps the whole law and yet stumbles at just one point is guilty of breaking all of it. ¹¹For he who said, "Do not commit adultery,"ᵇ also said, "Do not murder."ᶜ If you do not commit adultery but do commit murder, you have become a lawbreaker.

¹²Speak and act as those who are going to be judged by the law that gives freedom, ¹³because judgment without mercy will be shown to anyone who has not been merciful. Mercy triumphs over judgment!

Faith and Deeds ¹⁴What good is it, my brothers, if a man claims to have faith but has no deeds? Can such faith save him? ¹⁵Suppose a brother or sister is without clothes and daily food. ¹⁶If one of you says to him, "Go, I wish you well; keep warm and well fed," but does nothing about his physical needs, what good is it? ¹⁷In the same way, faith by itself, if it is not accompanied by action, is dead.

¹⁸But someone will say, "You have faith; I have deeds."

Show me your faith without deeds, and I will show you my faith by what I do.

ᵃ8 Lev. 19:18 ᵇ11 Exodus 20:14; Deut. 5:18 ᶜ11 Exodus 20:13; Deut. 5:17

JAMES 1:19–25

Have you ever heard anyone say, "I've just got a nasty temper"? They seem to think that having a "nasty temper" is a valid excuse for anything they do when angry. Well, it isn't. James says, "Everyone should be quick to listen, slow to speak and slow to become angry" (James 1:19). Anger isn't part of the "righteous life that God desires" (James 1:20). So how do you control a bad temper? You start by making sure you're living a good, moral life. Then you don't just listen to God's Word, you put it into practice. Put God first in your life, and your temper won't get the best of you. Or show you at your worst!

actions speak louder than words

Direct Line

James 2:14

¹⁹You believe that there is one God. Good! Even the demons believe that—and shudder.

²⁰You foolish man, do you want evidence that faith without deeds is useless[a]? ²¹Was not our ancestor Abraham considered righteous for what he did when he offered his son Isaac on the altar? ²²You see that his faith and his actions were working together, and his faith was made complete by what he did. ²³And the scripture was fulfilled that says, "Abraham believed God, and it was credited to him as righteousness,"[b] and he was called God's friend. ²⁴You see that a person is justified by what he does and not by faith alone.

²⁵In the same way, was not even Rahab the prostitute considered righteous for what she did when she gave lodging to the spies and sent them off in a different direction? ²⁶As the body without the spirit is dead, so faith without deeds is dead.

Taming the Tongue   Not many of you should presume to be teachers, my brothers, because you know that we who teach will be judged more strictly. ²We all stumble in many ways. If anyone is never at fault in what he says, he is a perfect man, able to keep his whole body in check.

³When we put bits into the mouths of horses to make them obey us, we can turn the whole animal. ⁴Or take ships as an example. Although they are so large and are driven by strong winds, they are steered by a very small rudder wherever the pilot wants to go. ⁵Likewise the tongue is a small part of the body, but it makes great boasts. Consider what a great forest is set on fire by a small spark. ⁶The tongue also is a fire, a world of evil among the parts of the body. It corrupts the whole person, sets the whole course of his life on fire, and is itself set on fire by hell.

⁷All kinds of animals, birds, reptiles and creatures of the sea are being tamed and have been tamed by man, ⁸but no man can tame the tongue. It is a restless evil, full of deadly poison.

⁹With the tongue we praise our Lord and Father, and with it we curse men, who have been made in God's likeness. ¹⁰Out of the same mouth come praise and cursing. My brothers, this should not be. ¹¹Can both fresh water and salt[c] water flow from the same spring? ¹²My brothers, can a fig tree bear olives, or a grapevine bear figs? Neither can a salt spring produce fresh water.

Two Kinds of Wisdom   ¹³Who is wise and understanding among you? Let him show it by his good life, by deeds done in the humility that comes from wisdom. ¹⁴But if you harbor bitter envy and selfish ambition in your hearts, do not boast about it or deny the truth. ¹⁵Such "wisdom" does not come down from heaven but is earthly, unspiritual, of the devil. ¹⁶For where you have envy and selfish ambition, there you find disorder and every evil practice.

¹⁷But the wisdom that comes from heaven is first of all pure; then peace-loving, considerate, submissive, full of mercy and good fruit, impartial and sincere. ¹⁸Peacemakers who sow in peace raise a harvest of righteousness.

Submit Yourselves to God   What causes fights and quarrels among you? Don't they come from your desires that battle within you? ²You want something but don't get it. You kill and covet, but you cannot have what you want. You quarrel and fight. You do not have, because you do not ask God. ³When you ask, you do not receive, because you ask with wrong motives, that you may spend what you get on your pleasures.

⁴You adulterous people, don't you know that friendship with the world is hatred toward God? Anyone who chooses to be a friend of the world be-

---

[a]20 Some early manuscripts *dead*   [b]23 Gen. 15:6   [c]11 Greek *bitter* (see also verse 14)

Dear Sam,
    Everyone else uses language I'm not allowed to use. Where does it say in the Bible that certain words or "dirty" jokes are bad?

Mitch in Minneapolis

Dear Sam, Inc.

100 Advice Lane, Anywhere, USA

Dear Mitch,
    Please take time to read James 3:3-12. James has some terrific insights on the tongue. In part of the passage he compares the tongue to a tiny spark that can destroy a giant forest. While humans can control almost all wild animals, they still can't control the tongue.
    We are supposed to praise God and encourage those around us. But James says that praising and cursing from the same tongue is like fresh and salt water coming from the same spring. It just can't happen.
    You will find that if you start using bad language, before long that language will pop out even when you don't want it to. If you listen to and tell dirty stories, before long those kinds of thoughts will fill your mind. What do you think God would rather you filled your mind with: praise and good thoughts? Or bad language and dirty jokes? I think the answer is pretty clear.

Sam

comes an enemy of God. ⁵Or do you think Scripture says without reason that the spirit he caused to live in us envies intensely?*ᵃ* ⁶But he gives us more grace. That is why Scripture says:

"God opposes the proud
but gives grace to the humble."*ᵇ*

⁷Submit yourselves, then, to God. Resist the devil, and he will flee from you. ⁸Come near to God and he will come near to you. Wash your hands, you sinners, and purify your hearts, you double-minded. ⁹Grieve, mourn and wail. Change your laughter to mourning and your joy to gloom. ¹⁰Humble yourselves before the Lord, and he will lift you up.

¹¹Brothers, do not slander one another. Anyone who speaks against his brother or judges him speaks against the law and judges it. When you judge the law, you are not keeping it, but sitting in judgment on it. ¹²There is only one Lawgiver and Judge, the one who is able to save and destroy. But you—who are you to judge your neighbor?

> Come near to God and he will come near to you (James 4:8).

Boasting About Tomorrow   ¹³Now listen, you who say, "Today or tomorrow we will go to this or that city, spend a year there, carry on business and make money." ¹⁴Why, you do not even know what will happen tomorrow. What is your life? You are a mist that appears for a little while and then vanishes. ¹⁵Instead, you ought to say, "If it is the Lord's will, we will live and do this or that." ¹⁶As it is, you boast and brag. All such boasting is evil. ¹⁷Anyone, then, who knows the good he ought to do and doesn't do it, sins.

Warning to Rich Oppressors   Now listen, you rich people, weep and wail because of the misery that is coming upon you. ²Your wealth has rotted, and moths have eaten your clothes. ³Your gold and silver are corroded. Their corrosion will testify against you and eat your flesh like fire. You have hoarded wealth in the last days. ⁴Look! The wages you failed to pay the workmen who mowed your fields are crying out against you. The cries of the harvesters have reached the ears of the Lord Almighty. ⁵You have lived on earth in luxury and self-indulgence. You have fattened yourselves in the day of slaughter.*ᶜ* ⁶You have condemned and murdered innocent men, who were not opposing you.

Patience in Suffering   ⁷Be patient, then, brothers, until the Lord's coming. See how the farmer waits for the land to yield its valuable crop and how patient he is for the autumn and spring rains. ⁸You too, be patient and stand firm, because the Lord's coming is near. ⁹Don't grumble against each other, brothers, or you will be judged. The Judge is standing at the door!

¹⁰Brothers, as an example of patience in the face of suffering, take the prophets who spoke in the name of the Lord. ¹¹As you know, we consider blessed those who have persevered. You have heard of Job's perseverance and have seen what the Lord finally brought about. The Lord is full of compassion and mercy.

¹²Above all, my brothers, do not swear—not by heaven or by earth or by anything else. Let your "Yes" be yes, and your "No," no, or you will be condemned.

The Prayer of Faith   ¹³Is any one of you in trouble? He should pray. Is anyone happy? Let him sing songs of praise. ¹⁴Is any one of you sick? He should call the elders of the church to pray over him and anoint him with oil in the name

---

ᵃ5 Or that God jealously longs for the spirit that he made to live in us; or that the Spirit he caused to live in us longs jealously   *ᵇ6 Prov. 3:34*   *ᶜ5 Or yourselves as in a day of feasting*

of the Lord. [15]And the prayer offered in faith will make the sick person well; the Lord will raise him up. If he has sinned, he will be forgiven. [16]Therefore confess your sins to each other and pray for each other so that you may be healed. The prayer of a righteous man is powerful and effective.

[17]Elijah was a man just like us. He prayed earnestly that it would not rain, and it did not rain on the land for three and a half years. [18]Again he prayed, and the heavens gave rain, and the earth produced its crops.

[19]My brothers, if one of you should wander from the truth and someone should bring him back, [20]remember this: Whoever turns a sinner from the error of his way will save him from death and cover over a multitude of sins.

IT'S NOT FAIR!

You do what's right, and still things turn out rotten.
You help a friend who fell off his bike, miss the bus to
the big game and get kicked off the team. Or you're
accused of something you didn't do, and your parents ground you. How can that be fair?

Peter wrote this letter to Christians who were being
treated unfairly. They were good citizens who obeyed
the law, but they were being persecuted anyway.
Some lost their jobs and homes, and some even lost
their lives. Peter wrote to show them how to triumph
when life is unfair.

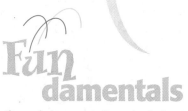

Fundamentals

*If people have to suffer, what's the
use of living (1 Peter 1)?*

*One teacher picks on you, so you
just don't do the work he assigns
(1 Peter 2:16-25).*

*Have you ever had a teacher mock
you because you're a Christian
(1 Peter 4:12-19)?*

FAST FACTS

*Peter was the leader of
Jesus' 12 disciples.*

*Peter wrote this letter around
A.D. 63, shortly before his execution in Rome.*

*By this time Christianity was an
illegal religion.*

*Nero, who was emperor from A.D.
54 to 68, burned many Christians
alive.*

*Peter wrote this letter to help
Christians face persecution and suffering.*

1 Peter, an apostle of Jesus Christ,

To God's elect, strangers in the world, scattered throughout Pontus, Galatia, Cappadocia, Asia and Bithynia, [2]who have been chosen according to the foreknowledge of God the Father, through the sanctifying work of the Spirit, for obedience to Jesus Christ and sprinkling by his blood:

Grace and peace be yours in abundance.

Praise to God for a Living Hope [3]Praise be to the God and Father of our Lord Jesus Christ! In his great mercy he has given us new birth into a living hope through the resurrection of Jesus Christ from the dead, [4]and into an inheritance that can never perish, spoil or fade—kept in heaven for you, [5]who through faith are shielded by God's power until the coming of the salvation that is ready to be revealed in the last time. [6]In this you greatly rejoice, though now for a little while you may have had to suffer grief in all kinds of trials. [7]These have come so that your faith—of greater worth than gold, which perishes even though refined by fire—may be proved genuine and may result in praise, glory and honor when Jesus Christ is revealed. [8]Though you have not seen him, you love him; and even though you do not see him now, you believe in him and are filled with an inexpressible and glorious joy, [9]for you are receiving the goal of your faith, the salvation of your souls.

> In his great mercy he has given us . . . an inheritance that can never perish, spoil or fade (1 Peter 1:3-4).

[10]Concerning this salvation, the prophets, who spoke of the grace that was to come to you, searched intently and with the greatest care, [11]trying to find out the time and circumstances to which the Spirit of Christ in them was pointing when he predicted the sufferings of Christ and the glories that would follow. [12]It was revealed to them that they were not serving themselves but you, when they spoke of the things that have now been told you by those who have preached the gospel to you by the Holy Spirit sent from heaven. Even angels long to look into these things.

Be Holy [13]Therefore, prepare your minds for action; be self-controlled; set your hope fully on the grace to be given you when Jesus Christ is revealed. [14]As obedient children, do not conform to the evil desires you had when you lived in ignorance. [15]But just as he who called you is holy, so be holy in all you do; [16]for it is written: "Be holy, because I am holy."[a]

[17]Since you call on a Father who judges each man's work impartially, live your lives as strangers here in reverent fear. [18]For you know that it was not with perishable things such as silver or gold that you were redeemed from the empty way of life handed down to you from your forefathers, [19]but with the precious blood of Christ, a lamb without blemish or defect. [20]He was chosen before the creation of the world, but was revealed in these last times for your sake. [21]Through him you believe in God, who raised him from the dead and glorified him, and so your faith and hope are in God.

[22]Now that you have purified yourselves by obeying the truth so that you have sincere love for your brothers, love one another deeply, from the heart.[b] [23]For you have been born again, not of perishable seed, but of imperishable, through the living and enduring word of God. [24]For,

> "All men are like grass,
>   and all their glory is like the flowers of the field;
>   the grass withers and the flowers fall,
> [25]   but the word of the Lord stands forever."[c]

And this is the word that was preached to you.

[a]16 Lev. 11:44,45; 19:2; 20:7   [b]22 Some early manuscripts *from a pure heart*   [c]25 Isaiah 40:6-8

Therefore, rid yourselves of all malice and all deceit, hypocrisy, envy, and slander of every kind. ²Like newborn babies, crave pure spiritual milk, so that by it you may grow up in your salvation, ³now that you have tasted that the Lord is good.

The Living Stone and a Chosen People ⁴As you come to him, the living Stone—rejected by men but chosen by God and precious to him— ⁵you also, like living stones, are being built into a spiritual house to be a holy priesthood, offering spiritual sacrifices acceptable to God through Jesus Christ. ⁶For in Scripture it says:

> "See, I lay a stone in Zion,
>   a chosen and precious cornerstone,
> and the one who trusts in him
>   will never be put to shame."*ᵃ*

⁷Now to you who believe, this stone is precious. But to those who do not believe,

> "The stone the builders rejected
>   has become the capstone,*ᵇ*"*ᶜ*

⁸and,

> "A stone that causes men to stumble
>   and a rock that makes them fall."*ᵈ*

They stumble because they disobey the message—which is also what they were destined for.

⁹But you are a chosen people, a royal priesthood, a holy nation, a people belonging to God, that you may declare the praises of him who called you out of darkness into his wonderful light. ¹⁰Once you were not a people, but now you are the people of God; once you had not received mercy, but now you have received mercy.

¹¹Dear friends, I urge you, as aliens and strangers in the world, to abstain from sinful desires, which war against your soul. ¹²Live such good lives among the pagans that, though they accuse you of doing wrong, they may see your good deeds and glorify God on the day he visits us.

Submission to Rulers and Masters ¹³Submit yourselves for the Lord's sake to every authority instituted among men: whether to the king, as the supreme authority, ¹⁴or to governors, who are sent by him to punish those who do wrong and to commend those who do right. ¹⁵For it is God's will that by doing good you should silence the ignorant talk of foolish men. ¹⁶Live as free men, but do not use your freedom as a cover-up for evil; live as servants of God. ¹⁷Show proper respect to everyone: Love the brotherhood of believers, fear God, honor the king.

¹⁸Slaves, submit yourselves to your masters with all respect, not only to those

---

Direct Line

1 PETER 2:9–10

How are you different from kids who aren't Christians? No, I know you don't have a third eye or six toes on each foot. And no one expects you to dress like your great grandpa. Hey, it's OK to look and act like a teenager. Still, Peter expects you to be different: "Now you are the people of God" (1 Peter 2:10). You belong to God. Being "different" as a Christian means making sure that everything you do reflects in a positive manner on God. Be a teen. And be a kind, thoughtful and honest person. Be a teen. And act toward your friends of both sexes with integrity. Be a teen. Be God's teen, the very best person you can be.

ᵃ6 Isaiah 28:16   *ᵇ7* Or *cornerstone*   *ᶜ7* Psalm 118:22
ᵈ8 Isaiah 8:14

who are good and considerate, but also to those who are harsh. ¹⁹For it is commendable if a man bears up under the pain of unjust suffering because he is conscious of God. ²⁰But how is it to your credit if you receive a beating for doing wrong and endure it? But if you suffer for doing good and you endure it, this is commendable before God. ²¹To this you were called, because Christ suffered for you, leaving you an example, that you should follow in his steps.

> ²²"He committed no sin,
>   and no deceit was found in his mouth."ᵃ

²³When they hurled their insults at him, he did not retaliate; when he suffered, he made no threats. Instead, he entrusted himself to him who judges justly. ²⁴He himself bore our sins in his body on the tree, so that we might die to sins and live for righteousness; by his wounds you have been healed. ²⁵For you were like sheep going astray, but now you have returned to the Shepherd and Overseer of your souls.

Wives and Husbands Wives, in the same way be submissive to your husbands so that, if any of them do not believe the word, they may be won over without words by the behavior of their wives, ²when they see the purity and reverence of your lives. ³Your beauty should not come from outward adornment, such as braided hair and the wearing of gold jewelry and fine clothes. ⁴Instead, it should be that of your inner self, the unfading beauty of a gentle and quiet spirit, which is of great worth in God's sight. ⁵For this is the way the holy women of the past who put their hope in God used to make themselves beautiful. They were submissive to their own husbands, ⁶like Sarah, who obeyed Abraham and called him her master. You are her daughters if you do what is right and do not give way to fear.

⁷Husbands, in the same way be considerate as you live with your wives, and treat them with respect as the weaker partner and as heirs with you of the gracious gift of life, so that nothing will hinder your prayers.

Suffering for Doing Good ⁸Finally, all of you, live in harmony with one another; be sympathetic, love as brothers, be compassionate and humble. ⁹Do not repay evil with evil or insult with insult, but with blessing, because to this you were called so that you may inherit a blessing. ¹⁰For,

> "Whoever would love life
>   and see good days
> must keep his tongue from evil
>   and his lips from deceitful speech.
> ¹¹He must turn from evil and do good;
>   he must seek peace and pursue it.
> ¹²For the eyes of the Lord are on the righteous
>   and his ears are attentive to their prayer,
> but the face of the Lord is against those who do
>   evil."ᵇ

¹³Who is going to harm you if you are eager to do good? ¹⁴But even if you should suffer for what is right, you are blessed. "Do not fear what they fearᶜ; do not be frightened."ᵈ ¹⁵But in your hearts set apart Christ as Lord. Always be prepared to give an answer to everyone who asks you to give the reason for the hope that you have. But do this with gentleness and respect, ¹⁶keeping a clear conscience, so that those who speak maliciously against your good behavior in Christ may be ashamed of their slander. ¹⁷It is better, if it is God's will, to suffer for doing good than for doing evil. ¹⁸For Christ died

---

ᵃ22 Isaiah 53:9 ᵇ12 Psalm 34:12-16 ᶜ14 Or *not fear their threats* ᵈ14 Isaiah 8:12

for sins once for all, the righteous for the unrighteous, to bring you to God. He was put to death in the body but made alive by the Spirit, [19]through whom[a] also he went and preached to the spirits in prison [20]who disobeyed long ago when God waited patiently in the days of Noah while the ark was being built. In it only a few people, eight in all, were saved through water, [21]and this water symbolizes baptism that now saves you also—not the removal of dirt from the body but the pledge[b] of a good conscience toward God. It saves you by the resurrection of Jesus Christ, [22]who has gone into heaven and is at God's right hand—with angels, authorities and powers in submission to him.

Living for God   Therefore, since Christ suffered in his body, arm yourselves also with the same attitude, because he who has suffered in his body is done with sin. [2]As a result, he does not live the rest of his earthly life for evil human desires, but rather for the will of God. [3]For you have spent enough time in the past doing what pagans choose to do—living in debauchery, lust, drunkenness, orgies, carousing and detestable idolatry. [4]They think it strange that you do not plunge with them into the same flood of dissipation, and they heap abuse on you. [5]But they will have to give account to him who is ready to judge the living and the dead. [6]For this is the reason the gospel was preached even to those who are now dead, so that they might be judged according to men in regard to the body, but live according to God in regard to the spirit.

[7]The end of all things is near. Therefore be clear minded and self-controlled so that you can pray. [8]Above all, love each other deeply, because love covers over a multitude of sins. [9]Offer hospitality to one another without grumbling. [10]Each one should use whatever gift he has received to serve others, faithfully administering God's grace in its various forms. [11]If anyone speaks, he should do it as one speaking the very words of God. If anyone serves, he should do it with the strength God provides, so that in all things God may be praised through Jesus Christ. To him be the glory and the power for ever and ever. Amen.

Suffering for Being a Christian   [12]Dear friends, do not be surprised at the painful trial you are suffering, as though something strange were happening to you. [13]But rejoice that you participate in the sufferings of Christ, so that you may be overjoyed when his glory is revealed. [14]If you are insulted because of the name of Christ, you are blessed, for the Spirit of glory and of God rests on you. [15]If you suffer, it should not be as a murderer or thief or any other kind of criminal, or even as a meddler. [16]However, if you suffer as a Christian, do not be ashamed, but praise God that you bear that name. [17]For it is time for judgment to begin with the family of God; and if it begins with us, what will the outcome be for those who do not obey the gospel of God? [18]And,

---

Direct Line

1 PETER 4:12–19

You "borrow" your mom's bracelet, lose it, and when she asks if you've seen it, you say, "Bracelet? What bracelet?" Then your best friend walks in waving the bracelet and says, "Hey, Hillary, you left this in my locker." Oh, well. At least you suffer through your punishment without complaining. But don't expect to be praised for it. On the other hand, if you suffer because of your Christian commitment and accept it cheerfully, that merits praise. There's no reason to be ashamed if some teacher puts you down for what you believe or if some of the other teens call you a goody-goody. Don't be ashamed, be proud. You're being a follower of Jesus.

---

[a]18,19 Or *alive in the spirit,* [19]*through which*   [b]21 Or *response*

"If it is hard for the righteous to be saved,
     what will become of the ungodly and the sinner?"[a]

[19]So then, those who suffer according to God's will should commit them-selves to their faithful Creator and continue to do good.

To Elders and Young Men   To the elders among you, I appeal as a fel-low elder, a witness of Christ's sufferings and one who also will share in the glory to be revealed: [2]Be shepherds of God's flock that is under your care, serving as overseers—not because you must, but because you are will-ing, as God wants you to be; not greedy for money, but eager to serve; [3]not lording it over those entrusted to you, but being examples to the flock. [4]And when the Chief Shepherd appears, you will receive the crown of glory that will never fade away.

[5]Young men, in the same way be submissive to those who are older. All of you, clothe yourselves with humility toward one another, because,

"God opposes the proud
     but gives grace to the humble."[b]

[6]Humble yourselves, therefore, under God's mighty hand, that he may lift you up in due time. [7]Cast all your anxiety on him because he cares for you.

[8]Be self-controlled and alert. Your en-emy the devil prowls around like a roar-ing lion looking for someone to devour. [9]Resist him, standing firm in the faith, be-cause you know that your brothers throughout the world are undergoing the same kind of sufferings.

[10]And the God of all grace, who called you to his eternal glory in Christ, after you have suffered a little while, will him-self restore you and make you strong, firm and steadfast. [11]To him be the pow-er for ever and ever. Amen.

Final Greetings   [12]With the help of Silas,[c] whom I regard as a faithful brother, I have written to you briefly, encouraging you and testifying that this is the true grace of God. Stand fast in it.

[13]She who is in Babylon, chosen to-gether with you, sends you her greetings, and so does my son Mark. [14]Greet one another with a kiss of love.

Peace to all of you who are in Christ.

1 PETER 5:7

Worrying isn't much fun. Test coming up? You get cramps and a cold sweat. Mom goes to visit Grandpa? You lie awake wondering if her plane crashed or if a hurricane struck Nebraska. Peter has a suggestion for worriers: Let God worry about it for you. "Cast all your anxiety on him because he cares for you" (1 Peter 5:7). Study for your test. But after that, let God do the worrying. Hug Mom and wave good-by. Say a prayer, and let God take over. At rest inside, you'll do better on your test. And you'll sleep better at night too.

Direct Line

[a]*18* Prov. 11:31   [b]*5* Prov. 3:34   [c]*12* Greek *Silvanus*, a variant of *Silas*

book of 2 Peter

DIFFERENT BELIEFS.

You know kids with beliefs that are different from yours. Some won't say the pledge of allegiance. Some won't go to doctors but say God will heal them. Sometimes these kids may try to convince you that what you believe is wrong. They can be convincing too—so convincing it may be hard to know who's right.

Peter's first letter was about persecution from non-Christians. This second letter is about danger from false teachers who claim to be believers. Peter shows you how to know what teachers and teachings are false.

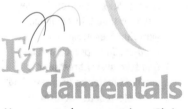

Fundamentals

How can you be sure you're a Christian (2 Peter 1:3-11)?

How can you tell if someone isn't teaching the truth (2 Peter 2)?

Will this world last forever (2 Peter 3:10-16)?

FAST FACTS

Peter wrote this letter of warning just before his execution in Rome.

Heresy is any teaching that contradicts the Bible or promotes sinful living.

Jude and 2 Timothy also warn about the dangers of false teaching.

The day of the Lord here refers to history's end, when Jesus will return and God will punish evil.

Simon Peter, a servant and apostle of Jesus Christ,

To those who through the righteousness of our God and Savior Jesus Christ have received a faith as precious as ours:

²Grace and peace be yours in abundance through the knowledge of God and of Jesus our Lord.

Making One's Calling and Election Sure   ³His divine power has given us everything we need for life and godliness through our knowledge of him who called us by his own glory and goodness. ⁴Through these he has given us his very great and precious promises, so that through them you may participate in the divine nature and escape the corruption in the world caused by evil desires.

⁵For this very reason, make every effort to add to your faith goodness; and to goodness, knowledge; ⁶and to knowledge, self-control; and to self-control, perseverance; and to perseverance, godliness; ⁷and to godliness, brotherly kindness; and to brotherly kindness, love. ⁸For if you possess these qualities in increasing measure, they will keep you from being ineffective and unproductive in your knowledge of our Lord Jesus Christ. ⁹But if anyone does not have them, he is nearsighted and blind, and has forgotten that he has been cleansed from his past sins.

¹⁰Therefore, my brothers, be all the more eager to make your calling and election sure. For if you do these things, you will never fall, ¹¹and you will receive a rich welcome into the eternal kingdom of our Lord and Savior Jesus Christ.

Prophecy of Scripture   ¹²So I will always remind you of these things, even though you know them and are firmly established in the truth you now have. ¹³I think it is right to refresh your memory as long as I live in the tent of this body, ¹⁴because I know that I will soon put it aside, as our Lord Jesus Christ has made clear to me. ¹⁵And I will make every effort to see that after my departure you will always be able to remember these things.

¹⁶We did not follow cleverly invented stories when we told you about the power and coming of our Lord Jesus Christ, but we were eyewitnesses of his majesty. ¹⁷For he received honor and glory from God the Father when the voice came to him from the Majestic Glory, saying, "This is my Son, whom I love; with him I am well pleased."ᵃ ¹⁸We ourselves heard this voice that came from heaven when we were with him on the sacred mountain.

¹⁹And we have the word of the prophets made more certain, and you will do well to pay attention to it, as to a light shining in a dark place, until the day dawns and the morning star rises in your hearts. ²⁰Above all, you must understand that no prophecy of Scripture came about by the prophet's own interpretation. ²¹For prophecy never had its origin in the will of man, but men spoke from God as they were carried along by the Holy Spirit.

ᵃ*17* Matt. 17:5; Mark 9:7; Luke 9:35

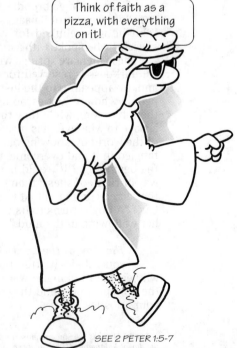

SEE 2 PETER 1:5-7

False Teachers and Their Destruction But there were also false prophets among the people, just as there will be false teachers among you. They will secretly introduce destructive heresies, even denying the sovereign Lord who bought them—bringing swift destruction on themselves. ²Many will follow their shameful ways and will bring the way of truth into disrepute. ³In their greed these teachers will exploit you with stories they have made up. Their condemnation has long been hanging over them, and their destruction has not been sleeping.

⁴For if God did not spare angels when they sinned, but sent them to hell,ᵃ putting them into gloomy dungeonsᵇ to be held for judgment; ⁵if he did not spare the ancient world when he brought the flood on its ungodly people, but protected Noah, a preacher of righteousness, and seven others; ⁶if he condemned the cities of Sodom and Gomorrah by burning them to ashes, and made them an example of what is going to happen to the ungodly; ⁷and if he rescued Lot, a righteous man, who was distressed by the filthy lives of lawless men ⁸(for that righteous man, living among them day after day, was tormented in his righteous soul by the lawless deeds he saw and heard)— ⁹if this is so, then the Lord knows how to rescue godly men from trials and to hold the unrighteous for the day of judgment, while continuing their punishment.ᶜ ¹⁰This is especially true of those who follow the corrupt desire of the sinful natureᵈ and despise authority.

Bold and arrogant, these men are not afraid to slander celestial beings; ¹¹yet even angels, although they are stronger and more powerful, do not bring slanderous accusations against such beings in the presence of the Lord. ¹²But these men blaspheme in matters they do not understand. They are like brute beasts, creatures of instinct, born only to be caught and destroyed, and like beasts they too will perish.

¹³They will be paid back with harm for the harm they have done. Their idea of pleasure is to carouse in broad daylight. They are blots and blemishes, reveling in their pleasures while they feast with you.ᵉ ¹⁴With eyes full of adultery, they never stop sinning; they seduce the unstable; they are experts in greed—an accursed brood! ¹⁵They have left the straight way and wandered off to follow the way of Balaam son of Beor, who loved the wages of wickedness. ¹⁶But he was rebuked for his wrongdoing by a donkey—a beast without speech—who spoke with a man's voice and restrained the prophet's madness.

¹⁷These men are springs without water and mists driven by a storm. Blackest darkness is reserved for them. ¹⁸For they mouth empty, boastful words and, by appealing to the lustful desires of sinful human nature, they entice people who are just escaping from those who live in error. ¹⁹They promise them freedom, while they themselves are slaves of depravity—for a man is a slave to whatever has mastered him. ²⁰If they have escaped the corruption of the world by knowing our Lord and Savior Jesus Christ and are again entangled in it and overcome, they are worse off at the end than they were at the beginning. ²¹It would have been better for them not to have known the way of righteousness, than to have known it and then to turn their backs on the sacred command that was passed on to them. ²²Of them the proverbs are true: "A dog returns to its vomit,"ᶠ and, "A sow that is washed goes back to her wallowing in the mud."

The Day of the Lord Dear friends, this is now my second letter to you. I have written both of them as reminders to stimulate you to wholesome thinking. ²I want you to recall the words spoken in the past by the holy prophets and the command given by our Lord and Savior through your apostles.

ᵃ4 Greek *Tartarus*   ᵇ4 Some manuscripts *into chains of darkness*   ᶜ9 Or *unrighteous for punishment until the day of judgment*   ᵈ10 Or *the flesh*   ᵉ13 Some manuscripts *in their love feasts*   ᶠ22 Prov. 26:11

Dear Sam,

I learned about evolution in school.
What does the Bible say about evolution?

Sanford in San Marcos

100 Advice Lane, Anywhere, USA

Dear Sanford,

The Bible doesn't talk about evolution. But it does emphasize over and over again the most important fact about creation: God did it. There is no conflict between science and the Biblical view of creation. Conflict only begins when a view of the beginning of the world leaves out God as Creator.

Sincere Christians have struggled with this issue for many years, and they have come to vastly different conclusions. But don't let those different conclusions distract you from the main truth of the Bible: a loving God, a powerful God is also a Creator God. No part of this world—from small, squishy, one-celled animals to complex human beings—is here by chance.

Many years ago Peter predicted that people would forget the fact that God created the universe (2 Peter 3:3-5). Take a close look at this passage. Then go to a library and check out a book or two that discusses the differing theories and God's involvement in the beginnings of the universe. But whatever you read, keep in mind what Peter said, and don't forget: God did it.

Sam

³First of all, you must understand that in the last days scoffers will come, scoffing and following their own evil desires. ⁴They will say, "Where is this 'coming' he promised? Ever since our fathers died, everything goes on as it has since the beginning of creation." ⁵But they deliberately forget that long ago by God's word the heavens existed and the earth was formed out of water and by water. ⁶By these waters also the world of that time was deluged and destroyed. ⁷By the same word the present heavens and earth are reserved for fire, being kept for the day of judgment and destruction of ungodly men.

⁸But do not forget this one thing, dear friends: With the Lord a day is like a thousand years, and a thousand years are like a day. ⁹The Lord is not slow in keeping his promise, as some understand slowness. He is patient with you, not wanting anyone to perish, but everyone to come to repentance.

¹⁰But the day of the Lord will come like a thief. The heavens will disappear with a roar; the elements will be destroyed by fire, and the earth and everything in it will be laid bare.ᵃ

¹¹Since everything will be destroyed in this way, what kind of people ought you to be? You ought to live holy and godly lives ¹²as you look forward to the day of God and speed its coming.ᵇ That day will bring about the destruction of the heavens by fire, and the elements will melt in the heat. ¹³But in keeping with his promise we are looking forward to a new heaven and a new earth, the home of righteousness.

¹⁴So then, dear friends, since you are looking forward to this, make every effort to be found spotless, blameless and at peace with him. ¹⁵Bear in mind that our Lord's patience means salvation, just as our dear brother Paul also wrote you with the wisdom that God gave him. ¹⁶He writes the same way in all his letters, speaking in them of these matters. His letters contain some things that are hard to understand, which ignorant and unstable people distort, as they do the other Scriptures, to their own destruction.

¹⁷Therefore, dear friends, since you already know this, be on your guard so that you may not be carried away by the error of lawless men and fall from your secure position. ¹⁸But grow in the grace and knowledge of our Lord and Savior Jesus Christ. To him be glory both now and forever! Amen.

Direct Line

2 PETER 3:10–16

What's the latest theory on how the world will end? A new ice age? Global warming? A comet crashing into the earth? An ozone hole so wide we'll all be sunburned to death? And when is this to happen? Fifty thousand years? Five million? Peter says Jesus *will* return. God will sweep away this earth to make room for a whole new creation. The Genesis flood is history's reminder that God does judge sin. Peter's vision helps to put lots of things into perspective. Never mind the doomsayers. But remember that this world is doomed, and don't get so involved in it that you forget to live for Jesus.

ᵃ10 Some manuscripts *be burned up* ᵇ12 Or *as you wait eagerly for the day of God to come*

Introduction

to the

book of 1 John

A CLOSE FRIEND.

Wouldn't it be great to feel as close to God as you do to your best friend? Or maybe you feel that close already. If you do, you already understand the important things John has to say in this letter.

John's first letter is about "fellowship." The word means "sharing": being close to God and other Christians. John says the keys to fellowship with God are love and obedience. If you love God, you'll stay close to him and pay attention to his Word. As you obey the Lord, you sense him near and learn to love him even more.

FAST FACTS

John the apostle wrote this letter.

John outlived all Jesus' other disciples. He probably wrote this in A.D. 90.

After A.D. 81 it was official policy to persecute Christians.

Many were executed for being Christians. Others lost their property.

John reminds you that if you love each other the church will be strong despite persecution.

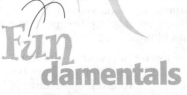

Fundamentals

You say you never sin? You just make mistakes sometimes? Really (1 John 1:5-10)?

Will you go to heaven just because you believe in Jesus? You don't have to obey him (1 John 2:3-11)?

Why shouldn't Christians be like everyone else (1 John 2:15-17)?

What is love (1 John 3:16-24)?

1

The Word of Life That which was from the beginning, which we have heard, which we have seen with our eyes, which we have looked at and our hands have touched—this we proclaim concerning the Word of life. ²The life appeared; we have seen it and testify to it, and we proclaim to you the eternal life, which was with the Father and has appeared to us. ³We proclaim to you what we have seen and heard, so that you also may have fellowship with us. And our fellowship is with the Father and with his Son, Jesus Christ. ⁴We write this to make our*ᵃ* joy complete.

Walking in the Light ⁵This is the message we have heard from him and declare to you: God is light; in him there is no darkness at all. ⁶If we claim to have fellowship with him yet walk in the darkness, we lie and do not live by the truth. ⁷But if we walk in the light, as he is in the light, we have fellowship with one another, and the blood of Jesus, his Son, purifies us from all*ᵇ* sin.

⁸If we claim to be without sin, we deceive ourselves and the truth is not in us. ⁹If we confess our sins, he is faithful and just and will forgive us our sins and purify us from all unrighteousness. ¹⁰If we claim we have not sinned, we make him out to be a liar and his word has no place in our lives.

2

My dear children, I write this to you so that you will not sin. But if anybody does sin, we have one who speaks to the Father in our defense—Jesus Christ, the Righteous One. ²He is the atoning sacrifice for our sins, and not only for ours but also for*ᶜ* the sins of the whole world.

³We know that we have come to know him if we obey his commands. ⁴The man who says, "I know him," but does not do what he commands is a liar, and the truth is not in him. ⁵But if anyone obeys his word, God's love*ᵈ* is truly made complete in him. This is how we know we are in him: ⁶Whoever claims to live in him must walk as Jesus did.

⁷Dear friends, I am not writing you a new command but an old one, which you have had since the beginning. This old command is the message you have heard. ⁸Yet I am writing you a new command; its truth is seen in him and you, because the darkness is passing and the true light is already shining.

⁹Anyone who claims to be in the light but hates his brother is still in the darkness. ¹⁰Whoever loves his brother lives in the light, and there is nothing in him*ᵉ* to make him stumble. ¹¹But whoever hates his brother is in the darkness and walks around in the darkness; he does not know where he is going, because the darkness has blinded him.

¹² I write to you, dear children,
  because your sins have been
    forgiven on account of his
      name.
¹³ I write to you, fathers,
  because you have known him
    who is from the beginning.
I write to you, young men,
  because you have overcome the
    evil one.
I write to you, dear children,
  because you have known the
    Father.

1 JOHN 1:5–10

Direct Line

John warns you to be honest about your faults. If you "claim to be without sin" (1 John 1:8), you don't fool others. But you will end up deceiving yourself. To stay close to God you have to be honest with yourself, even more than with others. You can't take your sister's sweater and then lie about it or say you're going one place and then go another. And then pretend it isn't wrong. If you find yourself doing things like this, please face the fact that you are sinning. Confess your sin to God, and he'll forgive you. He'll even cleanse you so you can start doing what's right. If you don't stop deceiving yourself, you'll never be really close to the Lord.

ᵃ4 Some manuscripts your ᵇ7 Or every ᶜ2 Or He is the one who turns aside God's wrath, taking away our sins, and not only ours but also ᵈ5 Or word, love for God ᵉ10 Or it

[14]I write to you, fathers,
> because you have known him who is from the beginning.
I write to you, young men,
> because you are strong,
> and the word of God lives in you,
> and you have overcome the evil one.

Do Not Love the World [15]Do not love the world or anything in the world. If anyone loves the world, the love of the Father is not in him. [16]For everything in the world—the cravings of sinful man, the lust of his eyes and the boasting of what he has and does—comes not from the Father but from the world. [17]The world and its desires pass away, but the man who does the will of God lives forever.

Warning Against Antichrists [18]Dear children, this is the last hour; and as you have heard that the antichrist is coming, even now many antichrists have come. This is how we know it is the last hour. [19]They went out from us, but they did not really belong to us. For if they had belonged to us, they would have remained with us; but their going showed that none of them belonged to us.

[20]But you have an anointing from the Holy One, and all of you know the truth.[a] [21]I do not write to you because you do not know the truth, but because you do know it and because no lie comes from the truth. [22]Who is the liar? It is the man who denies that Jesus is the Christ. Such a man is the antichrist—he denies the Father and the Son. [23]No one who denies the Son has the Father; whoever acknowledges the Son has the Father also.

[24]See that what you have heard from the beginning remains in you. If it does, you also will remain in the Son and in the Father. [25]And this is what he promised us—even eternal life.

[26]I am writing these things to you about those who are trying to lead you astray. [27]As for you, the anointing you received from him remains in you, and you do not need anyone to teach you. But as his anointing teaches you about all things and as that anointing is real, not counterfeit—just as it has taught you, remain in him.

Children of God [28]And now, dear children, continue in him, so that when he appears we may be confident and unashamed before him at his coming.

[29]If you know that he is righteous, you know that everyone who does what is right has been born of him.

3 How great is the love the Father has lavished on us, that we should be called children of God! And that is what we are! The reason the world does not know us is that it did not know him. [2]Dear friends, now we are children of God, and what we will be has not yet been made known. But we know that when he appears,[b] we shall be like him, for we shall see him as he is. [3]Everyone who has this hope in him purifies himself, just as he is pure.

[4]Everyone who sins breaks the law; in fact, sin is lawlessness. [5]But you know that he appeared so that he might take away our sins. And in him is no sin. [6]No one who lives in him keeps on sinning. No one who continues to sin has either seen him or known him.

[7]Dear children, do not let anyone lead you astray. He who does what is right is righteous, just as he is righteous. [8]He who does what is sinful is of the devil, because the devil has been sinning from the beginning. The reason the Son of God ap-

> How great is the
> love the Father
> has lavished
> on us, that we
> should be called
> children of God
> (1 John 3:1)!

---

[a]20 Some manuscripts *and you know all things*   [b]2 Or *when it is made known*

peared was to destroy the devil's work. [9]No one who is born of God will continue to sin, because God's seed remains in him; he cannot go on sinning, because he has been born of God. [10]This is how we know who the children of God are and who the children of the devil are: Anyone who does not do what is right is not a child of God; nor is anyone who does not love his brother.

Love One Another   [11]This is the message you heard from the beginning: We should love one another. [12]Do not be like Cain, who belonged to the evil one and murdered his brother. And why did he murder him? Because his own actions were evil and his brother's were righteous. [13]Do not be surprised, my brothers, if the world hates you. [14]We know that we have passed from death to life, because we love our brothers. Anyone who does not love remains in death. [15]Anyone who hates his brother is a murderer, and you know that no murderer has eternal life in him.

[16]This is how we know what love is: Jesus Christ laid down his life for us. And we ought to lay down our lives for our brothers. [17]If anyone has material possessions and sees his brother in need but has no pity on him, how can the love of God be in him? [18]Dear children, let us not love with words or tongue but with actions and in truth. [19]This then is how we know that we belong to the truth, and how we set our hearts at rest in his presence [20]whenever our hearts condemn us. For God is greater than our hearts, and he knows everything.

[21]Dear friends, if our hearts do not condemn us, we have confidence before God [22]and receive from him anything we ask, because we obey his commands and do what pleases him. [23]And this is his command: to believe in the name of his Son, Jesus Christ, and to love one another as he commanded us. [24]Those who obey his commands live in him, and he in them. And this is how we know that he lives in us: We know it by the Spirit he gave us.

Test the Spirits   Dear friends, do not believe every spirit, but test the spirits to see whether they are from God, because many false prophets have gone out into the world. [2]This is how you can recognize the Spirit of God: Every spirit that acknowledges that Jesus Christ has come in the flesh is from God, [3]but every spirit that does not acknowledge Jesus is not from God. This is the spirit of the antichrist, which you have heard is coming and even now is already in the world.

[4]You, dear children, are from God and have overcome them, because the one who is in you is greater than the one who is in the world. [5]They are from the world and therefore speak from the viewpoint of the world, and the

---

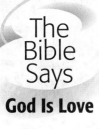

The Bible Says

God Is Love

Love is the key to understanding God and the life God wants you to live here on earth. One of the Bible's most beautiful passages about God's love (1 John 4:7–21) tells you:

* Love motivates all God does (1 John 4:16).
* Jesus proves God's love (1 John 4:9–10).
* God's love changes you so that you love him (1 John 4:19).
* God's love changes you so that you love others (1 John 4:20–21).

So don't let anyone tell you that Christianity is about lists of do's and don'ts that keep people from having fun. Christianity is all about love: God's love and your love for him and for others.

world listens to them. ⁶We are from God, and whoever knows God listens to us; but whoever is not from God does not listen to us. This is how we recognize the Spirit*a* of truth and the spirit of falsehood.

God's Love and Ours   ⁷Dear friends, let us love one another, for love comes from God. Everyone who loves has been born of God and knows God. ⁸Whoever does not love does not know God, because God is love. ⁹This is how God showed his love among us: He sent his one and only Son*b* into the world that we might live through him. ¹⁰This is love: not that we loved God, but that he loved us and sent his Son as an atoning sacrifice for*c* our sins. ¹¹Dear friends, since God so loved us, we also ought to love one another. ¹²No one has ever seen God; but if we love one another, God lives in us and his love is made complete in us.

¹³We know that we live in him and he in us, because he has given us of his Spirit. ¹⁴And we have seen and testify that the Father has sent his Son to be the Savior of the world. ¹⁵If anyone acknowledges that Jesus is the Son of God, God lives in him and he in God. ¹⁶And so we know and rely on the love God has for us.

God is love. Whoever lives in love lives in God, and God in him. ¹⁷In this way, love is made complete among us so that we will have confidence on the day of judgment, because in this world we are like him. ¹⁸There is no fear in love. But perfect love drives out fear, because fear has to do with punishment. The one who fears is not made perfect in love.

¹⁹We love because he first loved us. ²⁰If anyone says, "I love God," yet hates his brother, he is a liar. For anyone who does not love his brother, whom he has seen, cannot love God, whom he has not seen. ²¹And he has given us this command: Whoever loves God must also love his brother.

5 *Faith in the Son of God*   Everyone who believes that Jesus is the Christ is born of God, and everyone who loves the father loves his child as well. ²This is how we know that we love the children of God: by loving God and carrying out his commands. ³This is love for God: to obey his commands. And his commands are not burdensome, ⁴for everyone born of God overcomes the world. This is the victory that has overcome the world, even our faith. ⁵Who is it that overcomes the world? Only he who believes that Jesus is the Son of God.

⁶This is the one who came by water and blood—Jesus Christ. He did not come by water only, but by water and blood. And it is the Spirit who testifies, because the Spirit is the truth. ⁷For there are three that testify: ⁸the*d* Spirit, the water and the blood; and the three are in agreement. ⁹We accept man's testimony, but God's testimony is greater because it is the testimony of God, which he has given about his Son. ¹⁰Anyone who believes in the Son of God has this testimony in his heart. Anyone who does not believe God has made him out to be a liar, because he has not believed the testimony God has given about his Son. ¹¹And this is the testimony: God has given us eternal life, and this life is in his Son. ¹²He who has the Son has life; he who does not have the Son of God does not have life.

Concluding Remarks   ¹³I write these things to you who believe in the name of the Son of God so that you may know that you have eternal life. ¹⁴This is the confidence we have in approaching God: that if we ask anything according to his will, he hears

> He who has the Son has life; he who does not have the Son of God does not have life (1 John 5:12).

---

*a*6 Or *spirit*   *b*9 Or *his only begotten Son*   *c*10 Or *as the one who would turn aside his wrath, taking away*
*d*7,8 Late manuscripts of the Vulgate *testify in heaven: the Father, the Word and the Holy Spirit, and these three are one.* ⁸*And there are three that testify on earth: the* (not found in any Greek manuscript before the sixteenth century)

us. ¹⁵And if we know that he hears us—whatever we ask—we know that we have what we asked of him.

¹⁶If anyone sees his brother commit a sin that does not lead to death, he should pray and God will give him life. I refer to those whose sin does not lead to death. There is a sin that leads to death. I am not saying that he should pray about that. ¹⁷All wrongdoing is sin, and there is sin that does not lead to death.

¹⁸We know that anyone born of God does not continue to sin; the one who was born of God keeps him safe, and the evil one cannot harm him. ¹⁹We know that we are children of God, and that the whole world is under the control of the evil one. ²⁰We know also that the Son of God has come and has given us understanding, so that we may know him who is true. And we are in him who is true—even in his Son Jesus Christ. He is the true God and eternal life.

²¹Dear children, keep yourselves from idols.

Introduction

to the

book of 2 John

NOTES.

Everyone likes to pass notes in school. They don't have to be long notes or even say anything exciting. It's just a way of staying close to friends.

John's second letter is really just a note. It doesn't reveal any startling new doctrine. It expresses John's love and concern for others. The kind of love God wants you to have for your friends.

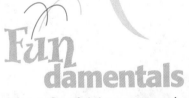

Fundamentals

What makes Christian parents and grandparents happiest (2 John 4)?

What's the key test of true or false teaching (2 John 7)?

FAST FACTS

The apostle John, who wrote the fourth Gospel, wrote this brief letter.

John reminds you what is important in life: you are to love one another and obey God's commandments.

Love means to put others first and actively try to serve them.

¹The elder,

To the chosen lady and her children, whom I love in the truth—and not I only, but also all who know the truth— ²because of the truth, which lives in us and will be with us forever:

³Grace, mercy and peace from God the Father and from Jesus Christ, the Father's Son, will be with us in truth and love.

⁴It has given me great joy to find some of your children walking in the truth, just as the Father commanded us. ⁵And now, dear lady, I am not writing you a new command but one we have had from the beginning. I ask that we love one another. ⁶And this is love: that we walk in obedience to his commands. As you have heard from the beginning, his command is that you walk in love.

⁷Many deceivers, who do not acknowledge Jesus Christ as coming in the flesh, have gone out into the world. Any such person is the deceiver and the antichrist. ⁸Watch out that you do not lose what you have worked for, but that you may be rewarded fully. ⁹Anyone who runs ahead and does not continue in the teaching of Christ does not have God; whoever continues in the teaching has both the Father and the Son. ¹⁰If anyone comes to you and does not bring this teaching, do not take him into your house or welcome him. ¹¹Anyone who welcomes him shares in his wicked work.

¹²I have much to write to you, but I do not want to use paper and ink. Instead, I hope to visit you and talk with you face to face, so that our joy may be complete.

¹³The children of your chosen sister send their greetings.

---

2 JOHN 4

Let's see. What's a great Christmas gift for a Christian mom and dad? Or a birthday present that keeps on giving all year long? John gives you a clue to the very best gift of all when he writes, "It has given me great joy to find some of your children walking in the truth." Talk about joy! There's no greater gift you can give Christian parents than to live a life that shows you're following Jesus.

Direct Line

to the

book of **3 John**

MORE NOTES.

You send a note to your friend across the room. She sends one back. You send hers back with more notes on it. It goes on and on. There's always more to tell each other!

The book of 3 John is a short note sent by John to Gaius, "my dear friend" (3 John 1). He writes to thank Gaius for his help, and he also wants to give him encouragement.

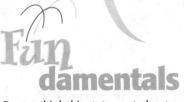

Fundamentals

Do you think this statement about Gaius could also be said about you (3 John 3)?

What should you imitate (3 John 11)?

What is better than a letter or note (3 John 13-14)?

FAST FACTS

This book was written by the apostle John around A.D. 90.

2 John 12 and 3 John 13-14 are almost the same.

John's letters are full of love and encouragement for the people to whom they were sent.

¹The elder,

To my dear friend Gaius, whom I love in the truth.

²Dear friend, I pray that you may enjoy good health and that all may go well with you, even as your soul is getting along well. ³It gave me great joy to have some brothers come and tell about your faithfulness to the truth and how you continue to walk in the truth. ⁴I have no greater joy than to hear that my children are walking in the truth.

⁵Dear friend, you are faithful in what you are doing for the brothers, even though they are strangers to you. ⁶They have told the church about your love. You will do well to send them on their way in a manner worthy of God. ⁷It was for the sake of the Name that they went out, receiving no help from the pagans. ⁸We ought therefore to show hospitality to such men so that we may work together for the truth.

⁹I wrote to the church, but Diotrephes, who loves to be first, will have nothing to do with us. ¹⁰So if I come, I will call attention to what he is doing, gossiping maliciously about us. Not satisfied with that, he refuses to welcome the brothers. He also stops those who want to do so and puts them out of the church.

> Do not imitate what is evil but what is good (3 John 11).

¹¹Dear friend, do not imitate what is evil but what is good. Anyone who does what is good is from God. Anyone who does what is evil has not seen God. ¹²Demetrius is well spoken of by everyone—and even by the truth itself. We also speak well of him, and you know that our testimony is true.

¹³I have much to write you, but I do not want to do so with pen and ink. ¹⁴I hope to see you soon, and we will talk face to face.

Peace to you. The friends here send their greetings. Greet the friends there by name.

Dear Sam,
Several of my friends are involved sexually. They kid me because I'm still a virgin. Is premarital sex wrong?

Diane in Duluth

100 Advice Lane, Anywhere, USA

Dear Sam, Inc.

Dear Diane,
Many people today will tell you, "If it feels good, do it!" But God has a different message. He tells you to save this special gift of sex for marriage.

Today more than ever before, the results of promiscuous sex are obvious: AIDS, herpes, pregnancy (with abortion often being the result) and STDs (sexually transmitted diseases). "If it feels good, do it" doesn't warn you about how these diseases may ravage your body.

God's laws are not there just to make life difficult for you. They are there for a reason. They are God's way to get the best in life. In 3 John 11, John tells you, "Do not imitate what is evil but what is good." Fill your life with good things: friendships with both girls and guys, lots of fun activities, positive interaction with your family, school (yes, school is good). Save sex for marriage, where God intended it and where it can be really good.

Sam

I n t r o d u c t i o n

to the

book of **Jude**

I'M SERIOUS!

Have you ever noticed that when your parents are
serious about something, they say it again and again.
"Sarah, clean your room." Then five minutes later,
"Sarah, clean your room." Hey, you just want to finish
your show. But oh, no, five minutes later, and they're
at it again. "Sarah, clean your room!"

Three New Testament books say, "Watch out for false
teachers," "Watch out for false teachers," "Watch out
for false teachers." Must be God is serious. Jude even
says he planned to write a different kind of letter, but
the Holy Spirit led him to write about false teachers
instead. Maybe we'd better listen!

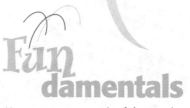

Fundamentals

*How can you recognize false teach-
ing (Jude 3-4)?*

*What are false teachers like
(Jude 5-16)?*

*It's kind of scary to think of false
teachers running around. How can
you protect yourself (Jude 17-23)?*

FAST FACTS

*Jude was a brother of James
and of Jesus. He was Mary
and Joseph's son.*

*The other two books about
false teachers are 2 Timothy
and 2 Peter.*

*Nineteen of Jude's 25 verses say
things also found in 2 Peter.*

*Jude quotes Jewish writings that
are not in the Bible (Jude 9,14-15).*

¹Jude, a servant of Jesus Christ and a brother of James,

To those who have been called, who are loved by God the Father and kept by*ᵃ* Jesus Christ:

²Mercy, peace and love be yours in abundance.

The Sin and Doom of Godless Men ³Dear friends, although I was very eager to write to you about the salvation we share, I felt I had to write and urge you to contend for the faith that was once for all entrusted to the saints. ⁴For certain men whose condemnation was written about*ᵇ* long ago have secretly slipped in among you. They are godless men, who change the grace of our God into a license for immorality and deny Jesus Christ our only Sovereign and Lord.

⁵Though you already know all this, I want to remind you that the Lord*ᶜ* delivered his people out of Egypt, but later destroyed those who did not believe. ⁶And the angels who did not keep their positions of authority but abandoned their own home—these he has kept in darkness, bound with everlasting chains for judgment on the great Day. ⁷In a similar way, Sodom and Gomorrah and the surrounding towns gave themselves up to sexual immorality and perversion. They serve as an example of those who suffer the punishment of eternal fire.

⁸In the very same way, these dreamers pollute their own bodies, reject authority and slander celestial beings. ⁹But even the archangel Michael, when he was disputing with the devil about the body of Moses, did not dare to bring a slanderous accusation against him, but said, "The Lord rebuke you!" ¹⁰Yet these men speak abusively against whatever they do not understand; and what things they do understand by instinct, like unreasoning animals—these are the very things that destroy them.

¹¹Woe to them! They have taken the way of Cain; they have rushed for profit into Balaam's error; they have been destroyed in Korah's rebellion.

¹²These men are blemishes at your love feasts, eating with you without the slightest qualm—shepherds who feed only themselves. They are clouds without rain, blown along by the wind; autumn trees, without fruit and uprooted—twice dead. ¹³They are wild waves of the sea, foaming up their shame; wandering stars, for whom blackest darkness has been reserved forever.

¹⁴Enoch, the seventh from Adam, prophesied about these men: "See, the Lord is coming with thousands upon thousands of his holy ones ¹⁵to judge everyone, and to convict all the ungodly of all the ungodly acts they have done in the ungodly way, and of all the harsh words ungodly sinners have spoken against him." ¹⁶These men are grumblers and faultfinders; they follow their own evil desires; they boast about themselves and flatter others for their own advantage.

ᵃ1 Or for; or in ᵇ4 Or men who were marked out for condemnation ᶜ5 Some early manuscripts Jesus

JUDE 3–23

According to Jude, a false teacher isn't the history teacher who promises you an essay test and then gives you multiple choice. False teachers are "godless men" (Jude 4) who look and sound religious but who lead you away instead of toward Jesus. Jude describes these false teachers and then gives instruction on how to avoid them (Jude 20–23): 1. Build your faith. Count on what the Bible says, not on what false teachers teach. 2. Pray in the Spirit. Let God's Spirit guide you. 3. Keep yourself in God's love. Stick to doing right while you're waiting for Jesus to come back. And be concerned about others. Do everything you can to help them get to know and love the Lord.

Direct Line

A Call to Persevere ¹⁷But, dear friends, remember what the apostles of our Lord Jesus Christ foretold. ¹⁸They said to you, "In the last times there will be scoffers who will follow their own ungodly desires." ¹⁹These are the men who divide you, who follow mere natural instincts and do not have the Spirit.

²⁰But you, dear friends, build yourselves up in your most holy faith and pray in the Holy Spirit. ²¹Keep yourselves in God's love as you wait for the mercy of our Lord Jesus Christ to bring you to eternal life.

²²Be merciful to those who doubt; ²³snatch others from the fire and save them; to others show mercy, mixed with fear—hating even the clothing stained by corrupted flesh.

Doxology ²⁴To him who is able to keep you from falling and to present you before his glorious presence without fault and with great joy— ²⁵to the only God our Savior be glory, majesty, power and authority, through Jesus Christ our Lord, before all ages, now and forevermore! Amen.

Introduction

to the

book of Revelation

HARD WORDS.

Sometimes when you don't understand a hard word, do you just ignore it and read on? Well, you can't ignore the hard words in this book of the Bible. There are just too many of them. And too many strange images: stars falling in the ocean and rivers turning to blood. What does it mean?

Even though Revelation uses difficult images and symbols, the message of the book is clear: This world will come to an end. Jesus will come back, and he'll punish evil. No matter how hard Satan and his forces struggle, Jesus will win. Then all will learn that both heaven and hell are real, for ever and ever.

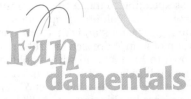

Fundamentals

What would you do if Jesus suddenly showed up tomorrow (Revelation 1:9-18)?

Will people give up when God starts to punish wickedness (Revelation 6)?

Will some people really go to hell (Revelation 20)?

What will heaven be like, anyway? Is it worth going there (Revelation 21–22)?

FAST FACTS

The apostle John wrote this last book of the Bible.

John was over 90 years old when he wrote it.

John was given his vision of Jesus on the prison island of Patmos.

John was exiled there by the Emperor Domitian for being a Christian.

Revelation shows you that God will surely triumph over evil.

Prologue   The revelation of Jesus Christ, which God gave him to show his servants what must soon take place. He made it known by sending his angel to his servant John, [2]who testifies to everything he saw—that is, the word of God and the testimony of Jesus Christ. [3]Blessed is the one who reads the words of this prophecy, and blessed are those who hear it and take to heart what is written in it, because the time is near.

Greetings and Doxology

[4]John,

To the seven churches in the province of Asia:

Grace and peace to you from him who is, and who was, and who is to come, and from the seven spirits[a] before his throne, [5]and from Jesus Christ, who is the faithful witness, the firstborn from the dead, and the ruler of the kings of the earth.

To him who loves us and has freed us from our sins by his blood, [6]and has made us to be a kingdom and priests to serve his God and Father—to him be glory and power for ever and ever! Amen.

> [7]Look, he is coming with the clouds,
>   and every eye will see him,
>   even those who pierced him;
>   and all the peoples of the earth will mourn because of him.
>   So shall it be! Amen.

[8]"I am the Alpha and the Omega," says the Lord God, "who is, and who was, and who is to come, the Almighty."

One Like a Son of Man

[9]I, John, your brother and companion in the suffering and kingdom and patient endurance that are ours in Jesus, was on the island of Patmos because of the word of God and the testimony of Jesus. [10]On the Lord's Day I was in the Spirit, and I heard behind me a loud voice like a trumpet, [11]which said: "Write on a scroll what you see and send it to the seven churches: to Ephesus, Smyrna, Pergamum, Thyatira, Sardis, Philadelphia and Laodicea."

[12]I turned around to see the voice that was speaking to me. And when I turned I saw seven golden lampstands, [13]and among the lampstands was someone "like a son of man,"[b] dressed in a robe reaching down to his feet and with a golden sash around his chest. [14]His head and hair were white like wool, as white as snow, and his eyes were like blazing fire. [15]His feet were like bronze glowing in a furnace, and his voice was like the sound of rushing waters. [16]In his right hand he held seven stars, and out of his mouth came a sharp double-edged sword. His face was like the sun shining in all its brilliance.

[17]When I saw him, I fell at his feet as though dead. Then he placed his right hand on me and said: "Do not be afraid. I am the First and the Last. [18]I am the Living

---

REVELATION 1:9–18

Remember how you thought of Jesus when you were a little kid? Warm and friendly and walking around in a long white nightgown? Probably many adult Christians still have that image of "gentle Jesus, meek and mild." So it's kind of shocking to read these verses and see John, stunned, fall on his face before an overwhelmingly powerful revelation of Jesus as God the Son. John probably never forgot this later revelation. You shouldn't either. Remember, Jesus isn't weak. He's the most powerful person in the whole universe. And he's on your side!

Direct Line

---

[a]4 Or *the sevenfold Spirit*   [b]13 Daniel 7:13

One; I was dead, and behold I am alive for ever and ever! And I hold the keys of death and Hades.

¹⁹"Write, therefore, what you have seen, what is now and what will take place later. ²⁰The mystery of the seven stars that you saw in my right hand and of the seven golden lampstands is this: The seven stars are the angels*a* of the seven churches, and the seven lampstands are the seven churches.

To the Church in Ephesus

"To the angel*b* of the church in Ephesus write:

These are the words of him who holds the seven stars in his right hand and walks among the seven golden lampstands: ²I know your deeds, your hard work and your perseverance. I know that you cannot tolerate wicked men, that you have tested those who claim to be apostles but are not, and have found them false. ³You have persevered and have endured hardships for my name, and have not grown weary.

⁴Yet I hold this against you: You have forsaken your first love. ⁵Remember the height from which you have fallen! Repent and do the things you did at first. If you do not repent, I will come to you and remove your lampstand from its place. ⁶But you have this in your favor: You hate the practices of the Nicolaitans, which I also hate.

⁷He who has an ear, let him hear what the Spirit says to the churches. To him who overcomes, I will give the right to eat from the tree of life, which is in the paradise of God.

To the Church in Smyrna

⁸"To the angel of the church in Smyrna write:

These are the words of him who is the First and the Last, who died and came to life again. ⁹I know your afflictions and your poverty—yet you are rich! I know the slander of those who say they are Jews and are not, but are a synagogue of Satan. ¹⁰Do not be afraid of what you are about to suffer. I tell you, the devil will put some of you in prison to test you, and you will suffer persecution for ten days. Be faithful, even to the point of death, and I will give you the crown of life.

¹¹He who has an ear, let him hear what the Spirit says to the churches. He who overcomes will not be hurt at all by the second death.

To the Church in Pergamum

¹²"To the angel of the church in Pergamum write:

These are the words of him who has the sharp, double-edged sword. ¹³I know where you live—where Satan has his throne. Yet you remain true to my name. You did not renounce your faith in me, even in the days of Antipas, my faithful witness, who was put to death in your city—where Satan lives.

¹⁴Nevertheless, I have a few things against you: You have people there who hold to the teaching of Balaam, who taught Balak to entice the Israelites to sin by eating food sacrificed to idols and by committing sexual

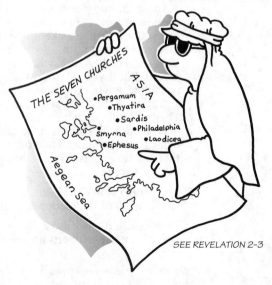

SEE REVELATION 2–3

---

a20 Or messengers   b1 Or messenger; also in verses 8, 12 and 18

immorality. [15]Likewise you also have those who hold to the teaching of the Nicolaitans. [16]Repent therefore! Otherwise, I will soon come to you and will fight against them with the sword of my mouth.

[17]He who has an ear, let him hear what the Spirit says to the churches. To him who overcomes, I will give some of the hidden manna. I will also give him a white stone with a new name written on it, known only to him who receives it.

To the Church in Thyatira

[18]"To the angel of the church in Thyatira write:

These are the words of the Son of God, whose eyes are like blazing fire and whose feet are like burnished bronze. [19]I know your deeds, your love and faith, your service and perseverance, and that you are now doing more than you did at first.

[20]Nevertheless, I have this against you: You tolerate that woman Jezebel, who calls herself a prophetess. By her teaching she misleads my servants into sexual immorality and the eating of food sacrificed to idols. [21]I have given her time to repent of her immorality, but she is unwilling. [22]So I will cast her on a bed of suffering, and I will make those who commit adultery with her suffer intensely, unless they repent of her ways. [23]I will strike her children dead. Then all the churches will know that I am he who searches hearts and minds, and I will repay each of you according to your deeds. [24]Now I say to the rest of you in Thyatira, to you who do not hold to her teaching and have not learned Satan's so-called deep secrets (I will not impose any other burden on you): [25]Only hold on to what you have until I come.

[26]To him who overcomes and does my will to the end, I will give authority over the nations—

> [27]'He will rule them with an iron scepter;
> he will dash them to pieces like pottery'[a]—

just as I have received authority from my Father. [28]I will also give him the morning star. [29]He who has an ear, let him hear what the Spirit says to the churches.

To the Church in Sardis

"To the angel[b] of the church in Sardis write:

These are the words of him who holds the seven spirits[c] of God and the seven stars. I know your deeds; you have a reputation of being alive, but you are dead. [2]Wake up! Strengthen what remains and is about to die, for I have not found your deeds complete in the sight of my God. [3]Remember, therefore, what you have received and heard; obey it, and repent. But if you do not wake up, I will come like a thief, and you will not know at what time I will come to you.

[4]Yet you have a few people in Sardis who have not soiled their clothes. They will walk with me, dressed in white, for they are worthy. [5]He who overcomes will, like them, be dressed in white. I will never blot out his name from the book of life, but will acknowledge his name before my Father and his angels. [6]He who has an ear, let him hear what the Spirit says to the churches.

To the Church in Philadelphia

[7]"To the angel of the church in Philadelphia write:

These are the words of him who is holy and true, who holds the key of David. What he opens no one can shut, and what he shuts no one can

---

[a]27 Psalm 2:9 [b]1 Or *messenger*; also in verses 7 and 14 [c]1 Or *the sevenfold Spirit*

open. [8]I know your deeds. See, I have placed before you an open door that no one can shut. I know that you have little strength, yet you have kept my word and have not denied my name. [9]I will make those who are of the synagogue of Satan, who claim to be Jews though they are not, but are liars—I will make them come and fall down at your feet and acknowledge that I have loved you. [10]Since you have kept my command to endure patiently, I will also keep you from the hour of trial that is going to come upon the whole world to test those who live on the earth.

[11]I am coming soon. Hold on to what you have, so that no one will take your crown. [12]Him who overcomes I will make a pillar in the temple of my God. Never again will he leave it. I will write on him the name of my God and the name of the city of my God, the new Jerusalem, which is coming down out of heaven from my God; and I will also write on him my new name. [13]He who has an ear, let him hear what the Spirit says to the churches.

To the Church in Laodicea

[14]"To the angel of the church in Laodicea write:

These are the words of the Amen, the faithful and true witness, the ruler of God's creation. [15]I know your deeds, that you are neither cold nor hot. I wish you were either one or the other! [16]So, because you are lukewarm—neither hot nor cold—I am about to spit you out of my mouth. [17]You say, 'I am rich; I have acquired wealth and do not need a thing.' But you do not realize that you are wretched, pitiful, poor, blind and naked. [18]I counsel you to buy from me gold refined in the fire, so you can become rich; and white clothes to wear, so you can cover your shameful nakedness; and salve to put on your eyes, so you can see.

[19]Those whom I love I rebuke and discipline. So be earnest, and repent. [20]Here I am! I stand at the door and knock. If anyone hears my voice and opens the door, I will come in and eat with him, and he with me.

[21]To him who overcomes, I will give the right to sit with me on my throne, just as I overcame and sat down with my Father on his throne. [22]He who has an ear, let him hear what the Spirit says to the churches."

The Throne in Heaven   After this I looked, and there before me was a door standing open in heaven. And the voice I had first heard speaking to me like a trumpet said, "Come up here, and I will show you what must take place after this." [2]At once I was in the Spirit, and there before me was a throne in heaven with someone sitting on it. [3]And the one who sat there had the appearance of jasper and carnelian. A rainbow, resembling an emerald, encircled the throne. [4]Surrounding the throne were twenty-four other thrones, and seated on them were twenty-four elders. They were dressed in white and had crowns of gold on their heads. [5]From the throne came flashes of lightning, rumblings and peals of thunder. Before the throne, seven lamps were blazing. These are the seven spirits[a] of God. [6]Also before the throne there was what looked like a sea of glass, clear as crystal.

In the center, around the throne, were four living creatures, and they were covered with eyes, in front and in back. [7]The first living creature was like a lion, the second was like an ox, the third had a face like a man, the fourth was like a flying eagle. [8]Each of the four living creatures had six wings and was covered with eyes all around, even under his wings. Day and night they never stop saying:

"Holy, holy, holy
is the Lord God Almighty,
who was, and is, and is to come."

[a]5 Or *the sevenfold Spirit*

⁹Whenever the living creatures give glory, honor and thanks to him who sits on the throne and who lives for ever and ever, ¹⁰the twenty-four elders fall down before him who sits on the throne, and worship him who lives for ever and ever. They lay their crowns before the throne and say:

> ¹¹ "You are worthy, our Lord and God,
>   to receive glory and honor and power,
> for you created all things,
>   and by your will they were created
>   and have their being."

The Scroll and the Lamb   Then I saw in the right hand of him who sat on the throne a scroll with writing on both sides and sealed with seven seals. ²And I saw a mighty angel proclaiming in a loud voice, "Who is worthy to break the seals and open the scroll?" ³But no one in heaven or on earth or under the earth could open the scroll or even look inside it. ⁴I wept and wept because no one was found who was worthy to open the scroll or look inside. ⁵Then one of the elders said to me, "Do not weep! See, the Lion of the tribe of Judah, the Root of David, has triumphed. He is able to open the scroll and its seven seals."

⁶Then I saw a Lamb, looking as if it had been slain, standing in the center of the throne, encircled by the four living creatures and the elders. He had seven horns and seven eyes, which are the seven spirits*ᵃ* of God sent out into all the earth. ⁷He came and took the scroll from the right hand of him who sat on the throne. ⁸And when he had taken it, the four living creatures and the twenty-four elders fell down before the Lamb. Each one had a harp and they were holding golden bowls full of incense, which are the prayers of the saints. ⁹And they sang a new song:

> "You are worthy to take the scroll
>   and to open its seals,
> because you were slain,
>   and with your blood you purchased men for God
>   from every tribe and language and people and nation.
> ¹⁰You have made them to be a kingdom and priests to serve our
>   God,
>   and they will reign on the earth."

ᵃ6 Or the sevenfold Spirit

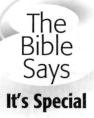

The Bible Says

It's Special

The book of Revelation is hard to understand. It's full of images and symbols. Many of the things it describes are great and terrible: stars plunge into the seas, mountains tremble, mysterious beasts emerge to lead humans in war against God.

Some people see Revelation as a description of what lies ahead for our world. Others say that Revelation is speaking of an attack on the Roman Empire in the author's day.

What is the best way to study this special book? Read it without trying to figure out every image. Try to imagine the wonderful and terrible events it describes. Read it with a growing confidence that God is in charge and that he will triumph over evil at history's end.

¹¹Then I looked and heard the voice of many angels, numbering thousands upon thousands, and ten thousand times ten thousand. They encircled the throne and the living creatures and the elders. ¹²In a loud voice they sang:

> "Worthy is the Lamb, who was slain,
> to receive power and wealth and wisdom and strength
> and honor and glory and praise!"

¹³Then I heard every creature in heaven and on earth and under the earth and on the sea, and all that is in them, singing:

> "To him who sits on the throne and to the Lamb
> be praise and honor and glory and power,
> for ever and ever!"

¹⁴The four living creatures said, "Amen," and the elders fell down and worshiped.

The Seals I watched as the Lamb opened the first of the seven seals. Then I heard one of the four living creatures say in a voice like thunder, "Come!" ²I looked, and there before me was a white horse! Its rider held a bow, and he was given a crown, and he rode out as a conqueror bent on conquest.

³When the Lamb opened the second seal, I heard the second living creature say, "Come!" ⁴Then another horse came out, a fiery red one. Its rider was given power to take peace from the earth and to make men slay each other. To him was given a large sword.

⁵When the Lamb opened the third seal, I heard the third living creature say, "Come!" I looked, and there before me was a black horse! Its rider was holding a pair of scales in his hand. ⁶Then I heard what sounded like a voice among the four living creatures, saying, "A quart*ᵃ* of wheat for a day's wages,*ᵇ* and three quarts of barley for a day's wages,*ᵇ* and do not damage the oil and the wine!"

⁷When the Lamb opened the fourth seal, I heard the voice of the fourth living creature say, "Come!" ⁸I looked, and there before me was a pale horse! Its rider was named Death, and Hades was following close behind him. They were given power over a fourth of the earth to kill by sword, famine and plague, and by the wild beasts of the earth.

⁹When he opened the fifth seal, I saw under the altar the souls of those who had been slain because of the word of God and the testimony they had maintained. ¹⁰They called out in a loud voice, "How long, Sovereign Lord, holy and true, until you judge the inhabitants of the earth and avenge our blood?" ¹¹Then each of them was given a white robe, and they were told to wait a little longer, until the number of their fellow servants and brothers who were to be killed as they had been was completed.

¹²I watched as he opened the sixth seal. There was a great earthquake. The sun turned black like sackcloth made of goat hair, the whole moon turned blood red, ¹³and the stars in the sky fell to earth, as late figs drop from a fig tree when shaken by a strong wind. ¹⁴The sky receded like a scroll, rolling up, and every mountain and island was removed from its place.

¹⁵Then the kings of the earth, the princes, the generals, the rich, the mighty, and every slave and every free man hid in caves and among the rocks of the mountains. ¹⁶They called to the mountains and the rocks, "Fall

REVELATION 6

QU∕ZZER

Q: What colors are associated with the four horsemen of Revelation?

BONUS: What does each horseman represent?

Answers on page 1621

ᵃ6 Greek *a choinix* (probably about a liter)   *ᵇ6* Greek *a denarius*

on us and hide us from the face of him who sits on the throne and from the wrath of the Lamb! ¹⁷For the great day of their wrath has come, and who can stand?"

7 *144,000 Sealed*   After this I saw four angels standing at the four corners of the earth, holding back the four winds of the earth to prevent any wind from blowing on the land or on the sea or on any tree. ²Then I saw another angel coming up from the east, having the seal of the living God. He called out in a loud voice to the four angels who had been given power to harm the land and the sea: ³"Do not harm the land or the sea or the trees until we put a seal on the foreheads of the servants of our God." ⁴Then I heard the number of those who were sealed: 144,000 from all the tribes of Israel.

⁵From the tribe of Judah 12,000 were sealed,
  from the tribe of Reuben 12,000,
  from the tribe of Gad 12,000,
⁶from the tribe of Asher 12,000,
  from the tribe of Naphtali 12,000,
  from the tribe of Manasseh 12,000,
⁷from the tribe of Simeon 12,000,
  from the tribe of Levi 12,000,
  from the tribe of Issachar 12,000,
⁸from the tribe of Zebulun 12,000,
  from the tribe of Joseph 12,000,
  from the tribe of Benjamin 12,000.

The Great Multitude in White Robes   ⁹After this I looked and there before me was a great multitude that no one could count, from every nation, tribe, people and language, standing before the throne and in front of the Lamb. They were wearing white robes and were holding palm branches in their hands. ¹⁰And they cried out in a loud voice:

> "Salvation belongs to our God,
>   who sits on the throne,
>   and to the Lamb."

¹¹All the angels were standing around the throne and around the elders and the four living creatures. They fell down on their faces before the throne and worshiped God, ¹²saying:

> "Amen!
> Praise and glory
> and wisdom and thanks and honor
> and power and strength
> be to our God for ever and ever.
> Amen!"

¹³Then one of the elders asked me, "These in white robes—who are they, and where did they come from?"

¹⁴I answered, "Sir, you know."

And he said, "These are they who have come out of the great tribulation; they have washed their robes and made them white in the blood of the Lamb. ¹⁵Therefore,

> "they are before the throne of God
>   and serve him day and night in his temple;
>   and he who sits on the throne will spread his tent over them.
> ¹⁶Never again will they hunger;
>   never again will they thirst.
> The sun will not beat upon them,
>   nor any scorching heat.

¹⁷For the Lamb at the center of the throne will be their
shepherd;
he will lead them to springs of living water.
And God will wipe away every tear from their eyes."

8 **The Seventh Seal and the Golden Censer** When he opened the seventh seal, there was silence in heaven for about half an hour.
²And I saw the seven angels who stand before God, and to them were given seven trumpets.

³Another angel, who had a golden censer, came and stood at the altar. He was given much incense to offer, with the prayers of all the saints, on the golden altar before the throne. ⁴The smoke of the incense, together with the prayers of the saints, went up before God from the angel's hand. ⁵Then the angel took the censer, filled it with fire from the altar, and hurled it on the earth; and there came peals of thunder, rumblings, flashes of lightning and an earthquake.

The Trumpets ⁶Then the seven angels who had the seven trumpets prepared to sound them.

⁷The first angel sounded his trumpet, and there came hail and fire mixed with blood, and it was hurled down upon the earth. A third of the earth was burned up, a third of the trees were burned up, and all the green grass was burned up.

⁸The second angel sounded his trumpet, and something like a huge mountain, all ablaze, was thrown into the sea. A third of the sea turned into blood, ⁹a third of the living creatures in the sea died, and a third of the ships were destroyed.

¹⁰The third angel sounded his trumpet, and a great star, blazing like a torch, fell from the sky on a third of the rivers and on the springs of water— ¹¹the name of the star is Wormwood.^a A third of the waters turned bitter, and many people died from the waters that had become bitter.

¹²The fourth angel sounded his trumpet, and a third of the sun was struck, a third of the moon, and a third of the stars, so that a third of them turned dark. A third of the day was without light, and also a third of the night.

¹³As I watched, I heard an eagle that was flying in midair call out in a loud voice: "Woe! Woe! Woe to the inhabitants of the earth, because of the trumpet blasts about to be sounded by the other three angels!"

9 The fifth angel sounded his trumpet, and I saw a star that had fallen from the sky to the earth. The star was given the key to the shaft of the Abyss. ²When he opened the Abyss, smoke rose from it like the smoke from a gigantic furnace. The sun and sky were darkened by the smoke from the Abyss. ³And out of the smoke locusts came down upon the earth and were given power like that of scorpions of the earth. ⁴They were told not to harm the grass of the earth or any plant or tree, but only those people who did not have the seal of God on their foreheads. ⁵They were not given power to kill them, but only to torture them for five months. And the agony they suffered was like that of the sting of a scorpion when it strikes a man. ⁶During those days men will seek death, but will not find it; they will long to die, but death will elude them.

⁷The locusts looked like horses prepared for battle. On their heads they wore something like crowns of gold, and their faces resembled human faces. ⁸Their hair was like women's hair, and their teeth were like lions' teeth. ⁹They had breastplates like breastplates of iron, and the sound of their wings was like the thundering of many horses and chariots rushing into battle.

Answers
*to Quizzer on
page 1619*

**A: White, red,
black and pale;
the colors
of their horses
(Revelation
6:2,4,5,8).**

**BONUS: They
represent
conquest, war,
famine and
death.**

^a*11* That is, Bitterness

¹⁰They had tails and stings like scorpions, and in their tails they had power to torment people for five months. ¹¹They had as king over them the angel of the Abyss, whose name in Hebrew is Abaddon, and in Greek, Apollyon.ᵃ

¹²The first woe is past; two other woes are yet to come.

¹³The sixth angel sounded his trumpet, and I heard a voice coming from the hornsᵇ of the golden altar that is before God. ¹⁴It said to the sixth angel who had the trumpet, "Release the four angels who are bound at the great river Euphrates." ¹⁵And the four angels who had been kept ready for this very hour and day and month and year were released to kill a third of mankind. ¹⁶The number of the mounted troops was two hundred million. I heard their number.

¹⁷The horses and riders I saw in my vision looked like this: Their breastplates were fiery red, dark blue, and yellow as sulfur. The heads of the horses resembled the heads of lions, and out of their mouths came fire, smoke and sulfur. ¹⁸A third of mankind was killed by the three plagues of fire, smoke and sulfur that came out of their mouths. ¹⁹The power of the horses was in their mouths and in their tails; for their tails were like snakes, having heads with which they inflict injury.

²⁰The rest of mankind that were not killed by these plagues still did not repent of the work of their hands; they did not stop worshiping demons, and idols of gold, silver, bronze, stone and wood—idols that cannot see or hear or walk. ²¹Nor did they repent of their murders, their magic arts, their sexual immorality or their thefts.

The Angel and the Little Scroll   Then I saw another mighty angel coming down from heaven. He was robed in a cloud, with a rainbow above his head; his face was like the sun, and his legs were like fiery pillars. ²He was holding a little scroll, which lay open in his hand. He planted his right foot on the sea and his left foot on the land, ³and he gave a loud shout like the roar of a lion. When he shouted, the voices of the seven thunders spoke. ⁴And when the seven thunders spoke, I was about to write; but I heard a voice from heaven say, "Seal up what the seven thunders have said and do not write it down."

⁵Then the angel I had seen standing on the sea and on the land raised his right hand to heaven. ⁶And he swore by him who lives for ever and ever, who created the heavens and all that is in them, the earth and all that is in it, and the sea and all that is in it, and said, "There will be no more delay! ⁷But in the days when the seventh angel is about to sound his trumpet, the mystery of God will be accomplished, just as he announced to his servants the prophets."

⁸Then the voice that I had heard from heaven spoke to me once more: "Go, take the scroll that lies open in the hand of the angel who is standing on the sea and on the land."

⁹So I went to the angel and asked him to give me the little scroll. He said to me,

---

Direct Line

REVELATION 9:20–21

Sometimes do you think that if God zapped people right away, every time they did something wrong, they'd reform? Like if every time you told a lie, you got a pain in your left foot. That would work, wouldn't it? Well, it might keep you from lying, but it wouldn't change you inside. That's something you can learn from this picture of God's terrible future judgment of those who refuse to believe. Despite their terror the survivors will not repent of their murders, magic, sexual immorality or thefts. The only chance people have to change is to hear and accept the gospel. Everyone has that chance today. When God's judgment day comes, it will be too late.

ᵃ11 *Abaddon* and *Apollyon* mean *Destroyer*.   ᵇ13 That is, projections

"Take it and eat it. It will turn your stomach sour, but in your mouth it will be as sweet as honey." [10]I took the little scroll from the angel's hand and ate it. It tasted as sweet as honey in my mouth, but when I had eaten it, my stomach turned sour. [11]Then I was told, "You must prophesy again about many peoples, nations, languages and kings."

11 *The Two Witnesses* I was given a reed like a measuring rod and was told, "Go and measure the temple of God and the altar, and count the worshipers there. [2]But exclude the outer court; do not measure it, because it has been given to the Gentiles. They will trample on the holy city for 42 months. [3]And I will give power to my two witnesses, and they will prophesy for 1,260 days, clothed in sackcloth." [4]These are the two olive trees and the two lampstands that stand before the Lord of the earth. [5]If anyone tries to harm them, fire comes from their mouths and devours their enemies. This is how anyone who wants to harm them must die. [6]These men have power to shut up the sky so that it will not rain during the time they are prophesying; and they have power to turn the waters into blood and to strike the earth with every kind of plague as often as they want.

[7]Now when they have finished their testimony, the beast that comes up from the Abyss will attack them, and overpower and kill them. [8]Their bodies will lie in the street of the great city, which is figuratively called Sodom and Egypt, where also their Lord was crucified. [9]For three and a half days men from every people, tribe, language and nation will gaze on their bodies and refuse them burial. [10]The inhabitants of the earth will gloat over them and will celebrate by sending each other gifts, because these two prophets had tormented those who live on the earth.

[11]But after the three and a half days a breath of life from God entered them, and they stood on their feet, and terror struck those who saw them. [12]Then they heard a loud voice from heaven saying to them, "Come up here." And they went up to heaven in a cloud, while their enemies looked on.

[13]At that very hour there was a severe earthquake and a tenth of the city collapsed. Seven thousand people were killed in the earthquake, and the survivors were terrified and gave glory to the God of heaven.

[14]The second woe has passed; the third woe is coming soon.

The Seventh Trumpet [15]The seventh angel sounded his trumpet, and there were loud voices in heaven, which said:

> "The kingdom of the world has become the kingdom of our
>   Lord and of his Christ,
>   and he will reign for ever and ever."

[16]And the twenty-four elders, who were seated on their thrones before God, fell on their faces and worshiped God, [17]saying:

> "We give thanks to you, Lord God Almighty,
>   the One who is and who was,
>   because you have taken your great power
>   and have begun to reign.
> [18]The nations were angry;
>   and your wrath has come.
>   The time has come for judging the dead,
>   and for rewarding your servants the prophets
>   and your saints and those who reverence your name,
>   both small and great—
>   and for destroying those who destroy the earth."

[19]Then God's temple in heaven was opened, and within his temple was seen the ark of his covenant. And there came flashes of lightning, rumblings, peals of thunder, an earthquake and a great hailstorm.

12 *The Woman and the Dragon* A great and wondrous sign appeared in heaven: a woman clothed with the sun, with the moon under her feet and a crown of twelve stars on her head. [2]She was pregnant and cried out in pain as she was about to give birth. [3]Then another sign appeared in heaven: an enormous red dragon with seven heads and ten horns and seven crowns on his heads. [4]His tail swept a third of the stars out of the sky and flung them to the earth. The dragon stood in front of the woman who was about to give birth, so that he might devour her child the moment it was born. [5]She gave birth to a son, a male child, who will rule all the nations with an iron scepter. And her child was snatched up to God and to his throne. [6]The woman fled into the desert to a place prepared for her by God, where she might be taken care of for 1,260 days.

[7]And there was war in heaven. Michael and his angels fought against the dragon, and the dragon and his angels fought back. [8]But he was not strong enough, and they lost their place in heaven. [9]The great dragon was hurled down—that ancient serpent called the devil, or Satan, who leads the whole world astray. He was hurled to the earth, and his angels with him.

[10]Then I heard a loud voice in heaven say:

> "Now have come the salvation and the power and the kingdom
>   of our God,
>   and the authority of his Christ.
> For the accuser of our brothers,
>   who accuses them before our God day and night,
>   has been hurled down.
> [11]They overcame him
>   by the blood of the Lamb
>   and by the word of their testimony;
>   they did not love their lives so much
>   as to shrink from death.
> [12]Therefore rejoice, you heavens
>   and you who dwell in them!
>   But woe to the earth and the sea,
>   because the devil has gone down to you!
>   He is filled with fury,
>   because he knows that his time is short."

[13]When the dragon saw that he had been hurled to the earth, he pursued the woman who had given birth to the male child. [14]The woman was given the two wings of a great eagle, so that she might fly to the place prepared for her in the desert, where she would be taken care of for a time, times and half a time, out of the serpent's reach. [15]Then from his mouth the serpent spewed water like a river, to overtake the woman and sweep her away with the torrent. [16]But the earth helped the woman by opening its mouth and swallowing the river that the dragon had spewed out of his mouth. [17]Then the dragon was enraged at the woman and went off to make war against the rest of her offspring—those who obey God's commandments and hold to the testimony of Jesus. **13** [1]And the dragon[a] stood on the shore of the sea.

The Beast out of the Sea And I saw a beast coming out of the sea. He had ten horns and seven heads, with ten crowns on his horns, and on each head a blasphemous name. [2]The beast I saw resembled a leopard, but had feet like those of a bear and a mouth like that of a lion. The dragon gave the beast his power and his throne and great authority. [3]One of the heads of the beast seemed to have had a fatal wound, but the fatal wound had been healed. The

---

[a]*1 Some late manuscripts *And I*

whole world was astonished and followed the beast. ⁴Men worshiped the dragon because he had given authority to the beast, and they also worshiped the beast and asked, "Who is like the beast? Who can make war against him?"

⁵The beast was given a mouth to utter proud words and blasphemies and to exercise his authority for forty-two months. ⁶He opened his mouth to blaspheme God, and to slander his name and his dwelling place and those who live in heaven. ⁷He was given power to make war against the saints and to conquer them. And he was given authority over every tribe, people, language and nation. ⁸All inhabitants of the earth will worship the beast—all whose names have not been written in the book of life belonging to the Lamb that was slain from the creation of the world.ᵃ

⁹He who has an ear, let him hear.

> ¹⁰If anyone is to go into captivity,
>   into captivity he will go.
> If anyone is to be killedᵇ with the sword,
>   with the sword he will be killed.

This calls for patient endurance and faithfulness on the part of the saints.

The Beast out of the Earth   ¹¹Then I saw another beast, coming out of the earth. He had two horns like a lamb, but he spoke like a dragon. ¹²He exercised all the authority of the first beast on his behalf, and made the earth and its inhabitants worship the first beast, whose fatal wound had been healed. ¹³And he performed great and miraculous signs, even causing fire to come down from heaven to earth in full view of men. ¹⁴Because of the signs he was given power to do on behalf of the first beast, he deceived the inhabitants of the earth. He ordered them to set up an image in honor of the beast who was wounded by the sword and yet lived. ¹⁵He was given power to give breath to the image of the first beast, so that it could speak and cause all who refused to worship the image to be killed. ¹⁶He also forced everyone, small and great, rich and poor, free and slave, to receive a mark on his right hand or on his forehead, ¹⁷so that no one could buy or sell unless he had the mark, which is the name of the beast or the number of his name.

¹⁸This calls for wisdom. If anyone has insight, let him calculate the number of the beast, for it is man's number. His number is 666.

The Lamb and the 144,000   Then I looked, and there before me was the Lamb, standing on Mount Zion, and with him 144,000 who had his name and his Father's name written on their foreheads. ²And I heard a sound from heaven like the roar of rushing waters and like a loud peal of thunder. The sound I heard was like that of harpists playing their harps. ³And they sang a new song before the throne and before the four living creatures and the elders. No one could learn the song except the 144,000 who had been redeemed from the earth. ⁴These are those who did not defile themselves with women, for they kept themselves pure. They follow the Lamb wherever he goes. They were purchased from among men and offered as firstfruits to God and the Lamb. ⁵No lie was found in their mouths; they are blameless.

The Three Angels   ⁶Then I saw another angel flying in midair, and he had the eternal gospel to proclaim to those who live on the earth—to every nation, tribe, language and people. ⁷He said in a loud voice, "Fear God and give him glory, because the hour of his judgment has come. Worship him who made the heavens, the earth, the sea and the springs of water."

ᵃ8 Or *written from the creation of the world in the book of life belonging to the Lamb that was slain*
ᵇ10 Some manuscripts *anyone kills*

⁸A second angel followed and said, "Fallen! Fallen is Babylon the Great, which made all the nations drink the maddening wine of her adulteries."

⁹A third angel followed them and said in a loud voice: "If anyone worships the beast and his image and receives his mark on the forehead or on the hand, ¹⁰he, too, will drink of the wine of God's fury, which has been poured full strength into the cup of his wrath. He will be tormented with burning sulfur in the presence of the holy angels and of the Lamb. ¹¹And the smoke of their torment rises for ever and ever. There is no rest day or night for those who worship the beast and his image, or for anyone who receives the mark of his name." ¹²This calls for patient endurance on the part of the saints who obey God's commandments and remain faithful to Jesus.

¹³Then I heard a voice from heaven say, "Write: Blessed are the dead who die in the Lord from now on."

"Yes," says the Spirit, "they will rest from their labor, for their deeds will follow them."

The Harvest of the Earth ¹⁴I looked, and there before me was a white cloud, and seated on the cloud was one "like a son of man"[a] with a crown of gold on his head and a sharp sickle in his hand. ¹⁵Then another angel came out of the temple and called in a loud voice to him who was sitting on the cloud, "Take your sickle and reap, because the time to reap has come, for the harvest of the earth is ripe." ¹⁶So he who was seated on the cloud swung his sickle over the earth, and the earth was harvested.

¹⁷Another angel came out of the temple in heaven, and he too had a sharp sickle. ¹⁸Still another angel, who had charge of the fire, came from the altar and called in a loud voice to him who had the sharp sickle, "Take your sharp sickle and gather the clusters of grapes from the earth's vine, because its grapes are ripe." ¹⁹The angel swung his sickle on the earth, gathered its grapes and threw them into the great winepress of God's wrath. ²⁰They were trampled in the winepress outside the city, and blood flowed out of the press, rising as high as the horses' bridles for a distance of 1,600 stadia.[b]

15 *Seven Angels With Seven Plagues* I saw in heaven another great and marvelous sign: seven angels with the seven last plagues— last, because with them God's wrath is completed. ²And I saw what looked like a sea of glass mixed with fire and, standing beside the sea, those who had been victorious over the beast and his image and over the number of his name. They held harps given them by God ³and sang the song of Moses the servant of God and the song of the Lamb:

> "Great and marvelous are your deeds,
> Lord God Almighty.
> Just and true are your ways,
> King of the ages.
> ⁴Who will not fear you, O Lord,
> and bring glory to your name?
> For you alone are holy.
> All nations will come
> and worship before you,
> for your righteous acts have been revealed."

⁵After this I looked and in heaven the temple, that is, the tabernacle of the Testimony, was opened. ⁶Out of the temple came the seven angels with the seven plagues. They were dressed in clean, shining linen and wore golden sashes around their chests. ⁷Then one of the four living creatures gave to the seven angels seven golden bowls filled with the wrath of God, who lives for

[a]14 Daniel 7:13   [b]20 That is, about 180 miles (about 300 kilometers)

ever and ever. ⁸And the temple was filled with smoke from the glory of God and from his power, and no one could enter the temple until the seven plagues of the seven angels were completed.

16 *The Seven Bowls of God's Wrath* Then I heard a loud voice from the temple saying to the seven angels, "Go, pour out the seven bowls of God's wrath on the earth."

²The first angel went and poured out his bowl on the land, and ugly and painful sores broke out on the people who had the mark of the beast and worshiped his image.

³The second angel poured out his bowl on the sea, and it turned into blood like that of a dead man, and every living thing in the sea died.

⁴The third angel poured out his bowl on the rivers and springs of water, and they became blood. ⁵Then I heard the angel in charge of the waters say:

"You are just in these judgments,
    you who are and who were, the Holy One,
    because you have so judged;
⁶for they have shed the blood of your saints and prophets,
    and you have given them blood to drink as they deserve."

⁷And I heard the altar respond:

"Yes, Lord God Almighty,
    true and just are your judgments."

⁸The fourth angel poured out his bowl on the sun, and the sun was given power to scorch people with fire. ⁹They were seared by the intense heat and they cursed the name of God, who had control over these plagues, but they refused to repent and glorify him.

¹⁰The fifth angel poured out his bowl on the throne of the beast, and his kingdom was plunged into darkness. Men gnawed their tongues in agony ¹¹and cursed the God of heaven because of their pains and their sores, but they refused to repent of what they had done.

¹²The sixth angel poured out his bowl on the great river Euphrates, and its water was dried up to prepare the way for the kings from the East. ¹³Then I saw three evil[a] spirits that looked like frogs; they came out of the mouth of the dragon, out of the mouth of the beast and out of the mouth of the false prophet. ¹⁴They are spirits of demons performing miraculous signs, and they go out to the kings of the whole world, to gather them for the battle on the great day of God Almighty.

¹⁵"Behold, I come like a thief! Blessed is he who stays awake and keeps his clothes with him, so that he may not go naked and be shamefully exposed."

¹⁶Then they gathered the kings together to the place that in Hebrew is called Armageddon.

¹⁷The seventh angel poured out his bowl into the air, and out of the temple came a loud voice from the throne, saying, "It is done!" ¹⁸Then there came flashes of lightning, rumblings, peals of thunder and a severe earthquake. No earthquake like it has ever occurred since man has been on earth, so tremendous was the quake. ¹⁹The great city split into three parts, and the cities of the nations collapsed. God remembered Babylon the Great and gave her the cup filled with the wine of the fury of his wrath. ²⁰Every island fled away and the mountains could not be found. ²¹From the sky huge hailstones of about a hundred pounds each fell upon men. And they cursed God on account of the plague of hail, because the plague was so terrible.

REVELATION 16

QU?ZZER

Q: Where will history's last battle be fought?

BONUS: Where is this location?

Answers on page 1629

---

[a]13 Greek *unclean*

The Woman on the Beast One of the seven angels who had the seven bowls came and said to me, "Come, I will show you the punishment of the great prostitute, who sits on many waters. ²With her the kings of the earth committed adultery and the inhabitants of the earth were intoxicated with the wine of her adulteries."

³Then the angel carried me away in the Spirit into a desert. There I saw a woman sitting on a scarlet beast that was covered with blasphemous names and had seven heads and ten horns. ⁴The woman was dressed in purple and scarlet, and was glittering with gold, precious stones and pearls. She held a golden cup in her hand, filled with abominable things and the filth of her adulteries. ⁵This title was written on her forehead:

MYSTERY
BABYLON THE GREAT
THE MOTHER OF PROSTITUTES
AND OF THE ABOMINATIONS OF THE EARTH.

⁶I saw that the woman was drunk with the blood of the saints, the blood of those who bore testimony to Jesus.

When I saw her, I was greatly astonished. ⁷Then the angel said to me: "Why are you astonished? I will explain to you the mystery of the woman and of the beast she rides, which has the seven heads and ten horns. ⁸The beast, which you saw, once was, now is not, and will come up out of the Abyss and go to his destruction. The inhabitants of the earth whose names have not been written in the book of life from the creation of the world will be astonished when they see the beast, because he once was, now is not, and yet will come.

⁹"This calls for a mind with wisdom. The seven heads are seven hills on which the woman sits. ¹⁰They are also seven kings. Five have fallen, one is, the other has not yet come; but when he does come, he must remain for a little while. ¹¹The beast who once was, and now is not, is an eighth king. He belongs to the seven and is going to his destruction.

¹²"The ten horns you saw are ten kings who have not yet received a kingdom, but who for one hour will receive authority as kings along with the beast. ¹³They have one purpose and will give their power and authority to the beast. ¹⁴They will make war against the Lamb, but the Lamb will overcome them because he is Lord of lords and King of kings—and with him will be his called, chosen and faithful followers."

¹⁵Then the angel said to me, "The waters you saw, where the prostitute sits, are peoples, multitudes, nations and languages. ¹⁶The beast and the ten horns you saw will hate the prostitute. They will bring her to ruin and leave her naked; they will eat her flesh and burn her with fire. ¹⁷For God has put it into their hearts to accomplish his purpose by agreeing to give the beast their power to rule, until God's words are fulfilled. ¹⁸The woman you saw is the great city that rules over the kings of the earth."

The Fall of Babylon After this I saw another angel coming down from heaven. He had great authority, and the earth was illuminated by his splendor. ²With a mighty voice he shouted:

"Fallen! Fallen is Babylon the Great!
    She has become a home for demons
and a haunt for every evil*a* spirit,
    a haunt for every unclean and detestable bird.
³For all the nations have drunk
    the maddening wine of her adulteries.

a2 Greek unclean

The kings of the earth committed adultery with her,
and the merchants of the earth grew rich from her excessive
luxuries."

[4]Then I heard another voice from heaven say:

"Come out of her, my people,
so that you will not share in her sins,
so that you will not receive any of her plagues;
[5]for her sins are piled up to heaven,
and God has remembered her crimes.
[6]Give back to her as she has given;
pay her back double for what she has done.
Mix her a double portion from her own cup.
[7]Give her as much torture and grief
as the glory and luxury she gave herself.
In her heart she boasts,
'I sit as queen; I am not a widow,
and I will never mourn.'
[8]Therefore in one day her plagues will overtake her:
death, mourning and famine.
She will be consumed by fire,
for mighty is the Lord God who judges her.

[9]"When the kings of the earth who committed adultery with her and shared her luxury see the smoke of her burning, they will weep and mourn over her. [10]Terrified at her torment, they will stand far off and cry:

" 'Woe! Woe, O great city,
O Babylon, city of power!
In one hour your doom has come!'

[11]"The merchants of the earth will weep and mourn over her because no one buys their cargoes any more— [12]cargoes of gold, silver, precious stones and pearls; fine linen, purple, silk and scarlet cloth; every sort of citron wood, and articles of every kind made of ivory, costly wood, bronze, iron and marble; [13]cargoes of cinnamon and spice, of incense, myrrh and frankincense, of wine and olive oil, of fine flour and wheat; cattle and sheep; horses and carriages; and bodies and souls of men.

[14]"They will say, 'The fruit you longed for is gone from you. All your riches and splendor have vanished, never to be recovered.' [15]The merchants who sold these things and gained their wealth from her will stand far off, terrified at her torment. They will weep and mourn [16]and cry out:

" 'Woe! Woe, O great city,
dressed in fine linen, purple and scarlet,
and glittering with gold, precious stones and pearls!
[17]In one hour such great wealth has been brought to ruin!'

"Every sea captain, and all who travel by ship, the sailors, and all who earn their living from the sea, will stand far off. [18]When they see the smoke of her burning, they will exclaim, 'Was there ever a city like this great city?' [19]They will throw dust on their heads, and with weeping and mourning cry out:

" 'Woe! Woe, O great city,
where all who had ships on the sea
became rich through her wealth!
In one hour she has been brought to ruin!
[20]Rejoice over her, O heaven!
Rejoice, saints and apostles and prophets!
God has judged her for the way she treated you.' "

²¹Then a mighty angel picked up a boulder the size of a large millstone and threw it into the sea, and said:

"With such violence
   the great city of Babylon will be thrown down,
      never to be found again.
²²The music of harpists and musicians, flute players and
         trumpeters,
   will never be heard in you again.
No workman of any trade
   will ever be found in you again.
The sound of a millstone
   will never be heard in you again.
²³The light of a lamp
   will never shine in you again.
The voice of bridegroom and bride
   will never be heard in you again.
Your merchants were the world's great men.
   By your magic spell all the nations were led astray.
²⁴In her was found the blood of prophets and of the saints,
   and of all who have been killed on the earth."

Hallelujah! After this I heard what sounded like the roar of a great multitude in heaven shouting:

"Hallelujah!
Salvation and glory and power belong to our God,
²   for true and just are his judgments.
He has condemned the great prostitute
   who corrupted the earth by her adulteries.
He has avenged on her the blood of his servants."

³And again they shouted:

"Hallelujah!
The smoke from her goes up for ever and ever."

⁴The twenty-four elders and the four living creatures fell down and worshiped God, who was seated on the throne. And they cried:

"Amen, Hallelujah!"

⁵Then a voice came from the throne, saying:

"Praise our God,
   all you his servants,
you who fear him,
   both small and great!"

⁶Then I heard what sounded like a great multitude, like the roar of rushing waters and like loud peals of thunder, shouting:

"Hallelujah!
   For our Lord God Almighty reigns.
⁷Let us rejoice and be glad
   and give him glory!
For the wedding of the Lamb has come,
   and his bride has made herself ready.
⁸Fine linen, bright and clean,
   was given her to wear."

(Fine linen stands for the righteous acts of the saints.)

⁹Then the angel said to me, "Write: 'Blessed are those who are invited to the wedding supper of the Lamb!' " And he added, "These are the true words of God."

¹⁰At this I fell at his feet to worship him. But he said to me, "Do not do it! I am a fellow servant with you and with your brothers who hold to the testimony of Jesus. Worship God! For the testimony of Jesus is the spirit of prophecy."

The Rider on the White Horse   ¹¹I saw heaven standing open and there before me was a white horse, whose rider is called Faithful and True. With justice he judges and makes war. ¹²His eyes are like blazing fire, and on his head are many crowns. He has a name written on him that no one knows but he himself. ¹³He is dressed in a robe dipped in blood, and his name is the Word of God. ¹⁴The armies of heaven were following him, riding on white horses and dressed in fine linen, white and clean. ¹⁵Out of his mouth comes a sharp sword with which to strike down the nations. "He will rule them with an iron scepter."ᵃ He treads the winepress of the fury of the wrath of God Almighty. ¹⁶On his robe and on his thigh he has this name written:

KING OF KINGS AND LORD OF LORDS.

> Hallelujah! For our Lord God Almighty reigns (Revelation 19:6).

¹⁷And I saw an angel standing in the sun, who cried in a loud voice to all the birds flying in midair, "Come, gather together for the great supper of God, ¹⁸so that you may eat the flesh of kings, generals, and mighty men, of horses and their riders, and the flesh of all people, free and slave, small and great."

¹⁹Then I saw the beast and the kings of the earth and their armies gathered together to make war against the rider on the horse and his army. ²⁰But the beast was captured, and with him the false prophet who had performed the miraculous signs on his behalf. With these signs he had deluded those who had received the mark of the beast and worshiped his image. The two of them were thrown alive into the fiery lake of burning sulfur. ²¹The rest of them were killed with the sword that came out of the mouth of the rider on the horse, and all the birds gorged themselves on their flesh.

20 *The Thousand Years*   And I saw an angel coming down out of heaven, having the key to the Abyss and holding in his hand a great chain. ²He seized the dragon, that ancient serpent, who is the devil, or Satan, and bound him for a thousand years. ³He threw him into the Abyss, and locked and sealed it over him, to keep him from deceiving the nations anymore until the thousand years were ended. After that, he must be set free for a short time.

⁴I saw thrones on which were seated those who had been given authority to judge. And I saw the souls of those who had been beheaded because of their testimony for Jesus and because of the word of God. They had not worshiped the beast or his image and had not received his mark on their foreheads or their hands. They came to life and reigned with Christ a thousand years. ⁵(The rest of the dead did not come to life until the thousand years were ended.) This is the first resurrection. ⁶Blessed and holy are those who have part in the first resurrection. The second death has no power over them, but they will be priests of God and of Christ and will reign with him for a thousand years.

Satan's Doom   ⁷When the thousand years are over, Satan will be released from his prison ⁸and will go out to deceive the nations in the four corners

ᵃ15 Psalm 2:9

of the earth—Gog and Magog—to gather them for battle. In number they are like the sand on the seashore. [9]They marched across the breadth of the earth and surrounded the camp of God's people, the city he loves. But fire came down from heaven and devoured them. [10]And the devil, who deceived them, was thrown into the lake of burning sulfur, where the beast and the false prophet had been thrown. They will be tormented day and night for ever and ever.

The Dead Are Judged [11]Then I saw a great white throne and him who was seated on it. Earth and sky fled from his presence, and there was no place for them. [12]And I saw the dead, great and small, standing before the throne, and books were opened. Another book was opened, which is the book of life. The dead were judged according to what they had done as recorded in the books. [13]The sea gave up the dead that were in it, and death and Hades gave up the dead that were in them, and each person was judged according to what he had done. [14]Then death and Hades were thrown into the lake of fire. The lake of fire is the second death. [15]If anyone's name was not found written in the book of life, he was thrown into the lake of fire.

21 **The New Jerusalem** Then I saw a new heaven and a new earth, for the first heaven and the first earth had passed away, and there was no longer any sea. [2]I saw the Holy City, the new Jerusalem, coming down out of heaven from God, prepared as a bride beautifully dressed for her husband. [3]And I heard a loud voice from the throne saying, "Now the dwelling of God is with men, and he will live with them. They will be his people, and God himself will be with them and be their God. [4]He will wipe every tear from their eyes. There will be no more death or mourning or crying or pain, for the old order of things has passed away."

[5]He who was seated on the throne said, "I am making everything new!" Then he said, "Write this down, for these words are trustworthy and true."

[6]He said to me: "It is done. I am the Alpha and the Omega, the Beginning and the End. To him who is thirsty I will give to drink without cost from the spring of the water of life. [7]He who overcomes will inherit all this, and I will be his God and he will be my son. [8]But the cowardly, the unbelieving, the vile, the murderers, the sexually immoral, those who practice magic arts, the idolaters and all liars— their place will be in the fiery lake of burning sulfur. This is the second death."

[9]One of the seven angels who had the seven bowls full of the seven last plagues came and said to me, "Come, I will show you the bride, the wife of the Lamb." [10]And he carried me away in the Spirit to a mountain great and high, and showed me the Holy City, Jerusalem, coming down out of heaven from God. [11]It shone with the glory of God, and its brilliance was like that of a very precious jewel, like a jasper, clear as crystal. [12]It had a great, high wall with twelve gates, and with twelve angels at the gates. On the gates were written the names of the twelve tribes of Israel. [13]There were three gates on the east, three on the north, three on

---

Direct Line

REVELATION 20:11–15

Most of the time death just doesn't seem real, does it? You know in your head that you'll die, but you don't feel it in your heart. Death is very real, something to take seriously. Especially what the Bible calls the "second death." The first death is biological. Your body dies, but your self-consciousness doesn't. You keep on being you for all eternity. You either spend that eternity with God in heaven or away from God in what Scripture calls "the lake of fire . . . the second death" (Revelation 20:14). You can't avoid the first death. But when you accept Christ, you are safe from the second death. Then, and forever.

the south and three on the west. ¹⁴The wall of the city had twelve foundations, and on them were the names of the twelve apostles of the Lamb.

¹⁵The angel who talked with me had a measuring rod of gold to measure the city, its gates and its walls. ¹⁶The city was laid out like a square, as long as it was wide. He measured the city with the rod and found it to be 12,000 stadia[a] in length, and as wide and high as it is long. ¹⁷He measured its wall and it was 144 cubits[b] thick,[c] by man's measurement, which the angel was using. ¹⁸The wall was made of jasper, and the city of pure gold, as pure as glass. ¹⁹The foundations of the city walls were decorated with every kind of precious stone. The first foundation was jasper, the second sapphire, the third chalcedony, the fourth emerald, ²⁰the fifth sardonyx, the sixth carnelian, the seventh chrysolite, the eighth beryl, the ninth topaz, the tenth chrysoprase, the eleventh jacinth, and the twelfth amethyst.[d] ²¹The twelve gates were twelve pearls, each gate made of a single pearl. The great street of the city was of pure gold, like transparent glass.

²²I did not see a temple in the city, because the Lord God Almighty and the Lamb are its temple. ²³The city does not need the sun or the moon to shine on it, for the glory of God gives it light, and the Lamb is its lamp. ²⁴The nations will walk by its light, and the kings of the earth will bring their splendor into it. ²⁵On no day will its gates ever be shut, for there will be no night there. ²⁶The glory and honor of the nations will be brought into it. ²⁷Nothing impure will ever enter it, nor will anyone who does what is shameful or deceitful, but only those whose names are written in the Lamb's book of life.

22 *The River of Life* Then the angel showed me the river of the water of life, as clear as crystal, flowing from the throne of God and of the Lamb ²down the middle of the great street of the city. On each side of the river stood the tree of life, bearing twelve crops of fruit, yielding its fruit every month. And the leaves of the tree are for the healing of the nations. ³No longer will there be any curse. The throne of God and of the Lamb will be in the city, and his servants will serve him. ⁴They will see his face, and his name will be on their foreheads. ⁵There will be no more night. They will not need the light of a lamp or the light of the sun, for the Lord God will give them light. And they will reign for ever and ever.

⁶The angel said to me, "These words are trustworthy and true. The Lord, the God of the spirits of the prophets, sent his angel to show his servants the things that must soon take place."

Jesus Is Coming ⁷"Behold, I am coming soon! Blessed is he who keeps the words of the prophecy in this book."

⁸I, John, am the one who heard and saw these things. And when I had heard and seen them, I fell down to worship at the feet of the angel who had been showing them to me. ⁹But he said to me, "Do not

REVELATION 21–22

What is heaven like? These chapters give you a glimpse. First, heaven isn't just a place. It's a whole new universe. The new earth won't revolve around a sun. It won't have to, because "the glory of God gives it light" (Revelation 21:23). Even more important is what heaven will mean for you. All your tears will be wiped away. Pain will be forgotten, a thing of the past. You won't even want to sin because you'll be truly good then. And best of all, God himself with be with you, and you will be with him. You can't really appreciate what heaven means now. But you'll sure appreciate it when you get there!

Direct Line

[a]16 That is, about 1,400 miles (about 2,200 kilometers) [b]17 That is, about 200 feet (about 65 meters) [c]17 Or high [d]20 The precise identification of some of these precious stones is uncertain.

do it! I am a fellow servant with you and with your brothers the prophets and of all who keep the words of this book. Worship God!"

[10]Then he told me, "Do not seal up the words of the prophecy of this book, because the time is near. [11]Let him who does wrong continue to do wrong; let him who is vile continue to be vile; let him who does right continue to do right; and let him who is holy continue to be holy."

[12]"Behold, I am coming soon! My reward is with me, and I will give to everyone according to what he has done. [13]I am the Alpha and the Omega, the First and the Last, the Beginning and the End.

[14]"Blessed are those who wash their robes, that they may have the right to the tree of life and may go through the gates into the city. [15]Outside are the dogs, those who practice magic arts, the sexually immoral, the murderers, the idolaters and everyone who loves and practices falsehood.

[16]"I, Jesus, have sent my angel to give you[a] this testimony for the churches. I am the Root and the Offspring of David, and the bright Morning Star."

[17]The Spirit and the bride say, "Come!" And let him who hears say, "Come!" Whoever is thirsty, let him come; and whoever wishes, let him take the free gift of the water of life.

[18]I warn everyone who hears the words of the prophecy of this book: If anyone adds anything to them, God will add to him the plagues described in this book. [19]And if anyone takes words away from this book of prophecy, God will take away from him his share in the tree of life and in the holy city, which are described in this book.

[20]He who testifies to these things says, "Yes, I am coming soon."

Amen. Come, Lord Jesus.

[21]The grace of the Lord Jesus be with God's people. Amen.

[a]16 The Greek is plural.

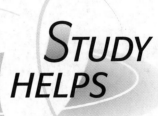

STUDY HELPS

Weights & Measures

What Do I Read?

Where Do I Look?

he figures of the table are calculated on the basis of a shekel equaling 11.5 grams, a cubit equaling 18 inches and an ephah equaling 22 liters. The quart referred to is either a dry quart (slightly larger than a liter) or a liquid quart (slightly smaller than a liter), whichever is applicable. The ton referred to in the footnotes is the American ton of 2,000 pounds.

This table is based upon the best available information, but it is not intended to be mathematically precise; like the measurement equivalents in the footnotes, it merely gives the approximate amounts and distances. Weights and measures differed somewhat at various times and places in the ancient world. There is uncertainty particularly about the ephah and the bath; further discoveries may give more light on these units of capacity.

		Biblical Unit	Approximate American Equivalent	Approximate Metric Equivalent
Weights	talent	(60 minas)	75 pounds	34 kilograms
	mina	(50 shekels)	1 1/4 pounds	0.6 kilogram
	shekel	(2 bekas)	2/5 ounce	11.5 grams
	pim	(2/3 shekel)	1/3 ounce	7.6 grams
	beka	(10 gerahs)	1/5 ounce	5.5 grams
	gerah		1/50 ounce	0.6 gram
Length	cubit		18 inches	0.5 meter
	span		9 inches	23 centimeters
	handbreadth		3 inches	8 centimeters
Capacity				
Dry Measure	cor homer	(10 ephahs)	6 bushels	220 liters
	lethek	(5 ephahs)	3 bushels	110 liters
	ephah	(10 omers)	3/5 bushel	22 liters
	seah	(1/3 ephah)	7 quarts	7.3 liters
	omer	(1/10 ephah)	2 quarts	2 liters
	cab	(1/18 ephah)	1 quart	1 liter
Liquid Measure	bath	(1 ephah)	6 gallons	22 liters
	hin	(1/6 bath)	4 quarts	4 liters
	log	(1/72 bath)	1/3 quart	0.3 liter

WHAT DO I READ TODAY?

The Bible contains exciting action, characters with whom you can identify, and help for all the good and not-so-good situations in your life. All you have to do is read to find it all.

1. If you are reading the Bible for the first time:
   - Begin by reading the Gospel of Mark or the Gospel of John in the New Testament.
   - After reading one of these gospels, read the book of Acts or the book of Romans.
   - After reading Acts or Romans, pick an Old Testament book like Genesis or perhaps Psalms.

2. If you want to read through the entire Bible in one year:
   - Read three chapters each day, Monday through Saturday, and five chapters on Sunday.

3. If you want to read through the entire Bible in two years:
   - Read two chapters each day, Sunday through Saturday.

The following chart covers every book and chapter of the Bible. To keep track of what you have read, mark off each chapter as you complete it.

GENESIS □ 1 □ 2 □ 3 □ 4 □ 5 □ 6 □ 7 □ 8 □ 9 □ 10 □ 11 □ 12 □ 13 □ 14 □ 15 □ 16 □ 17 □ 18 □ 19 □ 20 □ 21 □ 22 □ 23 □ 24 □ 25 □ 26 □ 27 □ 28 □ 29 □ 30 □ 31 □ 32 □ 33 □ 34 □ 35 □ 36 □ 37 □ 38 □ 39 □ 40 □ 41 □ 42 □ 43 □ 44 □ 45 □ 46 □ 47 □ 48 □ 49 □ 50

EXODUS □ 1 □ 2 □ 3 □ 4 □ 5 □ 6 □ 7 □ 8 □ 9 □ 10 □ 11 □ 12 □ 13 □ 14 □ 15 □ 16 □ 17 □ 18 □ 19 □ 20 □ 21 □ 22 □ 23 □ 24 □ 25 □ 26 □ 27 □ 28 □ 29 □ 30 □ 31 □ 32 □ 33 □ 34 □ 35 □ 36 □ 37 □ 38 □ 39 □ 40

LEVITICUS □ 1 □ 2 □ 3 □ 4 □ 5 □ 6 □ 7 □ 8 □ 9 □ 10 □ 11 □ 12 □ 13 □ 14 □ 15 □ 16 □ 17 □ 18 □ 19 □ 20 □ 21 □ 22 □ 23 □ 24 □ 25 □ 26 □ 27

NUMBERS □ 1 □ 2 □ 3 □ 4 □ 5 □ 6 □ 7 □ 8 □ 9 □ 10 □ 11 □ 12 □ 13 □ 14 □ 15 □ 16 □ 17 □ 18 □ 19 □ 20 □ 21 □ 22 □ 23 □ 24 □ 25 □ 26 □ 27 □ 28 □ 29 □ 30 □ 31 □ 32 □ 33 □ 34 □ 35 □ 36

DEUTERONOMY □ 1 □ 2 □ 3 □ 4 □ 5 □ 6 □ 7 □ 8 □ 9 □ 10 □ 11 □ 12 □ 13 □ 14 □ 15 □ 16 □ 17 □ 18 □ 19 □ 20 □ 21 □ 22 □ 23 □ 24 □ 25 □ 26 □ 27 □ 28 □ 29 □ 30 □ 31 □ 32 □ 33 □ 34

JOSHUA □ 1 □ 2 □ 3 □ 4 □ 5 □ 6 □ 7 □ 8 □ 9 □ 10 □ 11 □ 12 □ 13 □ 14 □ 15 □ 16 □ 17 □ 18 □ 19 □ 20 □ 21 □ 22 □ 23 □ 24

JUDGES □ 1 □ 2 □ 3 □ 4 □ 5 □ 6 □ 7 □ 8 □ 9 □ 10 □ 11 □ 12 □ 13 □ 14 □ 15 □ 16 □ 17 □ 18 □ 19 □ 20 □ 21

RUTH □ 1 □ 2 □ 3 □ 4

1 SAMUEL □ 1 □ 2 □ 3 □ 4 □ 5 □ 6 □ 7 □ 8 □ 9 □ 10 □ 11 □ 12 □ 13 □ 14 □ 15 □ 16 □ 17 □ 18 □ 19 □ 20 □ 21 □ 22 □ 23 □ 24 □ 25 □ 26 □ 27 □ 28 □ 29 □ 30 □ 31

2 SAMUEL □ 1 □ 2 □ 3 □ 4 □ 5 □ 6 □ 7 □ 8 □ 9 □ 10 □ 11 □ 12 □ 13 □ 14 □ 15 □ 16 □ 17 □ 18 □ 19 □ 20 □ 21 □ 22 □ 23 □ 24

1 KINGS ☐ 1 ☐ 2 ☐ 3 ☐ 4 ☐ 5 ☐ 6
☐ 7 ☐ 8 ☐ 9 ☐ 10 ☐ 11 ☐ 12 ☐ 13
☐ 14 ☐ 15 ☐ 16 ☐ 17 ☐ 18 ☐ 19
☐ 20 ☐ 21 ☐ 22

2 KINGS ☐ 1 ☐ 2 ☐ 3 ☐ 4 ☐ 5 ☐ 6
☐ 7 ☐ 8 ☐ 9 ☐ 10 ☐ 11 ☐ 12 ☐ 13
☐ 14 ☐ 15 ☐ 16 ☐ 17 ☐ 18 ☐ 19
☐ 20 ☐ 21 ☐ 22 ☐ 23 ☐ 24 ☐ 251

1 CHRONICLES ☐ 1 ☐ 2 ☐ 3 ☐ 4 ☐ 5
☐ 6 ☐ 7 ☐ 8 ☐ 9 ☐ 10 ☐ 11 ☐ 12
☐ 13 ☐ 14 ☐ 15 ☐ 16 ☐ 17 ☐ 18
☐ 19 ☐ 20 ☐ 21 ☐ 22 ☐ 23 ☐ 24
☐ 25 ☐ 26 ☐ 27 ☐ 28 ☐ 29

2 CHRONICLES ☐ 1 ☐ 2 ☐ 3 ☐ 4 ☐ 5
☐ 6 ☐ 7 ☐ 8 ☐ 9 ☐ 10 ☐ 11 ☐ 12
☐ 13 ☐ 14 ☐ 15 ☐ 16 ☐ 17 ☐ 18
☐ 19 ☐ 20 ☐ 21 ☐ 22 ☐ 23 ☐ 24
☐ 25 ☐ 26 ☐ 27 ☐ 28 ☐ 29 ☐ 30
☐ 31 ☐ 32 ☐ 33 ☐ 34 ☐ 35 ☐ 36

EZRA ☐ 1 ☐ 2 ☐ 3 ☐ 4 ☐ 5 ☐ 6
☐ 7 ☐ 8 ☐ 9 ☐ 10

NEHEMIAH ☐ 1 ☐ 2 ☐ 3 ☐ 4 ☐ 5
☐ 6 ☐ 7 ☐ 8 ☐ 9 ☐ 10 ☐ 11 ☐ 12
☐ 13

ESTHER ☐ 1 ☐ 2 ☐ 3 ☐ 4 ☐ 5 ☐ 6
☐ 7 ☐ 8 ☐ 9 ☐ 10

JOB ☐ 1 ☐ 2 ☐ 3 ☐ 4 ☐ 5 ☐ 6 ☐ 7
☐ 8 ☐ 9 ☐ 10 ☐ 11 ☐ 12 ☐ 13 ☐ 14
☐ 15 ☐ 16 ☐ 17 ☐ 18 ☐ 19 ☐ 20
☐ 21 ☐ 22 ☐ 23 ☐ 24 ☐ 25 ☐ 26
☐ 27 ☐ 28 ☐ 29 ☐ 30 ☐ 31 ☐ 32
☐ 33 ☐ 34 ☐ 35 ☐ 36 ☐ 37 ☐ 38
☐ 39 ☐ 40 ☐ 41 ☐ 42

PSALMS ☐ 1 ☐ 2 ☐ 3 ☐ 4 ☐ 5 ☐ 6
☐ 7 ☐ 8 ☐ 9 ☐ 10 ☐ 11 ☐ 12 ☐ 13
☐ 14 ☐ 15 ☐ 16 ☐ 17 ☐ 18 ☐ 19
☐ 20 ☐ 21 ☐ 22 ☐ 23 ☐ 24 ☐ 25
☐ 26 ☐ 27 ☐ 28 ☐ 29 ☐ 30 ☐ 31
☐ 32 ☐ 33 ☐ 34 ☐ 35 ☐ 36 ☐ 37
☐ 38 ☐ 39 ☐ 40 ☐ 41 ☐ 42 ☐ 43
☐ 44 ☐ 45 ☐ 46 ☐ 47 ☐ 48 ☐ 49
☐ 50 ☐ 51 ☐ 52 ☐ 53 ☐ 54 ☐ 55

☐ 56 ☐ 57 ☐ 58 ☐ 59 ☐ 60 ☐ 61
☐ 62 ☐ 63 ☐ 64 ☐ 65 ☐ 66 ☐ 67
☐ 68 ☐ 69 ☐ 70 ☐ 71 ☐ 72 ☐ 73
☐ 74 ☐ 75 ☐ 76 ☐ 77 ☐ 78 ☐ 79
☐ 80 ☐ 81 ☐ 82 ☐ 83 ☐ 84 ☐ 85
☐ 86 ☐ 87 ☐ 88 ☐ 89 ☐ 90 ☐ 91
☐ 92 ☐ 93 ☐ 94 ☐ 95 ☐ 96 ☐ 97
☐ 98 ☐ 99 ☐ 100 ☐ 101 ☐ 102 ☐ 103
☐ 104 ☐ 105 ☐ 106 ☐ 107 ☐ 108
☐ 109 ☐ 110 ☐ 111 ☐ 112 ☐ 113
☐ 114 ☐ 115 ☐ 116 ☐ 117 ☐ 118
☐ 119 ☐ 120 ☐ 121 ☐ 122 ☐ 123
☐ 124 ☐ 125 ☐ 126 ☐ 127 ☐ 128
☐ 129 ☐ 130 ☐ 131 ☐ 132 ☐ 133
☐ 134 ☐ 135 ☐ 136 ☐ 137 ☐ 138
☐ 139 ☐ 140 ☐ 141 ☐ 142 ☐ 143
☐ 144 ☐ 145 ☐ 146 ☐ 147 ☐ 148
☐ 149 ☐ 150

PROVERBS ☐ 1 ☐ 2 ☐ 3 ☐ 4 ☐ 5 ☐ 6
☐ 7 ☐ 8 ☐ 9 ☐ 10 ☐ 11 ☐ 12 ☐ 13
☐ 14 ☐ 15 ☐ 16 ☐ 17 ☐ 18 ☐ 19
☐ 20 ☐ 21 ☐ 22 ☐ 23 ☐ 24 ☐ 25
☐ 26 ☐ 27 ☐ 28 ☐ 29 ☐ 30 ☐ 31

ECCLESIASTES ☐ 1 ☐ 2 ☐ 3 ☐ 4 ☐ 5
☐ 6 ☐ 7 ☐ 8 ☐ 9 ☐ 10 ☐ 11 ☐ 12

SONG OF SONGS ☐ 1 ☐ 2 ☐ 3 ☐ 4
☐ 5 ☐ 6 ☐ 7 ☐ 8

ISAIAH ☐ 1 ☐ 2 ☐ 3 ☐ 4 ☐ 5 ☐ 6
☐ 7 ☐ 8 ☐ 9 ☐ 10 ☐ 11 ☐ 12 ☐ 13
☐ 14 ☐ 15 ☐ 16 ☐ 17 ☐ 18 ☐ 19
☐ 20 ☐ 21 ☐ 22 ☐ 23 ☐ 24 ☐ 25
☐ 26 ☐ 27 ☐ 28 ☐ 29 ☐ 30 ☐ 31
☐ 32 ☐ 33 ☐ 34 ☐ 35 ☐ 36 ☐ 37
☐ 38 ☐ 39 ☐ 40 ☐ 41 ☐ 42 ☐ 43
☐ 44 ☐ 45 ☐ 46 ☐ 47 48 ☐ 49 ☐ 50
☐ 51 ☐ 52 ☐ 53 ☐ 54 ☐ 55 ☐ 56
☐ 57 ☐ 58 ☐ 59 ☐ 60 ☐ 61 ☐ 62
☐ 63 ☐ 64 ☐ 65 ☐ 66

JEREMIAH ☐ 1 ☐ 2 ☐ 3 ☐ 4 ☐ 5 ☐ 6
☐ 7 ☐ 8 ☐ 9 ☐ 10 ☐ 11 ☐ 12 ☐ 13
☐ 14 ☐ 15 ☐ 16 ☐ 17 ☐ 18 ☐ 19
☐ 20 ☐ 21 ☐ 22 ☐ 23 ☐ 24 ☐ 25
☐ 26 ☐ 27 ☐ 28 ☐ 29 ☐ 30 ☐ 31
☐ 32 ☐ 33 ☐ 34 ☐ 35 ☐ 36 ☐ 37

☐ 38 ☐ 39 ☐ 40 ☐ 41 ☐ 42 ☐ 43
☐ 44 ☐ 45 ☐ 46 ☐ 47 ☐ 48 ☐ 49 50
☐ 51 ☐ 52

LAMENTATIONS ☐ 1 ☐ 2 ☐ 3 ☐ 4
☐ 5

EZEKIEL ☐ 1 ☐ 2 ☐ 3 ☐ 4 ☐ 5 ☐ 6
☐ 7 ☐ 8 ☐ 9 ☐ 10 ☐ 11 ☐ 12 ☐ 13
☐ 14 ☐ 15 ☐ 16 ☐ 17 ☐ 18 ☐ 19
☐ 20 ☐ 21 ☐ 22 ☐ 23 ☐ 24 ☐ 25
☐ 26 ☐ 27 ☐ 28 ☐ 29 ☐ 30 ☐ 31
☐ 32 ☐ 33 ☐ 34 ☐ 35 ☐ 36 ☐ 37
☐ 38 ☐ 39 ☐ 40 ☐ 41 ☐ 42 ☐ 43
☐ 44 ☐ 45 ☐ 46 ☐ 47 ☐ 48

DANIEL ☐ 1 ☐ 2 ☐ 3 ☐ 4 ☐ 5 ☐ 6
☐ 7 ☐ 8 ☐ 9 ☐ 10 ☐ 11 ☐ 12

HOSEA ☐ 1 ☐ 2 ☐ 3 ☐ 4 ☐ 5 ☐ 6
☐ 7 ☐ 8 ☐ 9 ☐ 10 ☐ 11 ☐ 12 ☐ 13
☐ 14

JOEL ☐ 1 ☐ 2 ☐ 3

AMOS ☐ 1 ☐ 2 ☐ 3 ☐ 4 ☐ 5 ☐ 6
☐ 7 ☐ 8 ☐ 9

OBADIAH ☐ Obadiah

JONAH ☐ 1 ☐ 2 ☐ 3 ☐ 4

MICAH ☐ 1 ☐ 2 ☐ 3 ☐ 4 ☐ 5 ☐ 6
☐ 7

NAHUM ☐ 1 ☐ 2 ☐ 3

HABAKKUK ☐ 1 ☐ 2 ☐ 3

ZEPHANIAH ☐ 1 ☐ 2 ☐ 3

HAGGAI ☐ 1 ☐ 2

ZECHARIAH ☐ 1 ☐ 2 ☐ 3 ☐ 4 ☐ 5
☐ 6 ☐ 7 ☐ 8 ☐ 9 ☐ 10 ☐ 11 ☐ 12
☐ 13 ☐ 14

MALACHI ☐ 1 ☐ 2 ☐ 3 ☐ 4

MATTHEW ☐ 1 ☐ 2 ☐ 3 ☐ 4 ☐ 5
☐ 6 ☐ 7 ☐ 8 ☐ 9 ☐ 10 ☐ 11 ☐ 12

☐ 13 ☐ 14 ☐ 15 ☐ 16 ☐ 17 ☐ 18
☐ 19 ☐ 20 ☐ 21 ☐ 22 ☐ 23 ☐ 24
☐ 25 ☐ 26 ☐ 27 ☐ 28

MARK ☐ 1 ☐ 2 ☐ 3 ☐ 4 ☐ 5 ☐ 6
☐ 7 ☐ 8 ☐ 9 ☐ 10 ☐ 11 ☐ 12 ☐ 13
☐ 14 ☐ 15 ☐ 16

LUKE ☐ 1 ☐ 2 ☐ 3 ☐ 4 ☐ 5 ☐ 6
☐ 7 ☐ 8 ☐ 9 ☐ 10 ☐ 11 ☐ 12 ☐ 13
☐ 14 ☐ 15 ☐ 16 ☐ 17 ☐ 18 ☐ 19
☐ 20 ☐ 21 ☐ 22 ☐ 23 ☐ 24

JOHN ☐ 1 ☐ 2 ☐ 3 ☐ 4 ☐ 5 ☐ 6
☐ 7 ☐ 8 ☐ 9 ☐ 10 ☐ 11 ☐ 12 ☐ 13
☐ 14 ☐ 15 ☐ 16 ☐ 17 ☐ 18 ☐ 19
☐ 20 ☐ 21

ACTS ☐ 1 ☐ 2 ☐ 3 ☐ 4 ☐ 5 ☐ 6
☐ 7 ☐ 8 ☐ 9 ☐ 10 ☐ 11 ☐ 12 ☐ 13
☐ 14 ☐ 15 ☐ 16 ☐ 17 ☐ 18 ☐ 19
☐ 20 ☐ 21 ☐ 22 ☐ 23 ☐ 24 ☐ 25
☐ 26 ☐ 27 ☐ 28

ROMANS ☐ 1 ☐ 2 ☐ 3 ☐ 4 ☐ 5 ☐ 6
☐ 7 ☐ 8 ☐ 9 ☐ 10 ☐ 11 ☐ 12 ☐ 13
☐ 14 ☐ 15 ☐ 16

1 CORINTHIANS ☐ 1 ☐ 2 ☐ 3 ☐ 4 ☐
5 ☐ 6 ☐ 7 ☐ 8 ☐ 9 ☐ 10 ☐ 11 ☐ 12
☐ 13 ☐ 14 ☐ 15 ☐ 16

2 CORINTHIANS ☐ 1 ☐ 2 ☐ 3 ☐ 4
☐ 5 ☐ 6 ☐ 7 ☐ 8 ☐ 9 ☐ 10 ☐ 11
☐ 12 ☐ 13

GALATIANS ☐ 1 ☐ 2 ☐ 3 ☐ 4 ☐ 5
☐ 6

EPHESIANS ☐ 1 ☐ 2 ☐ 3 ☐ 4 ☐ 5
☐ 6

PHILIPPIANS ☐ 1 ☐ 2 ☐ 3 ☐ 4

COLOSSIANS ☐ 1 ☐ 2 ☐ 3 ☐ 4

1 THESSALONIANS ☐ 1 ☐ 2 ☐ 3 ☐ 4
☐ 5

2 THESSALONIANS ☐ 1 ☐ 2 ☐ 3

1 TIMOTHY ☐ 1 ☐ 2 3 ☐ 4 ☐ 5 ☐ 6

2 TIMOTHY ☐ 1 ☐ 2 ☐ 3 ☐ 4

TITUS ☐ 1 ☐ 2 ☐ 3

PHILEMON ☐ Philemon

HEBREWS ☐ 1 ☐ 2 ☐ 3 ☐ 4 ☐ 5 ☐ 6
☐ 7 ☐ 8 ☐ 9 ☐ 10 ☐ 11 ☐ 12 ☐ 13

JAMES ☐ 1 ☐ 2 ☐ 3 ☐ 4 ☐ 5

1 PETER ☐ 1 ☐ 2 ☐ 3 ☐ 4 ☐ 5

2 PETER ☐ 1 ☐ 2 ☐ 3

1 JOHN ☐ 1 ☐ 2 ☐ 3 ☐ 4 ☐ 5

2 JOHN ☐ 2 John

3 JOHN ☐ 3 John

JUDE ☐ Jude

REVELATION ☐ 1 ☐ 2 ☐ 3 ☐ 4 ☐ 5 ☐
6 ☐ 7 ☐ 8 ☐ 9 ☐ 10 ☐ 11 ☐ 12 ☐
13 ☐ 14 ☐ 15 ☐ 16 ☐ 17 ☐ 18 ☐ 19
☐ 20 21 ☐ 22

WHERE DO I LOOK FOR THAT?

*T*his subject index will help you find just where you need to look to find information about a particular topic. Look through the list, and you'll probably find something you want to look up and read.

A

ABORTION
737, 788, 1579

ABUSE
19, 549, 796, 472, 1496

ADOPTION
737

ADVICE
91, 801, 1418, 1468

AIDS
133, 808, 1515, 1609

ALCOHOL
152, 464, 826, 977, 1496, 1522, 1535, 1602

AMBITIONS
331

ANGELS
448, 1152, 1566

ANGER
61, 356, 605, 796, 1275, 1281, 1583

ANIMALS
888

ARGUMENTS
1434, 1526, 1564

ASSURANCE OF SALVATION
1380, 1549

AUTHORITY
943

B

BIBLE AND DAILY LIFE
772, 801, 1161, 1224, 1259, 1557, 1561, 1583

BIBLE DIFFICULTIES
311, 372, 1269, 1387, 1404, 1460, 1461, 1550, 1618

BIBLE STUDY
340, 508, 576, 1152, 1611

BIBLE UNDERSTANDING
1077

BIBLE'S REVELATION
856

BIBLE'S TRUSTWORTHINESS
772, 951, 1077, 1104, 1276, 1324, 1374, 1557, 1597

BLAMING OTHERS
6, 1434

BLESSINGS
262, 1161, 1177, 1231

BROTHERS AND SISTERS
19, 33, 50, 60, 302, 574, 1342, 1434

C

CAREER
842

CELEBRATING
593

CELEBRATING GOD'S GIFTS
82, 593, 1485

CHANGE
60, 61, 608, 874, 1184

CHARACTER
77, 199, 879, 1402, 1442

CHEATING
35, 1220, 1546

CHOICES
6, 31, 52, 70, 77, 116, 140, 176, 225, 245, 283, 327, 335, 386, 508, 536, 589, 842, 977, 1002, 1063, 1138, 1162, 1227, 1327, 1343, 1527, 1529, 1573

CHRISTIAN LIVING
240, 375, 519, 537, 581, 727, 877, 929, 1209, 1331, 1431, 1461, 1468, 1478, 1482, 1493, 1513, 1534, 1551, 1570, 1575, 1590

CHRISTMAS
228

CHURCH
226, 283, 514, 1029, 1232, 1316, 1336, 1442, 1575

CLOTHES
178, 440, 507, 1442

COMFORT
25, 1298

COMMITMENT
283, 474, 519, 871, 1029, 1287, 1320, 1396, 1606

COMPARISONS
991, 1503, 1518

COMPLAINING
172, 1526, 1592

CONCEIT
50, 1401

CONFESSION
378, 706, 1306, 1600

CONFIDENCE
1441

CONFLICT
19, 33, 280, 302, 1342, 1488, 1564

CONSCIENCE
398, 1446, 1573

CONSEQUENCES
152, 176, 245, 1063, 1079, 1362, 1573

CONTENTMENT
172, 1528

CONVICTIONS
225, 1141, 1262, 1442, 1449

COURAGE
606, 1493

CREATION
2, 655, 888, 1455, 1476, 1597

CRITICISM
91, 1478, 1551

CROSS
951, 1314, 1327

D

DATING
28, 180, 236, 280, 282, 320, 380, 419, 580, 826, 863, 929, 1500, 1609

DEATH
617, 1154, 1361, 1491, 1541, 1632

DECISIONS
401, 417, 943, 1418, 1570, 1579

DEPRESSION
432

DISCIPLINE
382, 1507, 1578, 1579

DISCRIMINATION
See prejudice.

DISCOURAGEMENT
75, 1115

DISOBEDIENCE
234, 262, 340, 1199

DIVORCE
25, 324, 1091, 1283, 1298

DOING GOOD
61, 97, 307, 352, 589, 596, 877, 981, 1141, 1209, 1310, 1446, 1511, 1561

DO'S AND DON'TS
670, 1322

DOUBT
1276, 1387, 1549

E

EASTER
564, 1449

ECOLOGY
665

ENCOURAGEMENT
540, 856, 1074, 1575

END OF THE WORLD
1598, 1618

ENEMIES
97, 347

ENTERTAINMENT
1529

ENVY
See jealousy.

EVIL SPIRITS
1266, 1439

EVOLUTION
655, 1597

EXPRESSING FEELINGS
605, 617, 709, 747, 1275

F

FAILURE
1296

FAITH
26, 79, 81, 175, 467, 1141, 1154, 1263, 1296, 1320, 1336, 1387, 1396, 1449, 1458, 1555, 1597

FAITH AND WORKS
79, 537, 1029, 1493

FAITHFULNESS
877, 1269

FALSE TEACHERS
1611

FAMILY
302, 464, 503, 1094, 1115, 1247, 1342, 1378, 1434

FAMILY OF GOD
1316, 1472, 1518

FEAR
24, 43, 175, 606, 1276, 1424

FEAR OF GOD
247

FELLOWSHIP
1316, 1520, 1575

FLATTERY
551, 1538

FORGETTING GOD
220

FORGIVENESS
152, 176, 532, 570, 605, 687, 706, 874, 1067, 1281, 1306, 1339, 1409, 1446, 1457, 1463, 1549, 1564, 1572, 1573

FREEDOM
943

FRIENDS
180, 225, 280, 445, 529, 580, 605, 1162, 1482, 1495, 1500, 1527, 1538, 1564

FRIENDSHIP
298, 409, 436, 608, 617, 931, 1281, 1358, 1425, 1575

FUN
593, 1535

FUTURE
327, 1222, 1368, 1598, 1618

G

GIVING
132, 226, 228, 1364, 1417, 1501, 1561, 1606

GOD'S CHARACTER
879, 1209, 1224, 1352

GOD'S CONTROL
361, 888, 1366, 1434, 1439, 1506, 1593

GOD'S EXISTENCE
247, 670, 1417, 1455

GOD'S GREATNESS
1618

GOD'S IMAGE
665

GOD'S LAW
1468, 1511, 1515, 1572

GOD'S LOVE
1247, 1296, 1392, 1398, 1455, 1569, 1578, 1602

GOD'S NAME
72

GOD'S NATURE
72, 214, 232, 879, 981, 1158

GOD'S PRESENCE
24, 169, 1079, 1343, 1368, 1566, 1633

GOD'S PROMISES
15, 26, 373, 564, 856, 1177

GOD'S PROTECTION
448

GOD'S PROVISION
172, 428

GOD'S SON
1377

GOD'S WILL
1314, 1418, 1506, 1513

GOSSIP
319, 340, 354, 574, 853

GRADES
1487

GRIEF
617, 1541

GRUDGES
605, 1564

GUILT
6, 123, 242, 519, 532, 687, 706, 1115, 1446, 1573

H

HAPPINESS
747, 851

HEALING
541, 1019, 1506

HEALTH
133, 616, 1493

HEAVEN
1152, 1491, 1511, 1632, 1633

HELL
1293, 1632

HEROES
1331

HISTORY
1184

HOLIDAYS
82, 564, 879

HOLINESS
879

HOLY SPIRIT
1413, 1461, 1476, 1513, 1522, 1572

HOMOSEXUALITY
140, 144, 1515

HORMONES
419

HUMAN NATURE
551, 610, 788, 1468

HURT FEELINGS
853

HYPOCRISY
240

HYPOCRITES
1262

I

IDOLS
936, 1158

INSPIRATION OF SCRIPTURE
1557

J

JEALOUSY
50, 110, 173, 280, 347, 616, 1158, 1317, 1503

JESUS' DEATH
951

JESUS' NATURE
1377, 1532, 1614

JOY
747

JUDGING OTHERS
1281, 1478

JUDGMENT
232, 981, 1222, 1224, 1293, 1622

JUSTICE
1008

K

KINDNESS
1351

L

LAWS
222

LEADERSHIP
173, 290, 500, 576, 1550

LISTENING
1175, 1232

LONELINESS
608, 1298, 1496

LOOKS
282, 343, 589, 858, 1465, 1480

LOVE FOR GOD
222, 1322, 1409, 1455

LOVE FOR OTHERS
1008, 1241, 1247, 1322, 1345, 1351, 1398, 1442, 1501, 1602

LOVE, ROMANTIC
See romance.

LYING
351, 378, 436, 529, 1417, 1457, 1495, 1600

M

MAGIC
148, 1439

MAKING UP
1281

MARRIAGE
28, 38, 456, 580, 808, 871, 1283, 1500, 1540

MATERIALISM
31, 446, 847, 1008, 1317, 1528, 1552

MATURITY
849, 1570

MEMORIZING
169

MERCY
214, 616, 1463

MIRACLES
81, 541

MISTAKES
596, 977, 1409

MONEY
851, 1364, 1417, 1552

MOTIVES
173, 331, 398, 1383

MOVING
24, 608

N

NEIGHBORS
1351

O

OBEDIENCE
70, 79, 129, 222, 234, 242, 320, 529, 536, 580, 581, 1138, 1231, 1269, 1302, 1314

OBSTACLES
175

OCCULT
148, 230, 360, 1266, 1439

OLD PEOPLE
1551

OPINIONS
417

OUTSIDERS
931, 1425, 1472

OVERCOMING TEMPTATION
929, 1259, 1460, 1483, 1582

P

PARENTS
33, 178, 180, 230, 304, 320, 324, 328, 420, 464, 472, 507, 510, 529, 536, 549, 580, 1029, 1091, 1269, 1298, 1468, 1488, 1496, 1536, 1555, 1606

PARTICIPATION
201

PASSOVER
564

PATIENCE
849

PEACE
917

PEER PRESSURE
70, 225, 230, 375, 380, 507, 537, 727, 826, 877, 929, 1138, 1162, 1220, 1249, 1262, 1310, 1331, 1540, 1546, 1569, 1585

PENTECOST
1413

PERSECUTION
1015, 1431, 1549

PERSONAL EVANGELISM
931, 1094, 1115, 1307, 1449, 1482, 1500, 1611

PERSONAL RESPONSIBILITY
6, 123, 133, 386, 464, 503, 508, 581, 606, 929, 1029, 1091, 1220, 1227, 1488, 1507, 1527, 1535, 1546, 1570, 1579, 1590

POPULARITY
727, 931, 1249, 1262, 1482

PRAYER
22, 43, 262, 347, 373, 467, 529, 532, 584, 709, 1091, 1263, 1302, 1352, 1383, 1402, 1418, 1506, 1593

PREJUDICE
196, 1472, 1491, 1518

PRIDE
554, 1401

PRIORITIES
428, 446

PROCRASTINATION
401

PROMISES
15, 77, 199, 264, 324, 1495

PROPHECY
372, 951, 1104, 1241, 1324, 1368, 1598, 1618

PROVIDENCE
15, 361

PUNISHMENT
1067, 1079, 1184, 1293, 1457, 1507, 1515, 1544, 1592, 1622

R

RAPE
236, 380

REJECTING GOD
1287

REJECTION
25

RELYING ON GOD
541, 851, 936, 1002, 1222, 1259, 1266, 1511

REMEMBERING
116, 420

REPENTANCE
1199, 1306, 1549, 1622

REPUTATION
319, 574

RESOLUTIONS
596

RESTITUTION
162

RESURRECTION
1154, 1324, 1361, 1374, 1491, 1541

REVENGE
61, 97, 354, 358

REWARDS
994, 1463, 1477

RIDICULE
1476, 1592

RIGHT AND WRONG
162, 351, 382, 386, 398, 589, 727, 981, 994, 1002, 1079, 1184, 1220, 1446, 1460, 1468, 1511, 1513, 1535, 1540, 1561, 1573, 1582

ROMANCE
419, 863, 867, 871

RUNNING AWAY
19, 1199

S

SALVATION
450, 951, 1115, 1276, 1293, 1314, 1336, 1380, 1396, 1455, 1555, 1572

SATAN
508, 616, 1152, 1266, 1431

SCHOOL
24, 240, 474, 877, 929

SCIENCE
655

SECOND CHANCES
570, 874, 1067, 1409

SECOND COMING
372, 917, 1324, 1362, 1387

SECURITY
1222

SELF-CONTROL
356, 380, 826

SELF-EXAMINATION
116

SELF-IMAGE
106, 294, 335, 343, 589, 858, 991, 1401, 1424, 1441, 1477, 1480, 1503

SELFISHNESS
307

SELF-SACRIFICE
1327, 1398

SELF-WORTH
1485, 1487, 1503, 1550

SEX
52, 140, 152, 236, 311, 380, 419, 796, 808, 863, 867, 929, 1249, 1540, 1573, 1609

SIN
110, 311, 378, 570, 687, 706, 888, 1184, 1339, 1383, 1457, 1544

SISTERS AND BROTHERS
See brothers and sisters.

SPIRITUAL GIFTS
106, 1485

SPIRITUAL WARFARE
1152, 1431

SPIRITUALITY
474, 1431, 1493, 1534

STANDARDS
382, 1002, 1162, 1535

STRENGTHS
307

STRESS
445, 574

STRICTNESS
304, 328, 382

STUBBORNNESS
1161

SUFFERING
616, 1441, 1569, 1592

SUICIDE
1019, 1177

SWEARING
148, 240, 1585

SYMPATHY
617

T

TALENTS
106, 307, 540, 1401, 1487

TELEPHONES
1538

TEMPER
1583

TEMPTATION
508, 1483, 1569, 1582

THANKFULNESS
220, 228, 304, 1263

TIME
584, 1302

TRAGEDY
1506, 1573

TRUST
298, 510, 1227, 1458, 1501

TRUSTWORTHINESS
199, 264

TRUTHFULNESS
351, 436

U

UNBELIEF
670, 1366, 1396, 1458

UNFAIRNESS
55, 129, 152, 245, 340, 352, 358, 610,
994, 1327, 1358, 1536, 1544, 1578

UNITY
1404

V

VALUES
446, 847, 1008, 1138, 1162, 1220,
1227, 1249, 1310, 1442, 1552, 1600

W

WAITING
55, 428, 456, 849, 867

WAR
232

WEAKNESSES
294, 1199, 1503

WEALTH
1317, 1417, 1552

WISDOM
670, 801

WITCHES
360, 1266

WITNESSING
144, 217, 240, 375, 409, 450, 562,
1015, 1094, 1115, 1144, 1199, 1307,
1320, 1345, 1378, 1431, 1449, 1465,
1476, 1500

WOMEN
38, 290, 788, 842, 1359, 1550

WORDS, THE POWER OF
551, 853, 1074, 1585

WORKING
55, 503

WORRY
22, 1593

WORSHIP
474, 514, 570, 747

WRONG AND RIGHT
See right and wrong.

WRONGING OTHERS
162, 358

Y

YOUTH
562, 849, 1392, 1527

YOUTH GROUP
173, 201, 500, 1472